HISTORY OF MEDICINE

A Scandalously Short Introduction

Second Edition

For more than ten years Jacalyn Duffin's *History of Medicine* has been one of the leading texts used to teach medical and nursing students the history of their profession. It has also been widely read in history courses and by general readers. An accessible overview of medical history, this new edition is greatly expanded, including more information on medicine in the United States, Great Britain, and other European countries. The book continues to be organized conceptually around the major fields of medical endeavour such as anatomy, pharmacology, obstetrics, and psychiatry and has grown to include a new chapter on public health.

Years of pedagogic experience, medical developments, and reader feedback have led to new sections throughout the book on topics including bioethics, forensics, genetics, reproductive technology, clinical trials, and recent outbreaks of BSE, West Nile Virus, SARS, and anthrax. Up to date and offering pertinent examples and teaching tools such as a searchable online bibliography, *History of Medicine* continues to demonstrate the power of historical research to inform current health care practice and enhance cultural understanding.

JACALYN DUFFIN is a hematologist and historian who is Professor in the Hannah Chair of the History of Medicine at Queen's University.

HISTORY OF MEDICINE

A Scandalously Short Introduction

SECOND EDITION

Jacalyn Duffin

UNIVERSITY OF TORONTO PRESS
Toronto Buffalo London

© University of Toronto Press Incorporated 2010
Toronto Buffalo London
First edition published 1999
Reprinted 2000, 2001, 2004, 2006, 2008, 2009
www.utppublishing.com

Printed in Canada

ISBN 978-0-8020-9825-8 (cloth)
ISBN 978-0-8020-9556-5 (paper)

∞

Printed on acid-free and 100% post-consumer recycled paper with
vegetable-based inks

Library and Archives Canada Cataloguing in Publication

Duffin, Jacalyn
    History of medicine : a scandalously short introduction /
    Jacalyn Duffin. – 2nd ed.

    Includes bibliographical references and index.
    ISBN 978-0-8020-9825-2 (bound).   ISBN 978-0-8020-9556-5 (pbk.)

    1. Medicine – History. I. Title.

    RM131.D83 2010   610.9   C2009-907195-9

Excerpts of material written by L.M. Montgomery are published with the
permission of David Macdonald and Ruth Macdonald, who are the heirs of
L.M. Montgomery.

University of Toronto Press acknowledges the financial assistance to its
publishing program of the Canada Council for the Arts and the Ontario Arts
Council.

 Canada Council Conseil des Arts
for the Arts du Canada

 ONTARIO ARTS COUNCIL
CONSEIL DES ARTS DE L'ONTARIO

University of Toronto Press acknowledges the financial support for its publishing activities of the Government of Canada through the Book Publishing
Industry Development Program (BPIDP).

For my students
past, present, and future

Doc, I have an earache.

2000 B.C.	Here, eat this root.
1000 B.C.	That root is heathen, say this prayer.
1850 A.D.	Prayer is superstition, drink this potion.
1930	That potion is snake oil, swallow this pill.
1970	That pill is ineffective, take this antibiotic.
2000	That antibiotic is artifical, here, eat this root.

Anon, 'History of Medicine,' circulating on the Internet 1997–8

Contents

x   Contents

Suggestions for Further Reading (see bibliography website http://
histmed.ca)

Illustrations

Tables

Preface to the Second Edition

I wrote the first edition of this book in the late 1990s because my medical students repeatedly asked me to publish my lectures. I hesitated for a long time because of my limited expertise. They argued that it could serve as a guide for students, interested practitioners, and non-historian instructors wishing to incorporate history into health-care teaching. I hoped that it might also demystify medicine for students in other domains, such as history, philosophy, and sociology – although the thematic structure is unusual for a humanities course. But as soon as I began trying to turn those comfortably private, oral presentations into public print, I ran up against my own lack of erudition (as predicted) and was humbled by the numerous places where I risked falling into the very traps described in chapter 16. Without the security of fudging footnotes and scholarly apparatus, I began to feel exposed on alien turf – every sentence, a minefield; each choice of word, a little bomb waiting to explode.

Reviewers were kind, and 'Scandalous' enjoyed more success than I had imagined. Several readers wrote to suggest additions or correct errors. Although it was unabashedly aimed at Canadians, I was surprised (and perhaps the publisher was too) to discover that it found readers, course assigments, reprintings, and translation in the rest of North America, Europe, and Asia.

This new edition updates the book to include events of the past decade in both medicine and history; it also aims to serve a wider audience. Each chapter has been revised; the examples are broader and new sections have been added on many topics, including genetics, hospitals, bioethics, pharmaceuticals, biotechnology, Nazi medicine, and alternative medicines, with an entirely new chapter on public and international health. The examples from Canada are now joined by many more from other places, especially but not only Britain and the United States.

Around 2006, an additional challenge emerged: some students do not like this book because it is, well, a book. Teaching methods of lectures and readings are now called 'traditional.' Library stacks are echoing and empty, and shelves of books are being replaced with computer terminals. Scholars and medical practitioners – including me – conduct their research through the instant gratification of wondrous Google, information comes in concise bullets, and attentions spans are growing shorter.

Web mavens can rest assured that plans for an electronic edition are afoot; indeed, the Suggestions for Further Reading are already online. In the meantime, as a historian, I happily draw your attention to the remarkable, venerable technology of print on paper. Diverse, durable, portable, and lovely to hold, touch, and smell, books can go with you on canoe trips, or into the bath, without electricity or fear of shock. And in the end, unlike the disposible flux of a website, they stand as testimony to a moment in time and space, becoming historical sources themselves. Maybe books are an endangered species, but for nearly 600 years they conveyed so much medicine that it seems only right that a book should be the vehicle for its past.

Acknowledgments

Historical ideas, like diseases, can be both hereditary and communicable. In these pages, my mentor, Mirko Grmek, was able to see, just before he died, how he had passed on his historical and medical instruction; I am a grateful *heritière*. The infectious enthusiasm of my editors and their confidence in the outcome were essential catalysts for turning ideas into a book in the first place, and for embarking on this new edition; special thanks to Gerald Hallowell and Len Husband. Nor would there have been a book without the support of Queen's University and the unique teaching opportunities of the Hannah Chair generously endowed by Associated Medical Services.

I am indebted to many predecessors whose far more ambitious works resolved numerous problems, and I am grateful for the comments of practitioners, medical and historical, who were pestered to read portions of the work in its first iteration.

Many contributed by reading chapters, answering questions, offering creative suggestions, and helping with illustrations. For the first edition, Hannah Professors Paul Potter and Charles G. Roland, Cherrilyn Yalin, Martin Friedland, and an anonymous reviewer for the Press kindly commented on drafts of the entire manuscript. For their excellent advice on specific issues, I remain indebted to friends and colleagues: Ian Carr, the late Peter Cruse, Dale Dotten, Eleanor Enkin, Murray Enkin, Anita Johnston, and Felicity Pope. For similar help, I gladly acknowledge the generosity of Queen's colleagues Alex Bryans, Prakash Burra, Gerald Evans, Pamela Frid, Charles Graham,

Charles Hayter, R. Neil Hobbs, Steve Iscoe, Gerald Marks, Steven Pang, Terrie Romano, Joan Sherwood, Duncan G. Sinclair, Lucinda Walls, and James L. Wilson.

Over the last decade, several reviewers and colleagues described their uses of the book and their expectations of a new edition. In particular I thank Melanie Colpitts, Jayne Elliott, Heiner Fangerau, Bert Hansen, Geoff Hudson, Margaret Humphreys, Ross Kilpatrick, Joel Lexchin, Christopher Lyons, Pamela Miller, Sheila Pinchin, Susan Phillips, the late Roy Porter, Paul Potter, Ana Cecilia de Romo, Todd Savitt, Anne Smithers, Meryn Stuart, Lewis Tomalty, the wonderful staff of Bracken Library, and once again, as always, Robert David Wolfe and Cherrilyn Yalin.

My students are my teachers too, and the toughest critics. Their persistent requests for an introductory text made me finally decide to do what I had long resisted. For the first edition, several cheerfully read chapters in a test-drive exercise that shaped the finished version. They are former medical students, now doctors all, Hershel Berman, Matthew Bowes, Ruttan Bhardwaj, Darryl da Costa, Leigh Eckler, Kymm Feldman, Diana Fort, Fiona Mattatall, and Matteus Zurowski; and former graduate students Elaine Berman, Jennifer Marotta, and Megan Nichols. Without their inspiring belief in its future utility, the first edition would never have appeared.

For the second edition, another intrepid gang of Queen's students and young doctors offered thoughtful suggestions, criticisms, and inspiration, or they patiently read updated chapters. They include Courtney Casserly, Dan Finnigan, Rebekah Jacques, Raed Joundi, Ahmed Kayssi, Jessica Liauw, Melissa Pickles, Paul Uy, Mary-Clair Yelovich, and Julia Cameron Vendrig. May they find this new version useful – despite being a book! – it is for them with my gratitude.

Some readers will continue to notice errors; others will complain that I continue to ignore their favourite topics. I hope that they will let me know and help to make the next edition better.

HISTORY OF MEDICINE ·

A Scandalously Short Introduction

Second Edition

CHAPTER ONE

Introduction: Heroes and Villains in the History of Medicine*

My recommendation is that the doctor should be, plainly and unmistakably, a humanist.

– Robertson Davies, 'Can a Doctor Be a Humanist?' (1984)

The Heroes and Villains Game

In the early fall, the new medical students at Queen's University play a game called Heroes and Villains. Acting like an icebreaker at a party, the game introduces three components of their education: the library, the information literacy course, and the history of medicine. The students divide into teams to work with one or two partners of their choice. From an online worksheet, they choose a name from medicine's past (see table 1.1). The task is to find something written *by* that historical figure (a primary source) and something written *about* the figure (a secondary source), and to decide whether the person is a hero, a villain, or both. The students then prepare to present their findings to the class and write a brief report with a bibliography. Prizes are promised.

The list of potential heroes and villains includes figures from antiquity, Nobel laureates, women, and local worthies. There is nothing special about our list; an endless number of alternatives could be cre-

*Learning objectives for this book are found on p. 449.

Table 1.1
'Heroes' and 'villains' in medical history – game worksheet

Divide work among members of your team.
Use the catalogue and the reference tools of the librar(y)(ies) to find:
1. at least one item written by each person
2. something about each person
Is the person a 'hero,' a 'villain,' or both? *Why*?
Think about objectives (below) and hand in brief written conclusions *with references*.
Reports can be written by the whole team together or by groups within the team.

Abbott, Maude
Apgar, Virginia
Aretaeus of Cappadocia
Arnaldus of Villanova
Austin, J. L. 'Blimey'
Avicenna (Ibn Sina)
Baltimore, David
Banting, Frederick
Barry, James Miranda
Beaumont, W.R.
Bernard, Claude
Bethune, Norman
Blackwell, Elizabeth
Caius, John
Carrel, Alexis
Celsus
Chadwick, Edwin
Charcot, Jean Martin
Chisholm, Brock
Domagk, Gerhard
Egas-Moniz, A.A.C.
Erasistratus
Esquirol, J.E. Dominique
Freud, Sigmund
Gadjusek, D. Carleton
Galen
Gallo, Robert

Grenfell, Wilfred
Hahnemann, Samuel
Halsted, William
Harvey, William
Herophilus
Hildegard of Bingen
Hippocrates
Hunter, John
Hunter, William
Jackson, Mary Percy
Jenner, Edward
Kelsey, Frances Oldham
Koprowski, Hilary
Krugman, Saul
Kubler-Ross, Elisabeth
Lexchin, Joel
Mackenzie, James
MacMurchy, Helen
Maimonides
McBride, William
McKenzie, Robert Tait
Mitchell, Silas Weir
Morgentaler, Henry
Müller, P.H.
Neisser, Albert
Nelles (Pine), Susan
Nightingale, Florence

Olivieri, Nancy
Osler, William
Paracelsus
Pare, Ambroise
Pasteur, Louis
Pauling, Linus
Pinel, Philippe
Rhazes (Ibn Zakaria al-Raz)
Rush, Benjamin
Sarrazin, Michel
Simpson, James Young
Sims, James Marion
Smith-Shortt, Elizabeth
Soranus of Ephesus
Stopes, Marie
Stowe, Emily
Sydenham, Thomas
Trotula of Salerno
Trout, Jenny
Vesalius, Andreas
Virchow, Rudolf
Wagner-Jauregg, J.
Watson, James D.
Withering, William
Wright, Almroth

Learning Objectives
1. to distinguish the various types of monographs (single author, edited volume, posthumous collection, translation, facsimile etc.)
2. to search online catalogue for maximum effectiveness (author, subject, keyword)
3. to know the basics of controlled vocabularies
4. to understand the meaning of primary sources (books by) and secondary sources (books about).
5. to recognize that all history (even medical history) is a process of interpretation strongly influenced by the present.

ated to match the resources of other libraries and places. The whole-class session – nicknamed the 'debriefing' – usually takes place the following day. When the weather is fine, the class gathers on the lawn outside.

'Who would like to speak first?' I ask. Rare volunteers are immediately given the floor; often, however, my question meets with dead silence.

'Who chose Hippocrates?' I try next. Groans and pointing fingers identify a reluctant but usually grinning pair, who tell their classmates what they have learned about the Greek physician of 2,500 years ago. As they wrap up, I ask, 'Is he a hero or a villain?'

'Definitely a hero.'

'Why?' A variety of answers justify the opinion.

I play devil's advocate: 'Hippocrates seemed to forbid abortion and use of the knife; he taught medicine only to men.' But the students' judgment proves unshakable, and we move on to the next example.

After one or two of these enforced mini-presentations, volunteers clamour to tell of the remarkable personage whose life and work they have just studied. Time will not permit all topics to be covered. Sometimes, I must interrupt a speaker to give others a chance. (Once, two students spontaneously adopted the personas of their subjects and treated their classmates to the spectacle of Avicenna and Paracelsus debating the symbolic need to burn books.) The class of 2013 came with music, poetry, plays, and costumes.

As the hour flies by, I grow increasingly anxious that no one will win the prize and the whole point of the game will be missed. I begin asking for presentations on villainous figures who provoked famous controversies. But despite my best efforts at dredging up the shadier sides of these individual stories, the students keep resisting my attacks. Finally someone, perhaps an anonymous voice in the crowd, will answer the 'hero or villain' question with, 'It depends on how you look at it.'

'What did you say?' I ask. 'Louder.' Then I ask the whole class, 'What did she/he say?' The class repeats it. Then, amid laughter and clapping, the embarrassed student is conspicuously awarded the first prize, a book of Osler's writings, and I begin to relax.

Over the years, I have learned that medical students are intent on viewing their predecessors with unquestioning reverence, akin to religious awe. 'Yes, Hippocrates may have recommended never to use a knife, but he is a hero because he showed that disease had natural causes.' 'Yes, Alexis Carrel may have been a Nazi sympathizer, but he is a hero because he made it possible to transplant organs.' Even after the dramatic hints dished out in class, the majority of students will conclude their written assignments with heavy justifications for the view that their subject is a hero. In two decades of playing this game, only a handful of students have boldly proclaimed their subjects to be villains – though that judgment does not result in a prize either.

Few students question the premise of making value judgments about the past. But if one asks, 'Why are we doing this?' she also wins a prize, just like the student who says, 'It depends.' Understandably, first-year students want to find heroes in the past. Relieved to have survived the stiff competition for admission, they anticipate forty years or more in their chosen profession with optimism and idealism. On graduation day, most still remember the historical figure they researched in the first week of training. The game provides a historical role model, but it also draws attention to medicine's present and future too.

What's Important

It is of small consequence for the student to know that an obscure book upon a recondite subject, by an author with an unpronounceable name, was published at a particular date. On the other hand it is of considerable importance for the students to be familiar with … 'the climate of opinion' behind the intellectual deeds of a particular period.

– Cecilia Mettler, *History of Medicine*
(Philadelphia and Toronto: Blakiston, 1947), xii

The premise of the game Heroes and Villains is the premise of this book. Medical history, like all history, and like medical practice and medical science, is about questions and answers, evidence and interpretation. Some questions are better than others; some sources are more to be trusted than others; and some interpretations are stronger than others. Good historians are aware of the danger in projecting their own desires and values into historical scenarios and texts. History invites students to ponder why things came to be as they are and how they change. It challenges them to explain how something that is so wrong now could once have seemed right. And it reminds them of the future probability of having to relinquish the very ideas and 'facts' they are about to study. As a result, history is a brilliant instructor in the ideals of lifelong learning.

How to Use This Book

This book originated in teaching medical students and follows a structure organized around conceptual units of instruction. Many essays and books have been written on the reasons why history should be taught to medical students, and at least as many publications offer advice on how to do it effectively. On one level, this book represents just one of numerous methods. At Queen's University, instead of forming a separate course or seminar, history infiltrates the entire curriculum and is taught as an integral component of the various medical and scientific disciplines under study.

But the intended audience goes well beyond medical students to include general readers and students of any discipline, including humanities and social sciences. Unlike the usual history textbook, the structure does not follow an overriding chronology; the chapters are devoted to various disciplines of medical study appearing in an order that reflects the Queen's course. As a result, they can be read in any sequence. Chronology will be found within each chapter, together with a sampling of themes or questions that preoccupy historians and govern their current research. Some events are developed with reference to recent literature, while others are ignored. For those engaged in humanities education, the index will help to identify the themes that run across all chapters, such as gender, race, class, and historical period.

The goals of our program are the goals of this book: (1) to raise awareness of history (and the humanities as a whole) as a research discipline that enriches understanding of present-day medicine, and (2) to instil a sense of scepticism with regard to the 'dogma' of the rest of the curriculum.

These goals have been criticized for being insubstantial and unambitious; on occasion, they have also been viewed as pernicious. But we do not intend to turn future doctors into historians; rather, we offer them an additional, conceptual tool for learning about medicine. Medical students are intelligent. Even if they last studied humanities in high school, they soon grasp the thrill and adventure of a debate over questions and context. In reaching for these goals, students do indeed learn something about the past; however, they can select the events that seem most relevant to their personal lives and career plans. Names, dates, and factoids are less important than ideas. Good history relies on accurate reference to such details, but it is, above all, a way of thinking.

This book does not pretend to be comprehensive. It attempts a brief survey of the history of *western* medicine with reference to recent scholarly literature and current issues in health care, and with the recognition that practitioners can be of any sex, religion, race, or nationality. Several other weighty tomes provide far more information and many more pictures. The older sources are remarkably rich and should not be neglected (see Suggestions for Further Readings at the bibliography website http://histmed.ca).

Nor is the book's structure around medical fields particularly original. More than sixty years ago, Cecilia Mettler organized her textbook according to medical subjects and ideas.

In the first edition, Canadian examples were used often, partly because they did not appear in other sources; as examples, they are just as edifying as the more familiar cases from Britain and the United States. For this second edition, examples from other nations have been included. Instructors in other countries will find suitable equivalents in their own national histories. The suggestions for further reading are not exhaustive, but they will orient the interested reader to background on most of the material covered; sources specific to certain countries are listed separately.

The final chapter offers advice on how to research a question in the history of medicine. Once again, it is neither infallible nor comprehensive. The appendix provides some learning objectives for each chapter – so essential for medical curricula of the twenty-first century. The online resources include a few reference points for information on period, place, and ideas, including alternative health care and medicine in other times and places. Students often turn to the historian for information on these medical belief systems, which this book, being a history of our own dominant medicine, does not address; again the online resources give some direction to compensate for this failing.

Throughout and in keeping with the message of the Heroes and Villains game, I have tried to show that many interpretations exist for most elements of our past and that topics of interest go well beyond 'great men' and 'great discoveries' to include ideas, diseases, patients, institutions, and great mistakes. If the reader is left with some intriguing questions, then this book will have done its job.

Suggestions for Further Reading

At the bibliography website http://histmed.ca.

CHAPTER TWO

The Fabricated Body:
*History of Anatomy**

Anatomy is to physiology, as geography to history; it describes the theatre of events.

– Jean Fernel, *On the Natural Part of Medicine* (1542); cited in C. Sherrington,
The Endeavour of John Fernel (Cambridge: Cambridge University Press, 1946), 64

Anatomy is the study of the structure of the body. Today it seems integral to the study of medicine, but structural explanations of disease were long considered secondary to those of function (physiology). This chapter will explore the rise of anatomy from irrelevancy – even taboo – to its place as an institutional power in medical education.

The word 'anatomy' is derived from the Greek word *anatome*, meaning dissection. It still implies cutting, but also structure (morphology) – the shape, size, and relationships of body parts. It is also a metaphor for the analysis of any problem.

Medicine is the study of disease and its treatments. To understand disease, doctors focus on abnormalities of structure and function, which are the objects of the complementary disciplines of anatomy and physiology. Traditionally, these two domains have competed for curriculum time, laboratory space, and pride of place in the minds of practitioners. Of course, considerable overlap takes place between structure and function: a broken leg does not work very

*Learning objectives for this chapter are found on pp. 449–50.

well; neither does a heart with a hole in its septum. But abnormal structure does not always imply disease; for example, congenital deformities, such as having six toes or a large birthmark, are not intrinsically associated with suffering or shortened life. Similarly, abnormal function can be compatible with healthy living; for example, the carrier states of the hereditary conditions of thalassemia or sickle-cell disease are detectable, but they convey few consequences for affected individuals.

Medical cultures that emphasized the study of anatomy peaked centuries ago, in Alexandria, then declined, peaked again during the Renaissance, then declined, and peaked again in the last century. The present form of medical education still reflects this most recent heyday, but the perceived centrality of anatomy in modern medicine may be on the wane again.

Three themes recur throughout the history of anatomy:

1 Ambivalence, or 'approach-avoidance.' Should anatomical dissection be allowed or not? The desire to learn about illness often conflicted with religious or cultural aversions to the notion of cutting up dead bodies.
2 'The gift of art to medicine.' The expression of anatomical wisdom relied on visual forms of communication.
3 Anatomical study separate from medical wisdom. The pursuit of anatomy in art or science did not imply equal status in medicine.

Dissection and Anatomical Ideas in Antiquity

The elaborate burial practices of the ancient Egyptians provided frequent opportunities for the observation of body parts. Embalmers were adept at situating and extracting organs through tiny holes and slits in the body. Egyptian graphic art may have been stylized, but the statuary reveals a sensitive appreciation of surface and underlying structures. Unlike the embalmers and artists, however, the physicians do not appear to have used anatomy.

Our knowledge of ancient Egyptian medicine is based on a few surgical papyri (see chapter 10). Egyptian explanations of disease seem to have emphasized physiology, in which breath was the essence of

life. Blood vessels were hypothesized rather than known, and only
a few organs were connected with specific functions. Some organs
were associated with certain deities and used as hieroglyphics. For
instance, a stylized uterus, or *sa*, represented the goddess of childbirth. Because this symbol was bicornuate (had two horns), scholars
think that the model may have been animal rather than human. The
heart symbolized the soul. In illustrations for the *Book of the Dead*, the
heart of the deceased is weighed against the feather of truth; when
the two balance, the soul may pass on to the next world (see figure
2.1).

Ancient Greek sculpture reflects a preoccupation with the accurate portrayal of surface anatomy, with attention to the underlying
muscles and bones. Votive offerings left at temples by sick people
hoping for cures were fashioned from clay or stone to resemble
afflicted body parts – uterus, breasts, bladder, and limbs – sometimes
with anatomical derangements such as varicose veins.

Despite these artistic influences and their skill in observation,
Greek doctors were not especially interested in anatomy. Dissection
of human bodies was forbidden, and funeral practices centred on
cremation. Function was more important than structure. Explanation of illness relied on the four elements (earth, air, fire, and water)
and their four cognate humours inside the body (see chapter 3).
Given the laws and funeral customs, few opportunities arose for
examination of internal structures of humans. Exceptions are found
in Hippocratic treatises on fractures and dislocations, which reveal
extensive knowledge of bones and joints.

Illustration is essential to the teaching of anatomy, and the ban on
dissection did not extend to animals. The fourth-century B.C. philosopher and biologist Aristotle appears to have used large diagrams
when he taught the comparative anatomy of animals. Unfortunately
none of the original drawings has survived.

After about 300 B.C., the city of Alexandria permitted dissection
of the bodies of criminals, alive or dead. These public demonstrations were designed to horrify as much as instruct. That the practice
was reserved for criminals indicates the social ambivalence regarding
dissection, which could be seen as a desecration. Two Alexandrians,
Herophilus and Erasistratus, described minute structures, including

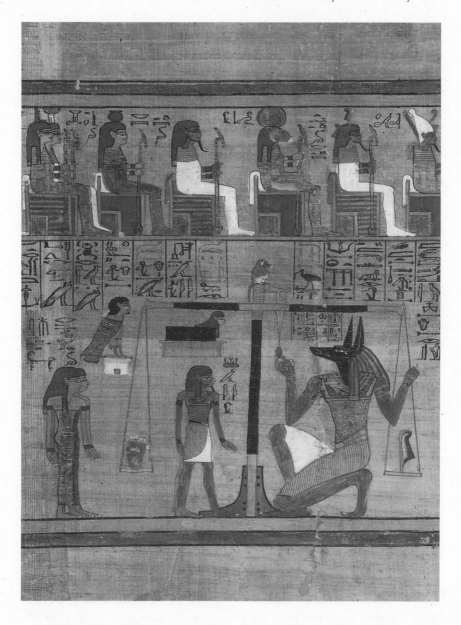

2.1   Weighing the heart. From the ancient Egyptian Book of the Dead, Papyrus of Ani, ca 1420 B.C. British Museum, London

lymph lacteals, the meninges, and vascular structures such as the *torcular herophili* (named after Herophilus). Like the early illustrations, none of their writings has survived. Our evidence for their work is based on other writers, including Galen, who lived some four hundred years later.

Galen on Herophilus

Herophilus 'attained the highest degree of accuracy in things which became known by dissection, and he obtained the greater part of his knowledge, not like the majority ... from irrational animals, but from human beings themselves.'

– Galen, second century A.D.; cited in H. von Staden,
Herophilus (Cambridge University Press, 1989), 143

Galen was born in 129 A.D. in Pergamum, on the Aegean coast of modern Turkey, but he lived much of his life in Rome. He deplored the laws that forbade human dissection; at least three of his many treatises were devoted to human anatomy, ostensibly as understood by the Alexandrians. Galen served as a physician to the gladiators, and he may have taken advantage of gaping wounds to observe internal structures. A great experimenter, he dissected animals, both living and dead, his preferred subjects being the pig and the monkey. He extrapolated from animals to humans and devised elaborate theories concerning anatomical structures, the motion of blood, and the origin and sustenance of life. Some observations were accurate for animals but missed their mark when applied to humans; for example, he ascribed five lobes to the liver and a vascular network in the brain called the *rete mirabile*.

Galen's writings are authoritative and bragging, and his teleological perspective allowed him to conceive of all structures as having been created for a purpose (see chapter 3). This confident philosophy corresponded well with the views of Christianity. As a result, his writings were the medical texts of choice for more than a thousand years. His immediate successors may have carried out some human dissection, but anatomies became rare and ritualized exercises for endorsing Galen's authority, not for seeking truth.

An anatomy lesson is the subject of a fourth-century A.D. wall painting from a Roman catacomb (Via Latina), discovered in 1957. The instructor sits a considerable distance from the cadaver. Neither he nor his students touches the body, which is prodded with a long pole as it lies on the ground as if to emphasize its base nature.

The oldest extant anatomical illustrations date from the early Middle Ages and are the work of Persian and Arab scholars, who preserved and transmitted the ancient Greek authors, illuminating the texts with stylized diagrams. The schematic figures squat in a froglike posture to expose the genitalia and the inner aspects of the limbs. Several drawings usually complete each series of five or six systems: vessels, muscles, nerves, organs, and bones (see figure 2.2). The practice extended into medieval Europe. The German medical historian Karl Sudhoff, who made a study of these drawings, concluded that their Greek precursors in Aristotle's work had probably come in similar series of five or six.

Medieval Treatises on the Body

In the thirteenth and fourteenth centuries, art and anatomy both experienced an awakening, fostered by legislative changes, the decline of religious teaching, and reactions to criminal violence or epidemic diseases. Municipalities, especially in Italy, were pressured to permit dissection in order to determine cause of death in cases of murder or other unusual situations (see table 2.1, page 18).

The rise of secular universities also contributed to the increase of dissection. In Christian tradition, the body was linked to sin and the temporal existence of the profane world. Learning about its inner workings was not only unnecessary but it could jeopardize salvation, because the literal interpretation of Scripture anticipated the resurrection of the soul within an intact body. As a result, the church did not condone dissection. Images of anatomies from the medieval period emphasize the barbarity of the act. Sometimes, the pope granted special dispensations for certain medical schools, such as Montpellier

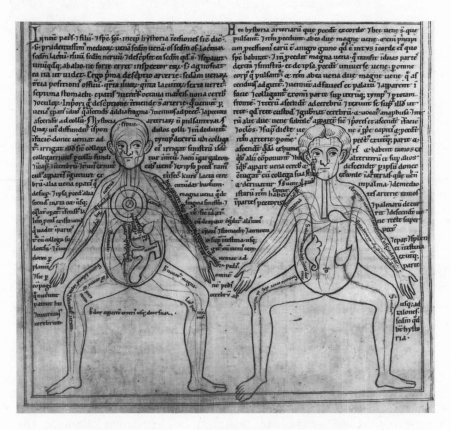

2.2   Five figure drawings, from a twelfth-century Bavarian manuscript. They are typical of those found in a number of Persian and Latin manuscripts of the Middle Ages. Bayerische Staatsbibliothek, CLM 120002, fols. 2v–3r

in southern France, but the subjects were executed criminals – or, on rare occasions, living criminals, who may have been sentenced to death by vivisection. Tension grew as schools yearned to practise dissection and the church refused; the resultant disorganization mirrored inconsistencies in the evolving power structure of society. Would-be anatomists were sometimes prosecuted.

Legal dissections were ritualized and infrequent – once or twice a year, for example; in some places, only once every five

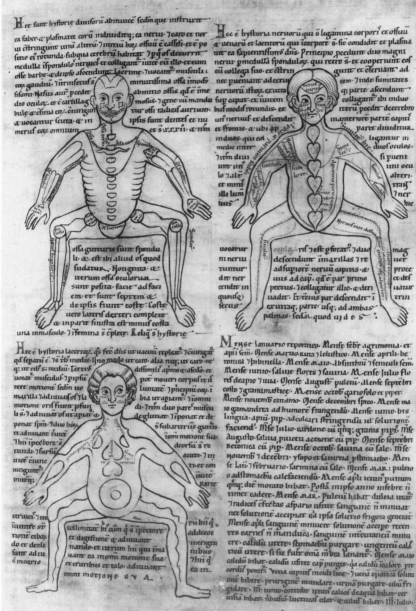

Table 2.1
Anatomy legislation in Europe, thirteenth to sixteenth centuries

Year	Place	Dissection permitted?
1207	Normandy	yes
1230	Saxony	no
1238	Sicily, Naples	yes
	Salerno (Frederick II)	yes – once every 5 years
1258	Bologna	yes – victims of aggression
1300	Vatican (Boniface VIII)	no
1302	Bologna	yes – autopsy for suspected poisoning
1308	Venice	yes – once a year
1315	Padua	yes – Mondino made public dissection
1319	Bologna	no – students arrested for dissecting
1366	Montpellier	yes – occasional dissections
1374	Montpellier	yes – once or twice a year
1391	Lerida, Spain	yes – one criminal every three years
1404	Vienna	yes – first public dissection
1540	Henry VIII England	yes – four times a year
1565	Elizabeth I England	yes – criminals after execution

years. The professor sat high above the scene, reading from a Latin edition of Galen. The demonstrators were often illiterate barbers, who dissected in conjunction with the lesson. (On barber-surgeons, see chapter 10.) As a result, the words of Galen could persist unchallenged. Differences between the cadaver and a Galenic ideal were explained by the imperfection of the (usually criminal) mortal (see figure 2.3).

One anatomist who broke with tradition was the Italian, Mondino dei Luzzi. He emphasized the need for anatomists to do their own dissection, but his teachings differed little from Galen. His 1316 treatise, the *Anathomia Mondini*, became the standard reference for the next 150 years. Its manuscript editions were not illustrated, but later versions were; however, when his work was first printed in 1478, it was already being superseded by newer treatises.

The artistic awakening of the late Middle Ages was applied to the portrayal of the body in several fourteenth-century anatomical treatises. In the *Chirurgia* (Surgery) of Henri de Mondeville, the image of the patient/cadaver is vertical and slightly more fluid than its rigid

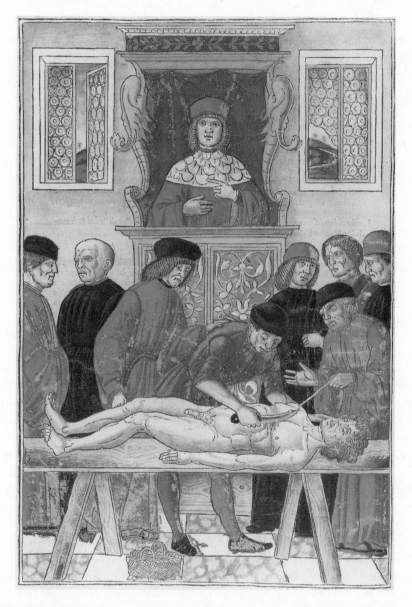

2.3   Fifteenth-century anatomy lesson. The professor reading from Galen sits high above the dissectors. From Johannes de Ketham, *Fasciculo di medicina*, 1493. Yale University Library

predecessors, as if captured in living action (see also chapter 10). The numerous images in the 1345 treatise of Guido de Vigevano (actually an illustrated edition of Mondino) display the anatomist himself conducting the dissection; however, the stylistic portrayal recalls the five-figure drawings from centuries before.

Sometimes the image of a 'zodiac man' was used to explain the relationship between the body and the external world and to indicate the auspicious times and sites to treat. These figures synthesized a large amount of information. Modifications were made to illustrate many potential injuries or diseases with the appropriate sites and methods of treatment: a 'wounds man,' a 'disease man,' and a 'bloodletting man.' Examples of these 'men' are found in the treatise *Fasciculus medicinae* (ca 1491) by Johannes de Ketham (see figures 2.4 and 2.5). Despite its apparent artistic and intellectual conservatism, the *Fasciculus* relied on one important innovation: printing. It could be said to mark a symbolic beginning of the anatomical Renaissance.

Art and Renaissance Anatomy

The Renaissance is a period in Western European history – roughly from 1400 to 1600 – when an artistic and intellectual awakening coincided with a reappreciation of the ancients. Many causes – economic, social, and demographic – can be cited for the Renaissance. From the perspective of medical history, one of the most intriguing and debated 'causes' is the fourteenth-century plague, which depopulated Europe and radically altered its economic structure (see chapter 7). Plague endorsed a certain scepticism toward Galen, who had not described it, and toward the church, because the 'good' seemed to die as readily as the 'sinful.' It also affected art. People became inured to the spectacle of corpses in the street, and the horror of human remains tended to fade. Prominent citizens took to having themselves portrayed on their future tombs as rotting corpses – *memento mori* – gruesome anatomical reminders of death, which not even the church could challenge. With this revival, or rebirth (*renaissance*), came a reappreciation of classical authors, art, and language, and a rediscovery of the beauty of the human body and the various modes of portraying it. If the exterior of the body could be glorified, it was a simple matter to extrapolate attention to its interior.

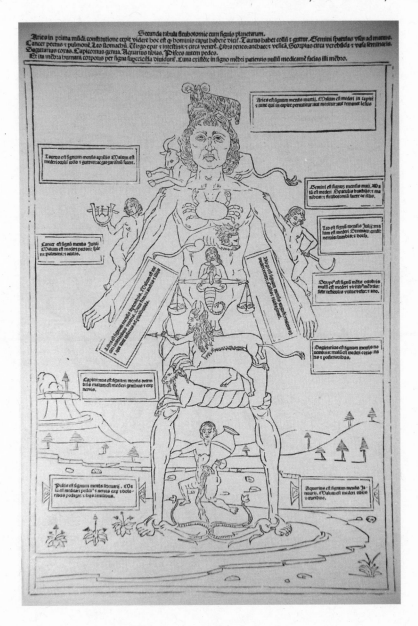

2.4 Zodiac man, Johannes de Ketham, *Fasciculus medicinae*, 1491[?], facsimile, Karl Sudhoff and Charles Singer, 1924

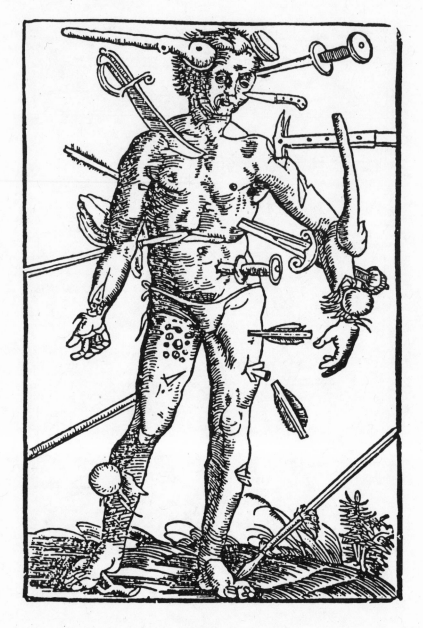

2.5   Wounds man, from Hans Gersdorff, *Feldbuch der Wundartznei*, 1517, facsimile, Wissenschaftliche Buchgesellschaft, 1967, xviii verso

Renaissance art contributed to anatomy, and artists conducted dissections. For example, Leonardo da Vinci – architect, painter, engineer, scientist, and philosopher – claimed to have dissected thirty bodies himself, although scholars now think it was fewer than ten. He planned a treatise of anatomy, maintaining that to elucidate the structure of the human body, several 'anatomies' must be conducted – one devoted to each structural system: bones, muscles, vessels, nerves, and organs. Two hundred pages of Leonardo's anatomical sketches and writings are kept in the Royal Library at Windsor Castle, England. His famous 'Vitruvian man' was drawn in the same year as the printing of Ketham's more static figures; the contrast between them demonstrates that anatomical detail preoccupied artists more than physicians.

Leonardo was interested in the finer points of structure for scientific and artistic reasons, but contemporary medicine remained ignorant or uninterested, and doctors continued to recite Galen as told by Mondino. Thirty years after Leonardo's drawings, yet another commentary on Mondino was published, by Giacomo Berengario da Carpi, who provided pleasing but stylistically simple woodcut images of cadavers, sometimes in the lifelike act of helping out with the dissection.

Why were medical practitioners less interested in anatomical wisdom than they are now? Doctors treated the sick for subjective illness, suffering, and dysfunction, but except for fractures and dislocations, most alterations in structure were impossible to fix. Consequently, trying to correlate disease with dead internal organs, which could be neither visualized nor altered during life, seemed to be a waste of time (see chapter 4). Clinicians did not reject dissection as an intellectual pursuit, so much as they found it lacking in practical application.

Vesalius and the *Fabrica* (The Structure of the Human Body)

The magnificent *De humani corporis fabrica* of Andreas Vesalius was published in 1543, fifty years after Leonardo's drawings. Born in Brussels in 1514, Vesalius studied medicine at Louvain, in modern-day Belgium, before travelling to France. In Paris he was taught by a professor who read Renaissance-style from Galen while prosectors dissected below. Vesalius later claimed to have dissected, boiled, and reassembled his first skeleton from the corpse of an executed criminal stolen from a gibbet. He moved on to Padua near Venice, where anatomy was more deeply integrated into medical studies than in Paris. Shortly after his arrival, he was awarded a doctorate in medicine. The following day, according to an oft-repeated legend, he was appointed 'professor' of surgery at the age of twenty-three. Vesalius then began anatomical teaching in earnest.

Not only did Vesalius conduct his own dissections, but he befriended artists of the nearby city states in Venice and Florence. Scholars have suggested that the contact was fostered by apothecary shops, where doctors went for their medicines and artists bought their pigments. Consequently, Vesalius obtained advice from talented artists, and therein lay his success.

In 1538 Vesalius published his first book, a sort of hors d'oeuvre that preceded his chef d'oeuvre by five years. Called the *Tabulae sex* (Six tables), this short book was astonishingly popular because it was illustrated with high-quality images. In keeping with long-standing tradition, it contained only six illustrations with narrative; reflecting Renaissance ideals, three ancient languages were used: Latin, Greek, and Hebrew. Despite the evident care taken in artistic preparation, some morphologic features and body proportions seem not quite right; the spine is a little too straight, the ribs shortened. More surprising are the residual Galenic features: a five-lobed liver and the *rete mirabile*! Surely, after all his personal experience, the young Vesalius knew that these structures did not exist. Why did he leave them there? Some historians think that it was a deliberate attempt to soften the reaction to his future work and spare himself the hostility of his older colleagues. The *Tabulae sex* sold out rapidly and was 'read to bits' as students hung the large images above their dissecting tables. Copies of the *Tabulae* are more scarce than original editions of the much bigger and more famous *Fabrica*.

On the title page of the 1543 *Fabrica*, Vesalius shows himself surrounded by a huge crowd at the Padua faculty; he is looking boldly at the reader while he dissects the corpse of a woman. The cadaver, he tells us, was the mistress of a monk; he and his students had acted quickly to remove identifying features before the body could be taken by the grieving cleric. The title page is full of symbolism. Below are the barbers, displaced from the table and squabbling. Cast off to the side are animals – dogs and monkeys, Galen's subjects and the source of his errors. Above, in the traditional place reserved for the recitation of Galen, is a skeleton. In the crowd are Vesalius's students and colleagues, including ancient savants, the bearded Realdo Colombo, who described the pulmonary circulation, and a youth writing or drawing, who, some think, may be the artist. Despite the emphasis on innovation, historian Andrew Cunningham has drawn attention to Vesalius's connections with the anatomists of antiquity; he found impressive clues, not only on the title page, that the anatomist was actually 'emulating' Galen. By his method, with its emphasis on personal exploration and vivisection, and despite his refutation of some Galenic anatomy, Vesalius 'was simply Galen restored to life,' a true Renaissance man (Cunningham 1997, 114). He also reminds us how early modern dissection continued to have ritualistic significance.

Who was Vesalius's artist? Similarities in the Mannerist style with the landscape background and architectural elements lead some to claim that it was the great Titian. The most likely candidate, according to a letter by Vesalius, is his fellow Belgian, Jan Stefan van Kalkar, who worked in Titian's studios. Another meticulous craftsman was probably engaged to sculpt the wood blocks from the original drawings. The blocks were then carried across the Alps for printing by the leading house of Johannes Oporinus in Basel, Switzerland.

The *Fabrica* contained not six drawings but seven books of many drawings each. The first book was devoted to the skeleton. The second featured the muscle men, the most famous series in the treatise, beginning with eight poses in the front view, including the *écorché*, a body with only the skin removed (see figure 2.6). Commentary explained what had been done to create each successive image by cutting the muscles at their origins to leave them dangling by their insertions. Ironic humour pervades the artwork: as the layers of muscle are removed, the poor cadaver became the worse for wear, moving from athletic exuberance to needing ropes and walls for support. The anatomical decay is reflected in the landscape background,

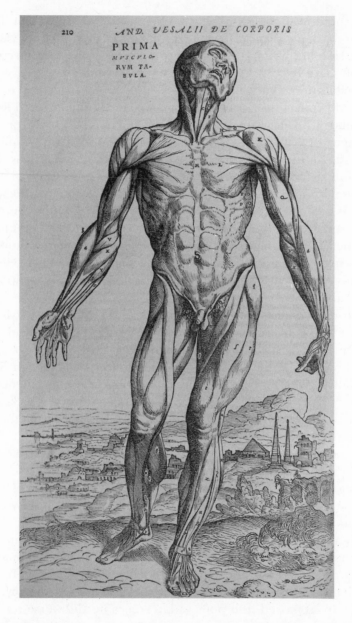

2.6   The *écorché*, one of the muscle men from Vesalius's *Fabrica* [1543], 2nd ed., 1555

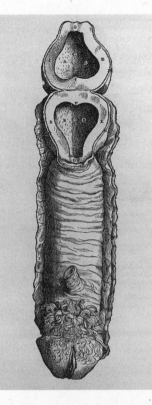

2.7   The vagina and vulva from Vesalius's *Fabrica* [1543], 2nd ed., 1555. The resemblence to the male organ is no accident. Vesalius was interested in homology, and the fallopian tubes had yet to be described.

which becomes increasingly barren as summer turns to winter. After the eighth pose, the whole process is repeated for the back view of the body.

The third book was devoted to the veins and arteries – gone was the *rete mirabile* of 1538. The fourth book described the nerves. The fifth explored the abdominal organs, with the liver's lobes reduced to two. It also included dissections of the genitalia, which have become the object of scholarly curiosity. The vulva, vagina, and uterus of the monk's defunct mistress are shown without adnexal attachments; the image resembles a penis, inviting speculation about a message of homology (see figure 2.7). The sixth book focused on the thoracic organs, and the seventh, on the brain.

Some anatomical inaccuracies can be identified in these images; for example, the rectus abdominus muscle extends too far up the rib cage. In contrast to its predecessors and many of its successors, however, Vesalius's achievement was unequalled. The *Fabrica* has become an object of veneration; first editions have been tracked down, and new translations made. Terence Cavanagh showed that placing the reversed muscle figures in a series creates a continuous landscape. Some scholars locate the scenery in the Eugenean Hills near Padua, where scores of doctors have travelled in search of the exact site.

Vesalius soon gave up academic life, and he successively went into the private service of various crowned heads: the Holy Roman Emperor Charles V, Philip II of Spain, and Henri II of France. He then seems to have left royal service to travel, only to die while on a pilgrimage to the Holy Land. His unmarked grave is thought to be on the small Mediterranean island of Zante, but circumstances surrounding his demise are obscure. The carved woodblocks for the illustrations of the *Fabrica* survived into the twentieth century and were used for an edition in 1934. But during the Second World War, they were destroyed in the bombing of Munich.

After the *Fabrica*, scientists began to pay more attention to structure. Several similar works followed, each an artistic achievement in itself. A series of brilliant dissections resulted in the discovery of hitherto forgotten or unknown body parts. In 1545, Charles E[s]tienne published an atlas that gave special attention to nerves and vessels. In 1561 Gabriele Fallopio (or Fallopius) described the inner ear, the cranial nerves, and the fallopian tubes that had been missing in the *Fabrica*. Bartolomeo Eustachio (or Eustachius) demonstrated the adrenals, the vena cavae, the sympathetic ganglions, and the inner ear, including the tube that bears his name. Girolamo Fabrizio da Aquapendente (or Hieronymous Fabricius) described the valves of the veins in 1603, and twenty years later Gaspare Aselli found the lymph lacteals while dissecting a living animal that was in the process of digestion. In 1747 Bernard Siegfried Weiss (or Albinus) published his celebrated atlas, which featured engravings of muscled and unmuscled human skeletons in a lush forest with other exotic marvels, including a rhinoceros. Anatomical amphitheatres offered demonstrations to an eager and cultivated public.

Notwithstanding these accomplishments, anatomy still had little to do with bedside medicine. The sixteenth- and seventeenth-century anatomists concentrated mostly on the discovery and artistic portrayal of the normal, or healthy, human form. They did not relate structure to disease. But early in the seventeenth century, scientists began to apply the new knowledge about structure to the study of function. Physiology, rather than medicine, was the first to find applications for the new anatomical research. For example, William Harvey discovered the circulation of blood by relying heavily (but not exclusively) on his teacher Fabrizio's demonstration of the valves in the veins (see chapter 3).

With the exceptions of Antonio Benivieni in the fifteenth century and Jean Fernel in the sixteenth, few writers were interested in *abnormal* anatomy until nearly a century and a half after the *Fabrica*. Théophile Bonet and Giovanni Battista Morgagni wrote massive compendia of anatomical pathology as a basis for disease; but their works were not illustrated (see chapter 4).

By the eighteenth century, dissection had become more respectable. A new philosophy of knowledge, called sensualism, was predicated on the view that all wisdom came from observation through the senses; observation was venerated, while theorizing was supposedly set aside. Anatomical studies could be seen to fit this new tradition. Artists painted distinguished anatomists at work surrounded by their students, a prime example being Rembrandt's famous painting of the lesson of Dr Tulp. Others created wax models, which became an important tool of medical education. Museums were founded to preserve elegant dissections and waxes for future reference. Spectacular remainders are the eighteenth-century collections of John and William Hunter in London and Glasgow, of Honoré Fragonard in Maisons Alfort outside Paris, of La Specola in Florence, and of the Mutter Museum in Philadelphia.

Observations in this early modern period sorted the body's architecture into ever smaller organs and planes, relying mostly on the naked eye. Meticulous examinations laid the foundations of embryology and comparative anatomy. Consideration was given to what might constitute the elementary 'unit' of living beings, and for many years

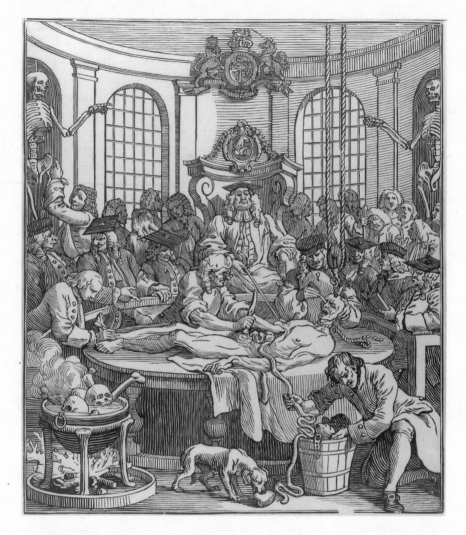

2.8   *The Reward of Cruelty.* Engraving by John Bell [prior to 1750], after William Hogarth. Yale University Library

Medical Mistrust of Anatomy

Others ... have pompously and speciously prosecuted the promoting of this art by searching into the bowels of dead and living creatures, as well sound as diseased ... but with how little success such endeavors have been or are likely to be attended I shall here in some measure make appear.

– Thomas Sydenham (ca 1668), cited in K. Dewhurst, *Medical History* 2 (1958): 3

All that anatomy can doe is only to shew us the gross and sensible parts of the body, or the vapid and dead juices all which, after the most diligent search, will be not much able to direct a physician how to cure a disease than how to make a man ... If anatomy shew us neither the causes nor cures of most diseases I think it is not very likely to bring any great advantages for removeing the pains and maladys of mankind.

– John Locke (ca 1668), cited in K. Dewhurst, *Medical History* 2 (1958): 3–4

And over a century later ...

Anatomy, though so carefully cultivated, has yet not supplied medicine with any truly important observations. One may scrupulously examine a corpse, yet the necessities on which life depends escape one ... Anatomy may cure a sword wound, but will prove powerless when the invisible dart of a particular miasma has penetrated beneath our skin.

– Louis Sebastien Mercier, *The Picture of Paris before and after the Revolution*, 1788. Trans. Wilfrid and Emilie Jackson (London: Routledge, 1929), 97

fibre was championed by careful observers, such as Giorgio Baglivi. A theory of tissues, rather than organs or fibres, began in the late eighteenth century, and continued with the advent of microscopy – an example of the reciprocal promotion of ideas and technology (see chapter 9). The notion of cells as the fundamental unit, often ascribed to Robert Hooke, did not emerge as a theory until much later with the work of Germans – zoologist Theodor Schwann, botanist Matthias Schleiden, and pathologist Rudolf Virchow. Cell theory found worthy opponents such as T.H. Huxley, whose heavy criticisms of 1853 are said to have done more to spread the idea in Britain than to defeat it. Again, knowledge and microscopic technology were mutually reinforcing; use of the microscope alone did not establish the theory; first cells had to be imagined, or 'envisaged.'

Despite these scientific successes, anatomy's relevance to medicine continued to be ill-defined. Why? First, aversion to human remains persisted. Eighteenth-century caricaturists such as William Hogarth derided dissection as a vile act, an appropriate 'reward for cruelty' (see figure 2.8) Second, even doctors who practised anatomy had difficulty imagining how to apply it; the same sensualism that celebrated anatomy made it an object of suspicion when it came to medicine. Doctors could not diagnose internal changes until the patient was dead; nor could they correct them. Diseases and diagnosis were based on symptoms (see chapter 4).

Anatomy Goes Medical

At the beginning of the nineteenth century, technology and a reconfiguration of disease concepts changed medical attitudes to anatomy. The diagnostic techniques of percussion and auscultation made it possible to detect structural changes inside the chest. Names and concepts of diseases changed from being subjective symptoms, such as hemoptysis and shortness of breath, to associated anatomical lesions, such as pulmonary effusion, pulmonary consolidation, and emphysema (see chapters 4 and 9).

As diseases became increasingly anatomical, medicine had to move in the same direction. Anatomy and dissection suddenly became not only interesting but essential for medical training. Chairs of anatomy, which had once been independent, became a feature of every well-dressed medical school. Pathological anatomy soon followed: the first British chair of pathological anatomy was awarded to Robert Carswell in 1828; the first French professorship went to Jean Cruveilhier in 1835. By 1848, twenty-five of the approximately forty medical schools in the United States offered instruction in dissection.

New problems soon arose because of the limited supply of bodies. Dissection may have become acceptable to academics, but the general public was not eager to see the corpses of its loved ones opened and displayed for instruction. Few places enjoyed legal mechanisms for obtaining anatomic material. In cities with large poorhouses and public hospitals, such as post-revolutionary Paris and New Orleans, unclaimed bodies were automatically given to medical educators. Elsewhere, cadavers were retrieved from cemeteries or were purchased on the sly.

The new occupation of 'resurrection man' emerged. Fabled in song and story, it satisfied the growing market for fresh bodies with the newly buried corpses of private citizens. Cages of iron, called 'mortsafes' were invented to protect wealthy corpses from body snatchers. The public was offended by the outrageous practice, and turned on the grave robbers' clients too. In the United States, physicians' homes and medical schools were mobbed and burned on several occasions. Cemeteries were guarded; following a burial, wealthy citizens posted sentries to protect family plots from violation. The Canadian medical teacher John Rolph, temporarily in exile at Rochester, New York, for his part in the 1837 Rebellion, had a former student in Toronto ship anatomical subjects across Lake Ontario in whisky barrels. To avoid middleman costs, medical students became adept at grave robbing; those in Kingston, Ontario, were notorious despoilers of patrician plots. Where medical schools operated in proximity to graveyards, the trade in human bodies could be brisk and ruthlessly competitive.

The inevitable happened: murder for the sale of corpses. Unknown numbers of disadvantaged people may have been killed to this end. Students and professors might have guessed the provenance of especially fresh or healthy-looking cadavers; however, in their eagerness both to dissect and to maintain supplies, they asked no questions. In the famous case of 1823, the Scotsmen William Burke and William Hare murdered at least sixteen people and sold the corpses to Robert

Table 2.2
Some nineteenth-century anatomy legislation

1831	Massachusetts
1832	England Warburton's Anatomy Act
1843	Canada (revised 1859 and 1864)
1844	Prussia
1854	New York
1865+	most U.S. states
1883	Pennsylvania
1983	Japan

Knox, anatomist at the leading medical school in Edinburgh. Knox took pains to remove the heads and other identifying features from the bodies as soon as he received them. First, the pair preyed on the poverty-stricken elderly tenants in Burke's home. Then they murdered a local prostitute, well known to the students; but the lads merrily dissected her corpse without comment. Only when Burke and Hare kidnapped a well-known boy with mental retardation, James Wilson ('Daft Jamie'), was suspicion aroused. A few days later, the body of Margery Docherty, a healthy woman who had been reported missing, was found in the anatomist's laboratory. Burke and Hare were charged with her murder. Hare was excused by testifying against his accomplice. Burke was hanged, his body dissected in public, and the remains displayed for hundreds of onlookers. His fate indicated that dissection was still a ghastly 'reward for cruelty'; his name is a synonym for murder. Neither Knox nor his students were charged, but the professor's career was in ruins.

Soon after, legislation restricted the sale of bodies and provided medical schools with access to unclaimed corpses in hospitals, prisons, and poorhouses (see table 2.2). France and Germany and other places in Europe had enacted legislation in the late eighteenth century. In Britain, the Anatomy Act became law nine years after the Burke and Hare affair. Massachusetts also moved early in this regard, but most American states revealed their chronic ambivalence to the issue by failing to pass legislation until after the Civil War. Canada's anatomy legislation was the special project of the colourful physician pioneer William 'Tiger' Dunlop. Recent scholarship examines the complexities of obtaining cadavers for medical education in Asian

countries, when the advent of Western medicine appeared to conflict
with cultural and religious practices. In Japan, it was only after the
expansion of Western-type medical schools in the 1970s that donation became acceptable; a law was passed in 1983.

Dissection slowly became acceptable to the public. Scenes of anatomy lessons relinquished their ghoulishness for an aura of solem-
nity, which symbolized the seriousness of medicine itself. Improved
techniques of preservation and injection of blood vessels enhanced
the longevity and utility of each corpse. Gender became an issue
as women entered medicine in the late nineteenth century. Many
schools believed that ladies were too delicate to confront corpses
or to look on naked male bodies, especially in the presence of living men, and some schools exempted women from dissection or
stipulated that they take their classes separately. Problems with the
supply of cadaveric material remained. The anatomy laws applied
most often to those disadvantaged by poverty or race. The idea of
donating one's body to science had yet to take hold, especially when
medical students were fond of joking about cadavers and skeletons
and had themselves photographed with the specimens in disrespectful poses (see figure 2.9). During the Third Reich, the corpses of
thousands of murdered Jews were sent to medical schools to satisfy the ostensible need for teaching and display. In 1998, investigations revealed that at least 1,377 bodies had been sent from Nazi
death camps to Vienna, where the professor Eduard Pernkopf
used them in preparing his sophisticated and widely used anatomical atlas. Anatomists, historians, librarians, and ethicists still debate
the appropriate uses and continued existence of this controversial
book.

But gradually the stigma was removed, and people became willing
to leave their bodies to science, in a new form of socially acceptable
charity. In the latter decades of the twentieth century, with the added
possibility of organ transplantation, donation was actively promoted
by governments and the general public. Historians have examined
this new impulse of fleshly gift giving as an indicator of attitudes to
science, education, and death. Most schools now mark the donation
with an annual service of thanksgiving and respect. At our medical
school, a special plot is kept for the remains in the local cemetery.

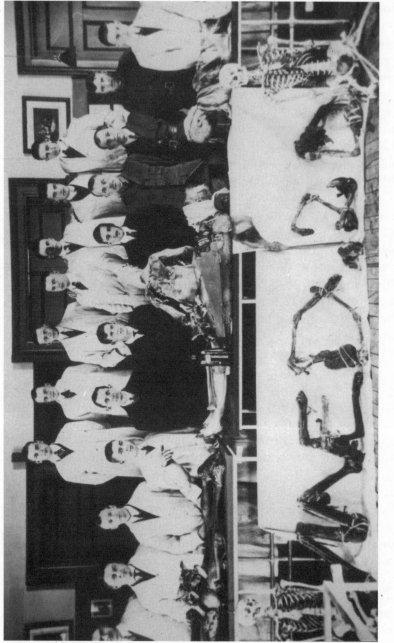

2.9   Queen's medical class of 1920 posing with anatomical parts. The words 'Med 20' are spelled in cadaver limbs. Friend-Vandewater Gallery, Botterell Hall, Queen's University. Photo by Queen's Medical Art and Photography Services

Anatomy Today: Basic Science or Hazing Ritual?

When health-care practitioners look back on the past that has just been described, it is difficult for them to see it as anything other than a logical series of progressive steps leading to openness and tolerance about the body that is the essence of medical wisdom and practice. For them, the body is a neutral and obvious assemblage of structural 'facts,' which should be available to all. Recently, cultural historians have shown that the story is not quite so straightforward. In a new trend called 'body history,' they challenge the idea of the human form as an immutable entity that is simply waiting to be discovered and explored. They have shown how its 'construction' was influenced by social and cultural pressures of time and place (see chapter 4). Instead of tracing a story about the 'fabric' of the body, historians are interested in how it may have been 'fabricated.'

For example, Londa Schiebinger pointed out that the shapes imputed by eighteenth-century anatomists to the female pelvis exaggerated natural proportions in a manner that emphasized women's role in childbearing. Similarly, Thomas Laqueur examined structural representations of femaleness as vehicles for the expression of political and cultural attitudes toward women. Sander Gilman and John Efron showed how anti-Semitism contributed to the 'normal' but deviant anatomies of Jews. Concepts of normalcy are culturally contingent; for example, excess weight can be a manifestation of health in one culture and a sign of illness in another. Other ideals of size and proportion, including height, skull capacity, and brain size, also have been influenced by notions of racial, cultural, and gender superiority. David Armstrong has shown that the constructing influences now include anatomy itself, which has become so pervasive in medical thought that many immaterial problems, such as illnesses, are reified as if they were material entities (see chapter 4). These ideas often spark opposition from anatomists who believe that they go too far.

If the history of anatomy is no longer quite as obvious as it once was, its future seems equally in doubt. Where exactly is anatomy going? Is it a pillar in the institutions of learning or has its time passed? Are we witnessing a new rise in the relative significance of function over

structure? Mounting evidence suggests that anatomy as an investigative discipline may be in decline once again.

After the hard-won legacy of Mondino and Vesalius, it is surprising
that medical students rarely do their own dissecting. Demonstrators
or prosectors prepare specimens in advance. Some demonstrators
are surgical residents who need refresher courses because their anatomy has been forgotten in the subsequent training. Why? Because
detailed anatomy is not reinforced by the general practice of medicine. In acknowledgment of this reality, the innovative schools at
McMaster University in Hamilton and at Calgary (founded in the late
1960s) have never taught anatomy through formal dissections.

Anatomy continues to hold departmental status in many health
science faculties; however, it has difficulty claiming to be a discrete
research discipline. Questions of morphology address ever smaller
components of the cell, and its molecules, often making it difficult
to distinguish anatomy from physiology. The publications of anatomy
professors rarely address the elucidation of gross or even microscopic
structure. At best, they investigate ultrastructure, growth, and function of embryos, cells, and genes. Often their research bears little
connection to anatomy at all. Department names are being changed
to include the words 'cell biology,' while the seemingly old-fashioned
museums are dubbed 'learning centres.' Cadavers are being replaced
by electronic models, accessible on the Internet or CD-ROM. One
example is the Visible Human Project, sponsored since 1986 by the
National Library of Medicine.

These observations are not meant to imply that study of body structure is irrelevant to medical practice or that it does not deserve a
prominent place early in medical training. On the contrary, illness is
felt and diagnosed within the body. But we can ask why anatomy continues as a form of academic organization if it is no longer a field of
active research. The once-shunned discipline is now establishment.
Even as the hours devoted to the study of anatomy are shrinking, the
long-contested privilege to dissect is not relinquished easily. Some
teachers lament its passing, pointing to the sensory and professional
advantages of handling a cadaver; our teachers dissected, we dissect,
and our students must dissect too.

Moreover – and in striking contrast to the past – society now *expects* future doctors to cut up dead bodies, even when they do not. While continuing to condone the practice, awestruck relatives and friends betray traces of retained revulsion when they ask medical students for the gory details: 'Ooooo! What's it like?' The same mix of fascination and horror greets the 'Body World' exhibitions of corpses plastinated by Gunther von Hagens; he claims to oppose elitism, hoping to demystify the body in health and disease and to educate through aesthetics. However, his grand public displays –sometimes called 'edutainment' – emerge from a tradition that stretches back to Vesalius and continues to provoke ethical comment. Are the poses disrespectful? Should anyone other than scientists gaze at the flayed dead?

Anatomy distinguishes doctors from others; it demarcates modern medicine, both intellectually and socially. Aside from its many other intrinsic merits, the study of anatomy is a symbolic rite of initiation that socializes members into a professional tradition.

Suggestions for Further Reading

At the bibliography website http://histmed.ca.

CHAPTER THREE

*Interrogating Life: History of Physiology**

We must never make experiments to confirm our ideas, but simply to control them.

– Claude Bernard, *An Introduction to the Study of Experimental Medicine* (1865), 38

Physiology is the study of the function of living beings. From a medical perspective, it stands both in relation and in opposition to anatomy, the study of structure. The word 'physiology,' derived from Greek, means the study of nature. It was used infrequently in antiquity by Galen and others; however, in modern times, it came to represent a separate discipline with well-defined methods. Throughout history, physiology has attempted to identify and classify the fundamental properties of life. It seeks to answer the question, What is life?

In the practice of analysing life, the functions of living beings have always been divided into smaller tasks, each a physiological process in itself. For example, nutrition can be divided into alimentation, mastication, swallowing, digestion, absorption, transportation, growth, repair, and excretion. Similarly, other functions – such as locomotion and reproduction – can be treated as ensembles of smaller tasks. In various permutations and combinations, these properties have always been the focus of physiology. Sometimes they were given different names or were grouped in different patterns, but in virtually every

*Learning objectives for this chapter are found on p. 450.

period the functions have been 'reified' until they became concrete objects or beings in themselves.

Four Recurrent Themes

This chapter will address four themes; three are dualistic. The first is about concepts of life: the relationship between *mechanism and vitalism*. Mechanism is the reduction of life to physical and chemical forces; it is sometimes related to materialism, which defines all existence in terms of tangible matter. Vitalism is the view that life is governed by forces peculiar only to living beings – forces which cannot be reduced to physical laws. The 'life force' of vitalism has often been associated with theological notions of spirit or soul, and its proponents have sometimes been devoutly religious. But this vital force of physiologists should not be equated with divine spirits. Neither mechanism nor vitalism satisfies all explanatory problems. When one mode of thinking dominates, a reactive swing back toward the other usually follows.

The second theme is about method of inquiry: it concerns the relationship between *teleology and empiricism*. The word 'teleology,' often defined as 'the doctrine of first [or final] causes,' refers to knowledge of purpose: the reason why something exists or happens; such questioning leads to the meaning of life and the possible existence of higher powers. 'Empiricism' refers to knowledge obtained through 'pure' observation without theoretical bias of higher purpose. Both methods deal with cause and effect. But teleology implies confidence in knowing the ultimate reason or purpose for a certain function; it therefore governs experiments and conclusions. Empirical methods, on the other hand, are supposedly confined only to observed events and their immediate (and equally observable) causes; they strive to control conditions and ignore higher purposes. Teleology was more influential in antiquity than it is today; a few centuries ago, it was devalued by scientists who preferred empirical methods and explanations as they established principles for experimentation on life. Virtually every problem in physiology could be reformulated with the question 'Why?' But the search for purpose is no longer the overtly stated aim of scientific experiments. Rather, the scientific method now purports to explore 'how' and confines experiments to observation of events in natural or manipulated environments (see positivism, below).

The third theme is the relationship between *speculation and experimentation,* which connects directly to the other two dualistic tensions just discussed. Speculation, often called 'armchair physiology,' refers to the style of physiology practised until modern times; it prized reasoning and observation over experimentation. The experimental *method* is relatively modern, but physiological experiments have been conducted for at least two thousand years. Nor should we think that speculation has no role in scientific investigation today.

The fourth and final theme is sociological: *the rise of physiology* as a separate discipline or profession. A desire to explain life has always been part of human character; in antiquity, however, a physiologist was most likely to be a philosopher. After the sixteenth century, a physiologist was an anatomist, or perhaps a doctor. In the nineteenth century, separate chairs and new departments of physiology were founded. Now, physiology is its own unique discipline with institutes, societies, journals, chairs, departments, and conferences. But we may be witnessing a decline in the generic all-purpose physiologist as subspecialties emerge. Psychology has invaded physiology, and it is through this window that I will bring the chapter back to the first theme of vitalism and mechanism.

All four themes enter into the philosophy of knowledge, called *positivism,* which appeared in the late eighteenth century and pervades scientific research today (see below).

An Overview of the History of Physiology

Throughout most of human history, physiology was far more important to medicine than was anatomy. Structure had little to do with concepts of disease, nor was it essential for explaining how bodies work (see chapter 2). To explain life functions, the Greeks embraced the notion of balance in four humours: black bile, yellow bile, phlegm, and blood (see figure 3.1). The four humours were cognates of, and combined the characteristics of, the four elements in the Greek 'periodic table': earth, air, fire, and water.

The power of this theory can be found in the works of many ancient writers, including Hippocrates and Galen. Its roots may extend to

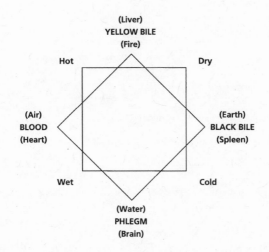

3.1   Schematic arrangement illustrating the properties and relationship of the four humours and four elements in Greek science. Mark Howes, Queen's University

an even older tradition, for the Ayurvedic writings of ancient India refer to three similar humours: *vayu* (air), *pitta* (bile), and *kapha* (phlegm). These three combined with other nutrients to form seven basic tissues, one of which was blood (*rakta*). However, our search for cognates runs the risk of perceiving similarities that may not exist. Historian Shigehisa Kuriyama points out that Greek and Chinese attempts to systematize the human body were radically different, although the observations were no less careful and the wisdom no less sound. He emphasizes the role of cultural priorities in analysis.

In addition to the four humours, the ancient Greeks also conceived of a life force (*enhormonta*, or *pneuma*) that permeated and sustained living beings. Much simplified, Galenic understanding of nutrition and circulation proceeded as follows: Food is consumed, absorbed, and transformed in the liver into blood with natural spirit (*pneuma physicon*). It passes to the lung, where it is imbued with air or vital spirit (*pneuma zoticon*). It then flows outward, in both arteries and veins, to all the organs including the brain, which adds animal spirit (*pneuma psychicon*), the source of motion. The health of an individual depends on the balance of humours and the strength of the life forces (see figure 3.2).

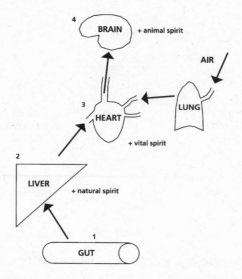

3.2   Schematic illustration of Galen's physiology. Mark Howes, Queen's University

Galen imagined that blood constantly flowed outward from the heart, like water in an irrigation ditch. To make the concept 'work,' he postulated the existence of pores in the heart. Incredulous observers wonder how Galen could have mistaken the anatomy of the heart and the direction of blood flow, but human dissections were largely forbidden during his time.

A Thought Experiment

Limit yourself to what Galen knew and the methods of investigation available to him. Then try to refute his theory.

Galen was not an 'armchair physiologist'; he performed many experiments on animals to determine the relative importance of the brain, heart, lungs, and liver. A teleological framework is evident in his writing – he attributed certain specific faculties to each body part:

attractive, retentive, alterative, repulsive, or eliminative. The following passage from his treatise *On the Natural Faculties* is derived from his description of an experiment to tie the ureters and the urethra. It displays both teleology and vitalism:

> In fact, those who are enslaved to their sects are not merely devoid of all knowledge, but they will not even stop to learn! Instead of listening as they ought, to the reasons why liquid can enter the bladder through the ureters, but is unable to go back the same way ... they refuse to learn; they even go so far as to scoff and maintain that the kidneys as well as many other things have been made by nature *for no purpose!* ...
>
> If we are not going to grant the kidneys a faculty for attracting this particular quality ... we shall discover no other reason. For surely as everyone sees that either the kidneys must attract the urine or the veins propel it. (Bk 1:13, 15)

In later centuries, Galen's physiology appealed to the Christian church. His references to the life force were conflated with the 'soul,' and his dogmatic formulations took on the aura of biblical edict. As a result, Galenic notions were repeated, commented on, and copied for generations. If doubts arose, they were not expressed until the fifteenth and sixteenth centuries (see chapter 2).

The overthrow of Galenic theories was gradual; some were repeatedly discredited before they were toppled. For example, the pulmonary circulation was first described by the Arab intellectual Ibn al-Nafis of Syria and Egypt. He refuted Galen by announcing that blood did not pass through pores in the cardiac septum but went from the right heart to the left through the lungs. His work was unknown in Europe until it was translated. Three hundred years later, the Spanish physician and cleric Michael Servetus also described pulmonary circulation in a religious treatise. Denounced as a heretic for his theological views by reformers, including John Calvin, Servetus was burned alive with his books in 1553. General acceptance of the notion of pulmonary circulation would take seventy more years.

The Advent of Mechanism

Despite the resilience of Galenic authority, attacks eventually arose on all sides. Galen's critics claimed that he had ignored effective therapies and failed to describe two important scourges of more recent times: plague and syphilis (see chapter 7). In 1628, the English physician William Harvey published his book *On the Motion of the Heart*, explaining how blood circulated through the lungs and the body.

Harvey's famous discovery was no accident. In addition to his precursors Ibn al-Nafis and Servetus, several preconditions had set the stage; some were anatomical, others conceptual. First, during his studies at Padua, Harvey had learned of the valves in the veins from anatomy teachers who had known of Vesalius. Anatomically, he knew that blood in the veins flowed toward the heart. Second, using mathematical calculations based on the pulse and the stroke volume, he reasoned that if blood did *not* circulate, the liver must manufacture 400 gallons (1,800 litres) of blood a day – vastly more, it seemed, than could be fabricated from average daily food intake. Third, Harvey was influenced by philosophical notions of cycles in nature and by the new mechanical pumps and fire engines in the world around him. He showed that the heart was a pump too.

Harvey appears to have hesitated more than a decade before publishing what would be seen as a radical revision of Galen. His argument relied on anatomical observations and calculations, using the experiments as proof, and it seemed removed from ancient theorizing or speculation. As a result, many cite his book as the beginning of modern experimental physiology. Yet his many animal experiments merely confirmed the prior reasoning; speculation was also important.

Following Harvey, others were inspired to seek mechanistic explanations for life functions. A numerical passion flowed into medicine from other disciplines preoccupied with finding simpler ways of describing events. Typifying the agenda of his era, Harvey's contemporary Galileo Galilei said, 'Measure all that is measurable and make those things measurable which have hitherto not been measured' (K. Rothschuh, *History of Physiology*, New York: Krieger, 1973, 76). In this new tradition, the Italian physician Santorio Santorio of Venice and Padua invented a pendulum machine to count the pulse. To measure body heat, he devised a large, unwieldy thermometer, an elaborate precursor of the smaller instruments that would enter clinical practice two centuries later. But the best known of Santorio's inventions was a metabòlic balance chair, in which he spent much time, often eating and sleeping there. By carefully weighing his ingesta and excreta, Santorio calculated a daily average loss of 1.25 kg in the form of 'insensible perspiration.'

René Descartes, the seventeenth-century French philosopher and mathematician, expressed the philosophic mood: without denying the existence of God, he explained bodily functions according to mechanical laws. To explain sensation and reaction, Descartes invoked small, rapidly moving particles – 'animal spirits' – which travelled in hollow nerves. Muscles contracted on hydraulic principles, swollen by the in-rush of animal spirits. Descartes knew of Harvey; in his theory, however, blood circulated not because it was pumped by the heart, but because it was heated in the heart to projectile expansion.

Descartes Compares a Sick Man to a Poorly Made Clock (in contrast to a healthy man and a well-made clock)

A sick man is in truth no less the creation of God than is man in full health ... A clock, composed of wheels and counterweights, is no less exactly obeying all the laws of nature when it is badly made and does not mark the time correctly than when it completely fulfills the intention of its maker; so also the human body may be considered as a machine, so built and composed of bones, nerves, muscles, veins, blood, and skin that even if there were no mind in it, it would not cease to move in all the ways it does at present when it is not moved under the direction of the will.

– Descartes, *Meditations* (1641), trans. Lawrence J. Lafleur
(Indianapolis and New York: Bobbs Merrill, 1960), 138–9

For Descartes, heat, not life force, was the major characteristic of life. He recognized the existence of a divinely created soul, which he equated with the mind and located in the pineal gland. This soul was distinct from bodily operations. Animals were alive, but they did not have souls. The separation of soul from body, expressed by Descartes (although he had predecessors), is often referred to as Cartesian 'mind-body dualism.' Ignoring the mind to focus on the body resulted in a number of scientific treatises that represented the body in mechanistic terms. Mind-body dualism also provoked debate over the relationships between anatomical structure, life experience, and illness. Critics soon challenged the inadequacies of dualism. In many ways, the controversy has yet to be resolved, although it is largely ignored in biomedical research. The medicine subtended by such a philosophy was called 'iatromechanism.'

Iatromechanists defined and described disease through physical analogies involving pumps, levers, springs, and pulleys. These physiologists also noticed that chemistry could mimic the living phenomena of fermentation, combustion, and decomposition. Because bodily processes could be described in similar terms, iatrochemistry became a specialized subset of early modern physiology. By the seventeenth century, sulphur, mercury, and salt had expanded the traditional four elements of the periodic table. All elements, old and new, participated in explanations of life and disease.

The English iatrochemist John Mayow, taking his lead from Descartes's equation of heat and life, studied living beings as units of combustion – a candle needs air to burn, just as animals need air to live. Placing a lit candle under a jar inverted in water, he used the rising level of water to measure the air consumed. He observed that the candle went out when about one-fifth of the air was gone and concluded that only some, not all, air could sustain burning. He repeated the experiment using a mouse instead of a candle and noticed that the mouse died when the same proportion of air had been consumed (see figure 3.3). Again he concluded that only some air was able to support life. But was 'breathable air' the same as 'burnable air'? To answer the question, he placed a mouse and a candle together in the jar. Both were extinguished faster than when they had been alone, and still only one-fifth of the air had been consumed. The 'breathable' and 'burnable' airs were identical. We know now that it is oxygen, which comprises roughly 20 per cent of air. Mayow thereby brought life closer to the combustion of inanimate objects.

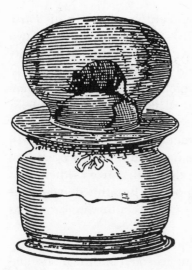

3.3 Mouse in a jar. From John Mayow, *Tractatus duo quorum*, 1668. The consumed air is measured by displacement of the membrane

During the late seventeenth and early eighteenth centuries, several physiologists reacted to what they considered exaggerated mechanism. Among them were the German Georg Stahl and the French physician Julien Offray de La Mettrie. Stahl, who began as a mechanist, provided the label 'phlogiston' for the combustible portion of air. It had been interesting, even useful, he said, to separate the soul from the body. But he soon found that the separation hindered investigation of certain problems, such as voluntary motion. Stahl thought that in emphasizing mechanics and matter, the iatromechanists had fostered a trend away from life itself. How, he asked, did attractive but simplistic analogies – describing the heart as a pump, or heat as a driving force – refute the existence of an underlying life force that moves the heart or generates heat? Mechanistic physiologists simply ignored these questions.

Stahl reintroduced the ancient concept of a life force in terms of a gaslike *anima* that resembled the newly discovered but invisible gravity of Isaac Newton. For Stahl, a lifeless body was a chemical soup that would simply decompose. The *anima* was the force that kept it alive, composed, in good repair, and moving. Eighteenth-century Europe divided into two camps physiologically speaking: the mechanistic and the vitalistic.

The Swiss physician-naturalist Albrecht von Haller was perhaps the most prolific physiologist of the eighteenth century. In his *Physiological Elements of the Human Body* (1757–66), he re-examined two well-known properties of life: sensibility (perception) and irritability (response). All living beings – plants and animals – were said to possess both. Study of these properties, which we would now call neurophysiology, became the central focus of life research for at least a century. Von Haller based his conclusions on anatomical observations, and he conducted animal experiments. Using similar methods, his Italian contemporary Lazzaro Spallanzani studied reproduction, concluding that all living beings were descended from others and that spontaneous generation did not occur. But the debate over spontaneous generation raged on for another century before it was put to rest by Louis Pasteur.

Arising from the earlier entities of phlogiston and combustible air, oxygen was the product of several interconnected and near simultaneous discoveries in the 1770s by scientists working in three different countries: Carl Wilhelm Scheele, Joseph Priestley, and Antoine-Laurent Lavoisier (see chapter 8). Soon it was generally accepted that all animal life required oxygen. Like a flame, life could be seen as combustion of carbon in the presence of oxygen. This idea corresponded well with the parallel notion of heat as life.

In 1780, the Italian Luigi Galvani made the startling observation that passing electric current through the leg of a frog could produce reflex movement. Electricity thus joined gravity and the life force as an invisible but powerful entity that produced movement.

Positivism and the Rise of Experimental Physiology

In the eighteenth century, physiologists had been preoccupied with the causes of life functions, but in the nineteenth century they turned to the more elemental definition of 'facts,' as defined by empirical methods. This trend was a product of the rise of positivism, a rigid extrapolation of the older sensualism, a philosophy of knowledge preoccupied with observation (see chapter 2).

Positive philosophy was named and described by Auguste Comte of France. He is often called 'the founder of sociology,' because he argued that social behaviours should also be subject to measurement and analysis. With their emphasis on numbers, the tenets of positivism had already been unarticulated ideals for many of his scientific contemporaries before his lessons were published.

With these tenets, positivism cast teleology, speculation, and to a certain extent vitalism outside the scientific method. Postmodern philosophy criticizes positivism, especially its confidence in the existence of immutable 'facts,' which are now seen as constructs susceptible to the biases of the observer (see, for example, Fleck 1979, and chapter 4). Nevertheless, physiology and medicine are still strongly positivistic, even if doctors and scientists have not heard of the philosophy.

Physiological research in the early nineteenth century continued to focus on anatomy to locate the site of biological processes and elucidate their nature. By the time anatomy became essential to medical

---

Tenets of Positivism

1. All knowledge evolves through three increasingly sophisticated stages:
   - *theological:* explanations based on gods or supernatural powers
   - *metaphysical:* explanations based on immaterial forces
   - *positive:* explanations based only on direct observations.
2. The most positive systems of knowledge are mathematics and astronomy; the least are biology and the social sciences.
3. A search for cause(s) of events is futile, because causes are unknowable.
4. Instead, positive knowledge stems from observed events or 'facts.'
5. Numbers should be used to describe observations to avoid subjective verbal metaphors that drag science back into metaphysics or theology.
6. Positivism seeks to establish laws through correlation of facts.

– Based on Auguste Comte, *Cours de philosophie positive* (1830–42), trans. Frederick Ferré (Indianapolis: Hackett, 1988)

education, physiologists were well placed to profit; however, medical anatomy was done on cadavers. Because a dead body was unsuitable for the study of life, physiologists conducted their observations on living animals, and not usually in medical schools. Increasingly, they opted to investigate by actively altering structure through surgery on animals. Historians, including Gerald Geison, have identified experimentation as the hallmark that demarcated physiology as a separate discipline.

In a few years of vigorous research following the French Revolution, François Xavier Bichat, a young genius from Lyons working in Paris, attempted to define the properties of life by exploring aspects of existence that disappeared with death. His methods were both anatomical (he adopted the notion of tissues as anatomical structures and used surgical methods) and philosophical (he classified life functions into two types: animal and organic). After a winter of frenzied investigation – during which he dissected six hundred corpses, taught at least two courses, and worked on several books – Bichat died of a sudden febrile illness at the age of thirty.

Inspired by Bichat, the French physician François Magendie vivisected unanesthetized animals to explore the properties of life. In some famously cruel experiments, he carefully related neurological function to structure. For example, he showed that sensory and motor nerve fibres travelled together in the whole nerve, except near the spinal cord, where sensory fibres occupied the dorsal root and motor fibres, the ventral. Priority for this discovery resulted in a dispute with Charles Bell of England, who also had experimented on motor function. Bell went on to make other observations, especially on cranial nerves and the facial palsy that bears his name. Magendie extended his investigations to circulation, digestion, and the effects of drugs and 'poisons,' including rabies virus in saliva (see chapter 5). He hesitated to draw sweeping conclusions from his work, but he dismissed the vital forces of his predecessors as arbitrary assumptions. Yet he too was unable to avoid certain vitalistic concepts in his interpretations.

Magendie founded one of the first periodicals of physiology (see table 3.1). Essays on life function had been published since scholarly

Table 3.1
First national periodicals and societies in physiology

Year	Country	Editor	Title/Society
1795	Germany	Reil	*Archiv für Physiologie*
1821	France	Magendie	*Journal de physiologie*
1828	France		Société de Biologie
1876	UK		The Physiological Society
1878	England	Foster	*Journal of Physiology*
1887	U.S.		American Physiological Society
1898	U.S.	Porter	*American Journal of Physiology*
1904	Germany		Deutsche Gesellschaft für Physiologie
1926	France		L'Association des Physiologistes
1929	Canada	Collip	*Canadian Journal of Research*
1936	Canada		Canadian Physiological Society
1950	worldwide		250 titles
1990	worldwide		thousands (or very few?)

journalism began, but the creation of periodicals devoted to physiology was a nineteenth-century development.

A materialistic view of life appealed to many of Magendie's contemporaries. In 1828 Friedrich Wöhler, working in Berlin, synthesized urea, a substance previously thought to be a product of living processes only. It was said that vitalism was dead: no special forces were needed to explain life, because all vital functions, like urea, would eventually be reproduced in the laboratory. The research of the German chemist Justus von Liebig and his colleagues at Giessen was devoted to similar chemical interpretations of life processes. Liebig synthesized chloroform (1830), studied fermentation, discovered the amino acid tyrosine (1846), and wrote an influential textbook on what he called 'animal chemistry.'

Not everyone agreed with the empirical spirit that had informed the investigations of Liebig and Magendie. A counter-movement, *Naturphilosophie*, emphasized intuition over empiricism and scorned experimentation. Its advocate, Friedrich von Schelling, described *Naturphilosophie* as speculation about life in terms of hierarchies and orders; it was based on the principle that nature was visible spirit, and spirit was invisible nature. Influenced by the ideas of the writer J.W. von Goethe, who had studied the morphology of plants, Schelling urged a search for similarities in life functions in order to uncover the general cosmic patterns governing nature. *Naturphilosophie* appealed to many prominent German physicians, including J.C. Reil, F. Blumenbach, and Johannes Müller. Müller's influential handbook of physiology blended these ideas with evidence from experimental science.

Features of *Naturphilosophie*

Nature is a hierarchy, ranging from plants, characterized by a vegetative preoccupation with reproduction; to insects and animals, characterized by their irritability; to humans, characterized by their sensibility.

Many histories recount how Schelling's *Nature Philosophy* 'retarded' the growth of 'real' science. But we might ask, Why did it develop when it did? Like many before him, Schelling was concerned with the mind-body problem. Even his critics seem to have regarded body organization as the product of an immaterial force – vital, spiritual, or creative. Both structure and function had to have some antecedent cause, yet the new positivistic experimentation rejected the search for causes as unwelcome teleological thinking. Ignoring causes and purposes to focus on minute properties because they could be measured struck Schelling as unscientific. A debate over these modes of reasoning about life began in earnest. At the time, few could predict which perspective would emerge victorious; however, overt teleology would soon be hounded from the scientific method.

The most famous physiologists of the mid-nineteenth century were Claude Bernard of France and Karl Friedrich Wilhelm Ludwig of Germany. Their work formed the methodological basis of today's experimental physiology. A student of Magendie, Bernard was educated as a doctor but spent his life in animal research, making many discoveries on the formation of glycogen and other life processes. His main contribution, however, was the elaboration of an approach to experimentation, now known as 'the scientific method.' Bernard would observe a phenomenon, localize it to an anatomical structure, and then surgically alter that structure in order to study its effects. His *Introduction to the Study of Experimental Physiology* (1865) laid out the philosophical and methodological principles of investigation. Bernard advocated isolating the event under study by *controlling* all conditions of the experiment. He endorsed the empirical view that everything needed to understand an event can be derived from rigorous observation of that event. Without denying a vital force, he claimed that only its consequences could be observed. His ideas are steeped in positivism and reflected in the epigraph to this chapter.

Bernard recognized that the living organism reacts to change in its environment to maintain a constant, or homeostatic, *milieu intérieur*. His work on both glycogen and diabetes was permeated with this ideal. At the end of his life, experimental physiology was greatly admired, especially in drug testing, but it was still peripheral to medical studies, which continued to be preoccupied with cadaveric research. Bernard never became a professor in a medical school; he worked at the Sorbonne and the Collège de France in Paris.

A Vignette

Bernard's home life was said to be unhappy because both his wife and daughter were antivivisectionists. My friend François Gallouin, also a physiologist, suggests that domestic discord may be beneficial to scientific work, since it favours long hours in the lab.

Germany poured uniquely large sums into education and purpose-built laboratories for scientific research. Soon it led the world in establishing physiological journals, chairs, departments, and laboratories, in a process called professionalization. In Berlin, Müller taught several scientists who went on to establish distinguished careers, including the Swiss histologist R.A. von Kolliker, the German neurologist Emil du Bois-Reymond, and the German pathologist Rudolf Virchow. But Karl Ludwig's institute at Leipzig was the mecca for physiology.

Ludwig was firmly convinced that physics and chemistry could explain all life functions. Politically he was a liberal; spiritually, an atheist. His social and philosophic views were associated with his reductionist science, providing yet more fodder for the debate over the nature of life. He analysed renal and cardiovascular physiology, inventing mechanical devices to measure the previously unmeasurable – the kymograph (1846), and the *Stromuhr* or 'stream clock' (1867), which monitored blood flow. Genealogies of Ludwig's many disciples illustrate his powerful influence on physiology in Russia, Italy, England, Scandinavia, and the United States.

The surgeon William Beaumont was the first American to attract international fame for physiological investigation of an unusual case. In 1822 he treated the abdominal gunshot wound of a French Canadian, Alexis St Martin. Because the wound healed with an external fistula (hole) to the stomach, Beaumont could experiment on St Martin's digestion by tying string around pieces of meat and other foods, inserting them through the fistula, and retrieving them after varied periods of time. So eager was he to maintain the investigations over the next decade that he often had St Martin live with him for up to two years at a time. But the patient grew tired of the arrangement and returned to his home at St Thomas, in Joliette County, Quebec. At the age of seventy-eight, he was reported to be healthy with his fistula still open, but he was apprehensive of scientific designs upon him. When he died in 1880, William Osler received a telegram from St Martin's family, warning him to stay away and describing a deliberate delay before the exceptionally deep burial of the body in an unmarked grave. They hoped that decomposition and depth would dissuade doctors from attempts to dissect it. In 1962, the Canadian Physiological Society placed a bronze plaque on the church wall of the cemetery to commemorate St Martin's contributions to science.

Physiology in the Twentieth Century

Once physiology became a separate discipline defined by its commitment to experimentation, its relevance to medicine increased. In

On Accident in Discovery

Chance favours the prepared mind.

– Saying attributed to Louis Pasteur, ca 1854, cited in R. Vallery-Radot, *Life of Pasteur*, trans. R.I. Devonshire (Garden City, NY: Garden City Publishing, 1927), 76–9

Many inventors and discoverers ascribe their findings to 'accident,' 'serendipity,' or 'chance.' First-hand accounts notwithstanding, historians and philosophers of science regard chance as a bit player rather than the *magister ludi.* Only when an observer knows that something is missing or needed is it likely to be found. An unexpected coincidence can bring a juxtaposition of circumstances to the attention of an observer who may be looking for something else. But a discovery will be made only if that observer has some insight or special knowledge – a 'lucky ticket' – that allows for correlation. The chance occurrence may have taken place many times in the past without a 'discovery.' For example, 'accidents' such as St Martin's had probably happened earlier, but it was Beaumont's awareness of research elsewhere that enabled him to take full advantage of that particular fistulous stomach. Patterns of scientific communication, the conscious development of a method, and the existence of laboratories – and even, to a certain extent, relative amounts of research funding – tend to diminish the role left to chance.

fact the two were mutually dependent: physiologists needed clinical medicine to understand how to operate and keep their animals alive; physicians needed physiology to shore up claims to being scientific. In Europe, the great physiologists had worked in scientific institutes rather than medical schools, even if they had trained as physicians. In North America, anatomy had been part of medical training from the founding of the earliest medical schools; however, physiology had to be introduced. William Osler described the integration of physiology into medicine as the 'growth of truth'; his career spanned this process.

Integrating physiology with medical education was a project of the late nineteenth and early twentieth centuries. In Britain and America, it involved the international efforts of a number of distinguished physician-scientists, many of whom had visited other countries for studies or meetings of their societies. They included John Burdon-Sanderson at Oxford, Michael Foster at Cambridge, Charles Brown-Sequard of Paris (and Harvard), and the Harvard-educated physician John C. Dalton, who in 1855 at the age of thirty became America's first professor of physiology. Dalton's appointment at Columbia's College of Physicians and Surgeons was remarkably early; most physiology chairs and professorships within medical schools came after 1870. For example, in 1871, physician Henry P. Bowditch became Harvard's first medical professor of physiology, although he had predecessors in other faculties. Four of the five founders of the American Physiological Society, including Bowditch, were doctors who had sojourned in Europe. In Canada, a short-lived veterinary school was created in Kingston simply to provide skills needed to sustain animal investigation in the local medical school. By the first decades of the twentieth century, physiology defined scientific medicine.

Unlike Beaumont, few physiologists could conduct research on humans who had survived interesting accidents. Following the premises of observing, tampering with, or even removing body parts to uncover their function, some, like Santorio, made use of their own bodies or those of student volunteers. Others co-opted the services of disadvantaged people bought or compelled to serve: patients, paupers, condemned criminals, soldiers, prostitutes, wet nurses, and the racially different. The abuses of Nazi doctors included so-called scientific experimentation on people without their consent in investigations that often ended in killing (see chapter 15). The horrifying discovery of these practices during the doctors' trial after the Second World War resulted in the Nuremberg Code (1947), which outlined the ethical basis for research on human subjects. A fuller expression of these principles came with the Declaration of Helsinki in 1964.

Mostly however, physiologists used animals, the choice influenced as much by availability and cost as by similarities to human beings. Rats, mice, rabbits, cats, dogs, monkeys, cattle, horses, sheep, pigs, ferrets, guinea pigs, and various birds, fish, reptiles, and bacteria had been used in experiments throughout the nineteenth century, even before the discovery of anesthesia mid-century. The perceived need to sacrifice the lives and well-being of animals to the demands of science met with vigorous opposition and the formation of antivivisection groups, often growing from long-established entities devoted to the prevention of cruelty to animals. The concept of animal rights arose in the late nineteenth century and was widely promoted in the 1960s by a group of intellectuals at Oxford University and Australian philosopher Peter Singer, author of *Animal Liberation* (1973). Extremists waged violent attacks on laboratories. The continued pressure from this movement resulted in national standards for laboratory animal care and systems for inspection and revision. It played into the rise of bioethics as a discipline (see chapter 6), and it sparked a counter-reaction among researchers, doctors, and patients who wanted to explain the benefits of animal research and allay the threats of activists; they established new organizations such as Partners in Research (Canada, 1988), Americans for Medical Progress (U.S., 1991), and the Coalition for Medical Progress (UK, 2003). This topic is still of great interest to historians and ethicists alike.

First awarded in 1901, the Nobel Prizes in medicine were also prizes in physiology; in general, they have been given for the reduction of life processes to physicochemical terms. That is, they display the triumph of mechanism. Cardiac contraction and circulation were now electrical as well as muscular. Respiration was no longer a phenomenon of the lungs alone, but a chemical event operating at the level of cells, subcellular organelles, and molecules (see chapter 8). In the early twentieth century, hormones and vitamins were identified as the enzymes of living processes – the former being an intrinsic product of the organism; the latter, extrinsic and synthesized by other organisms (see chapter 13). In 1944, nucleic acid was recognized as the chemical stuff of heredity by Nova Scotian Oswald T. Avery, putting the new field of genetics on a molecular basis (see chapter 4). From the 1950s, psychology and psychiatry both became increasingly physiological as perception and movement were described in mechanical terms that could be measured and manipulated. The advent of major tranquillizers (neuroleptics) that help people with schizophrenia to manage their symptoms seemed to further endorse a chemical theory of mind, as did the advent of lithium for bipolar disorders (see chapter 12). The rapid rise of physiology as a discipline was charted by Rothschuh through the attendance at international conferences – from 124 delegates representing eighteen countries at the first meeting in 1889, to 4,300 delegates from fifty-one countries by 1968.

But general physiology meetings are less well attended now relatively speaking. Physiologists specialize in a way their predecessors did not. Clusters of researchers – anatomists, physiologists, and physicians who are interested in structure, function, and their problems (disease) form epistemic communities around functional systems: circulatory, respiratory, reproductive, digestive, and above all neurological.

For one example, histories of neuroscience tell how investigation of the mind, brain, and nerves has a long tradition stretching back to the dawn of writing. This observation is true, but early researchers turned their attention to stomach and muscle as often as they examined the brain. Judging by the titles of books and journals, the word 'neuroscience' to designate a scientific field of inquiry emerged in the early 1960s. From a search of medical literature, the earliest indexed article using the word 'neuroscience' in its title was from 1967 (see figure 3.4). Various neuroscience societies formed and began holding annual meetings in the 1970s (the United States in 1971; Europe, 1977; Japan 1978). Journals using the word 'neuroscience' in their titles also date from the 1970s. Now neuroscience is so well established as a field that its *history* has also been institutionalized with a distinguished journal, founded in 1991, and an International Society for the History of Neurosciences founded in Montreal in 1995. In other words, the vast interdisciplinary domain of neuroscience emerged from redefinition and subspecialization of physiology writ large. The same could be said for many other systems-based forms of inquiry.

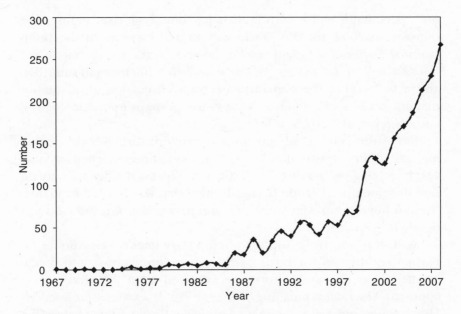

3.4   The rising frequency of the word 'neuroscience(s)' in titles of articles indexed in Medline, 1967–2008. Source: Medline, 2,603 results from title search 20 June 2009

The continued dominance of positivism means that our methods demand numbers, even for those aspects of life that seem entirely qualitative, not quantitative. No one doubts the relevance of quality of life, and the importance of spiritual and mental well-being in the overall functioning of the human body. Practitioners wish to consider these things in their research and practice. Because it is almost impossible to treat a problem scientifically without reformulating it in terms that can be measured, methods have been devised to express this qualitative information as a quantity. For example, new tools were invented to measure health-related quality of life, such as the Sickness Impact Profile (1975), the Quality of Life Index (1981), the McMaster Health Index Questionnaire (1982), the Quality of Well-Being Scale (1984), and the Edmonton Symptom Assessment Scale (1991). A journal on research into quality of life began in the early 1990s. These tools are widely used in clinical trials, which strive to include the effects of physical treatments on mind, thought, emotion, personality, spirituality, and behaviour. Positivism defines the domain: in 2007, for the fourteenth annual meeting of the International Society for Quality of Life Research, the words 'measure,' 'measuring,' or 'measurement' appeared over 700 times in some 370 abstracts. Without these quantitative tools, discussion of qualitative matters would seem vitalistic, speculative, perhaps even teleological, and consequently unscientific.

Here is the same mind-body problem that disturbed Stahl, Schelling, and others who are now known (and sometimes scorned) as vitalists. In relying on quantitative indices to express quality, we may do well to remember Claude Bernard's idea that most of life is qualitative: numbers simply facilitate our understanding of it, they do not define it.

Vitalism is not irrelevant to contemporary science. Hormones, in particular, offer an interesting bridge between vitalistic and mechanistic views. The word 'hormone,' derived from the Greek word ὁρμῶντα (hormonta, meaning 'I arouse' or 'I excite,' was used by Hippocrates and two millennia of other medical writers to describe the life force. 'Hormone,' as a modern scientific word, was coined in 1902 by the British physiologists W.M. Bayliss and E.H. Starling when they announced their discovery of secretin. In other words, when modern hormones were first conceived, they were deliberately identified as a chemical translation of the life force. Among the most recent of hormone finds are the endorphins discovered in the mid-1970s. Secreted in response to pleasurable events, they bind to internal receptors, which can also bind various narcotic drugs. More than any other substance, the endorphins seem to fit into a mechanical conception of the mind-body link. Similar excitement greeted the concepts of vitamins because they seemed to solve inscrutable mysteries of living chemistry. The intellectual fervour over each endocrine or vitamin discovery was reflected in the Nobel Prizes. (On insulin, see chapter 5; on sex hormones, chapter 11; on endocrinology and stress, chapter 12; and on vitamins, chapter 13.)

Western society celebrates explanations of motion, will, and thought in terms of chemistry and physics as the most important accomplishments in medicine and physiology. One well might ask why physicochemical discoveries attract fame and reward while other less reductionist observations are not celebrated. For example, why were the efforts of scientist Linus Pauling and the founders of International Physicians for the Prevention of Nuclear War (see chapter 6) awarded the Nobel Prize for peace, not medicine, although their actions may have prevented millions of deaths if not global annihilation? Does medicine's close identification with experimental physiology (and its attendant positivism) explain its difficulty with the less measurable social, cultural, environmental, and economic determinants of health? Is medicine's focus on cure rather than prevention a product of its link to experimental physiology? Does this link explain medical preference for biological and mechanical therapies over others?

Historians such as J.V. Pickstone have tried to connect philosophical attitudes in biological science to the political and religious views of individual scientists. Some correlations have been found, but no pervasive consensus can be reached. Indeed, convincing arguments suggest that all science partakes of both vitalism and mechanism, and both speculation and experimentation – what differs is the extent to which scientists are willing to admit it. Recognizing the pejorative connotations of 'vitalism,' one physician-historian characterized the debate between vitalists and mechanists as a fight between the 'modest' and the 'arrogant' (G. Canguilhem, *Connaissance de la vie*, Paris 1980, 86, 95, 99). Those who try to address aspects of life that cannot yet be expressed in 'scientific' terms are called vitalists, usually by others and not by themselves. Vitalists offend the reductionist mechanists by being perceived as too humble – possessed of a fatal modesty, *sophrosyne*, the opposite of *hubris* (F.J. Ingelfinger, 'Arrogance,'*New England J. Medicine* 303 [1980], 1507–11). In return, reductionists offend vitalists not only for arrogance (although that is part of it) but also for the necessary limitations that they impose on investigations, because certain conditions, such as attitude, personality, pleasure, and value, cannot be controlled or measured. Nobel laureate Peter Medawar wrote that biologists no longer need to invoke vital forces, and vitalistic ideas fall into the 'limbo of that which is disregarded' (P.B. Medawar and J.S. Medawar, *Aristotle to Zoos*, Harvard University Press, 1983, 277). But so-called vitalists refuse to disregard the as-yet-unmeasurable phenomena that may well constitute the most significant aspects of being alive.

Vignette: What Does Carlson Think of Vitalism? of Religion?

Both [Francis] Crick and [James] Watson [Nobel laureates 1962] had been influenced by Erwin Schrödinger's *What Is Life?*, a popularization of genetics seen from a physicist's perspective. Crick's approach to biology was quite different from Schrödinger's because Crick was an atheist and Schrödinger's perception of life was vitalistic. What Crick found of value, however, was Schrödinger's recognition that many of the uniquely biological properties, such as heredity, were amenable to an analysis that physicists had successfully used for the structure of inanimate matter.

– Elof Axel Carlson, 'Francis Crick,' in Daniel Fox et al.,
Nobel Laureates in Physiology or Medicine (New York: Garland, 1990), 111–12

Teleology may be unacceptable as a framework for the scientific exploration of life, but 'Why?' is the most seductive question we can ask of science (and of history!). Speculation will continue to thrive in the minds of creative scientists, and consequently thinking that gets labelled as 'vitalistic' cannot be suppressed. The concept of irreducible, complex processes still proves useful – even for those who pretend to repudiate vitalism – if only for providing a language to address the unexplained: What makes a DNA molecule unzip? Why are some of us sane and others insane? Why do we not decompose during life? Why are some physicochemical mixtures alive and some dead? It is fascinating to notice how often scientists who win the Nobel Prize eventually write philosophical essays in which they acknowledge questions that are not (yet) amenable to laboratory investigation as a stimulus to further research. (On reading this chapter my physiologist colleague Steven Iscoe observed how rarely award-winning humanists ever do the reverse!)

Suggestions for Further Reading

At the bibliography website http://histmed.ca.

CHAPTER FOUR

Science of Suffering:
History of Pathology*

Life is short, the Art long, opportunity fleeting, experience treacherous, judgment difficult.

– Hippocrates, *Aphorisms*, I, 1

Pathology as a System of Medical Knowledge

Medicine is not a science; rather, it is an applied technology or an art that makes extensive use of science. Medicine's claims to being scientific are anchored in pathology as the study of disease. Pathology, from the Greek words for 'suffering' and 'theory about,' is literally the study of suffering. But its meaning has narrowed to represent material knowledge about disease.

Humans have always tried to understand illness, injury, and death. In other words, pathology has always been practised, even if it was not explicitly named. Pathology is a system of knowledge used to draw conclusions about illness. It changed through the centuries, but in every time and place it was validated by current science and philosophy. Past pathologies may not resemble our own, but they have always acknowledged contemporary views of 'science.'

Functions of Pathology

Despite differences in content, the functions of pathology are uni-

*Learning objectives for this chapter are found on pp. 450–1.

versal. First, it is used to *explain* suffering, to account for why and how humans are subject to pain and death. 'Why me?' ask sick people. Illness demands a 'logical' explanation, rooted either in the cultural and spiritual ideas of sin and blame or in the more material and 'scientific' ideas of structure, function, heredity, contagion, and risk.

Second, pathology is used to *identify* or label the ailment from which a person suffers: the process of diagnosis. Doctors use signs that point – just like signs on the highway – to the diagnosis or prognosis. Good clinical skills convert symptoms into signs. A physical examination yields more signs. Signs are not simply the product of observation; they also contain knowledge. For example, the subjective symptom of squeezing chest pain becomes an objective sign of heart disease with the addition of medical knowledge.

This diagnostic function of pathology has an important corollary: in identifying that which is 'abnormal' or sick, pathology also defines the 'normal.' The line between normal and abnormal is conditioned by culture, religion, economics, race, class, gender, and other social and biological factors. Phenomena once thought to be 'abnormal,' or 'diseased,' are now considered variants of normal. Examples include visceroptosis (the drooping gut syndrome) and homosexuality (see chapters 10 and 12). Conversely, some newly recognized diseases were inconceivable as health problems only a short time ago. Examples include psychiatric problems, hypertension, carcinoma in situ, sleep apnea, fetal alcohol syndrome, chronic fatigue, compulsive swearing, and AIDS. Histories have been written on all these conditions (see bibliography website http://histmed.ca).

Third, pathology is used to *predict* outcomes. In some cultures, especially in antiquity, accurate prognosis was at least as important as the ability to diagnose or cure. Based on a few reliable signs relating to an individual, medical prediction resembled priestly divination: 'You will die on the seventh day.' Prognosis is still an important function of pathology, but it is now couched in statistics, derived from the experience of a cohort, defined by age, sex, diagnosis, and extent of lesion. For example, we speak of five-year survival, the 50 per cent mortality index, and risk factors.

Fourth, pathology is used to *justify* treatments. As we will see in chapter 5, most treatments were discovered through observation rather than reasoning (i.e., empirically). Therapeutic rationales were often applied post hoc; in some cases, they still are. They relate an apparently effective treatment to the scientific formulation of a problem. Sometimes, a remedy of choice persists while the explanation of how it works alters considerably.

Finally, pathology has been used to *prove* the reasonableness of an explanation, a diagnosis, or a course of action. Postmortem examination is the most obvious form of this function. In Europe, occasional records of autopsies for retrospective diagnosis can be traced to the late thirteenth century. Autopsy is still the ultimate challenge of our knowledge system. Was the diagnosis correct? Could anything else have been done? The widespread use of forensics in medicine and law increased after 1800, when diseases were linked to organic changes and when the number of lawsuits for malpractice began to rise.

Disease versus Illness

Humans still suffer from the illnesses that plagued our prehistoric and simian ancestors. The subjective aspects of being sick do not change – pain, fever, swelling, vomiting, diarrhea, deformity, injury, loss of weight, loss of blood, loss of function, loss of life. But medical ideas about illness change; they are what we call disease.

We tend to think of illness and disease as identical and use the words interchangeably. For this discussion, however, and following philosophers, the word 'illness' designates individual suffering; the word 'disease' pertains to ideas about the illness. 'Illness' exists as the real suffering felt by a person; 'disease' exists only as a theory constructed to explain the illness, its presumed cause, and its target. More than semantic, the distinction is useful in the philosophy of medical knowledge, or medical epistemology, the study of how we know what we think we know.

Medical knowledge is the ability to recognize and respond to disease.

A Thought Experiment about 'Illness' and 'Disease'

'Does smallpox exist?'

'No,' says the student aware of WHO's eradication of small-pox in 1979.

'Yes,' says the student, who knows that the planned destruction of the remaining vials of smallpox virus has been deferred once again.

'But,' comes the philosophic reply, 'do the vials contain "smallpox" or do they contain the virus, which, when introduced into a human being, produces the illness that we label "smallpox" disease?'

Does smallpox exist? Is it a disease? An entity? An illness? An idea?

Therefore, constructing, recognizing, and treating disease is its central enterprise. Disease concepts are 'built' from observations of many individual sufferings of a similar nature. They take into account the patient, the illness, and the presumed cause, but they are also influenced by the observer/doctor. Diseases are given characteristics (symptoms), names (diagnoses), life expectancies (course), anticipated outcomes (prognoses), and recommended treatments. A cause is implied in the concept constructed for a disease even when the cause is unknown.

The Hippocratic Triangle

The art has three factors, the disease, the patient, the physician. The physician is the servant of the art. The patient must cooperate with the physician in combatting the disease.

– Hippocrates, *Epidemics I*, 11

If diseases are intangible thoughts about various illnesses, then what single theory or definition can be found to define all diseases? In other words, what do all diseases have in common? So far, no single explanation has been found that successfully applies to every account of disease. However, one theory dominates medical practice – the organismic, or individual, theory of disease.

The organismic theory holds that diseases are bad, discontinuous, and affect individuals. From the perspective of an organism (individual), this theory is difficult to refute. By its very name, medicine subscribes to this ideal: diseases must be bad, because individuals turn to medicine to be rid of them. Medical education is aimed at how to recognize, cure, and prevent disease. Most medical accounts of disease have conformed to this view even if the authors had never heard of the theory.

Known as the 'medical model,' the organismic theory comfortably addresses the patient as target of the disease, but it offers little to explain the causes. Throughout history, two additional perspectives about cause have vied for dominance. The first is the ontological theory, which holds that the causes come from *outside* the patient, that diseases vary one from another, and that they exist separate from the patient. The word 'ontology' stems from nouns derived from the Greek verb 'to be'; it emphasizes the idea of disease as a separate 'being,' or entity. The second theory about the cause of disease is the physiological theory, which holds that causes emerge from *inside* the patient, that patients vary, and that diseases do not exist separate from patients.

These theories of disease can be used to analyse any account of illness and disease. A medical practitioner who approaches disease through the ontological theory will be concerned with what the patient has; conversely, a physiological perspective would emphasize who or what the patient is. Both cause-based theories have currency in modern medicine, and some disease descriptions use a combination of the two. At the end of this chapter, we will explore some criticisms of medical reasoning and another theory of disease that challenges the medical model.

Historical Overview of Pathology

Construction of disease concepts moved from spiritualistic accounts of nature, to careful bedside descriptions of illness, and then to the laboratory enterprise that is familiar to us today. The following pages briefly summarize the shift.

Supernatural Causes of Disease

At the beginning of Homer's epic poem *The Iliad* (which originated sometime before 700 B.C.), the Greeks suffer a deadly pestilence, but they do not understand its cause. Few details about the illness are provided. They consult an oracle, who proclaims the cause: the king has stolen the daughter of the priest of Apollo; the bereft father begs his god to punish all Greeks with a disease. Armed with this information, the crowd confronts the king, the daughter is released, and the pestilence goes away.

The Book of Job in the Bible also dates from the same period. It describes another illness with a supernatural cause. The devout Job has a fine family, good health, and great wealth, but Satan tells God that it is easy for Job to be devout because he has everything. To prove that Job is constant, God wagers with Satan, who then destroys Job's family, his wealth, and his health. Job suffers festering boils over his whole body, but he keeps his faith. After forty chapters of agony, God rewards him by restoring all his losses.

Both these accounts of illness conform to organismic and ontological views. The disease is bad and the sufferers want it to end. It is sent by remote powers to punish or to test them. The associated terror and misery are apparent, but the features of the illnesses seem unimportant, since few details are given. The professional healer or priest does not concentrate on symptoms but looks widely for signs to determine why the deity has sent the affliction. In this context, the patient's subjective opinion about the causes of the illness are given serious consideration, including the possibility that the disease may have moral, spiritual, or pedagogic functions. Treatment is the maintenance or restoration of integrity – righting wrongs, keeping faith.

Supernatural accounts of illness may have little currency in the modern science of pathology, but they continue to influence patients and policymakers. Diseases sometimes construed as punishments include AIDS, eating disorders, and the effects of drugs, smoking, and alcohol. On this view, some people are thought to deserve their illnesses, while others feel outraged at being sick without having committed a 'sinful' act. The healthy can accept their good fortune as a token of their superiority. Similarly, chronic ailments such as arthritis and multiple sclerosis are called 'trials' – tests of character – and people who suffer uncomplainingly are said to have 'the patience of Job.'

Pathology at the Bedside

Greco-Roman Antiquity: Disease = Natural Imbalance

In the West, medical writings began in approximately the fifth century B.C. with a self-conscious refutation of the supernatural origins of disease. The Greco-Roman world had a pantheon of gods and an extensive mythology, but it also recognized a natural world of four elements and a healthy balance in the human body of four humours within an individual's temperament (see chapter 3).

The seventy treatises that make up the Hippocratic Corpus contain writings on medical philosophy and duties, for example, *The Oath*. Some disease descriptions from this period are classic examples of clinical observation, because they are recognizable as conditions diagnosed today. But pathology also looms large in the case histories, the descriptions of diseases and wounds, and the aphorisms. These last are sentences that summarize knowledge, usually for the elaboration of signs – for example, 'In athletes a perfect condition that is at its highest pitch is treacherous' (*Aphorisms*, I, 3); 'Old men endure fasting most easily, then men of middle age, youths very badly, and worst of all children, especially those of a liveliness greater than the ordinary' (*Aphorisms*, I, 13); and '[In] acute pain of the ear with ... high fever ... younger patients die ... on the seventh day or even earlier; old men die much later' (*Prognostic*, XXII).

Hippocratic pathology followed the five themes described above: it described, predicted, interpreted, and justified diseases and their treatments in concert with the best science of the day – clinical observation and reasoning. A good example is the famous text *The Sacred Disease*, a masterful description of what we now call epilepsy. The name was derived from the even older view that the sufferer was possessed by demons or touched by gods. But the author began with a clear statement: 'It is not, in my opinion, any more divine or more sacred than other diseases, but has a natural cause, and its supposed divine origin is due to men's inexperience and to their wonder at its peculiar character' (*Sacred Disease*, I). The clinical symptoms were described in detail: falling, shaking, loss of consciousness, incontinence. Affected children sensing the onset of an attack ('aura') would run to their mothers for comfort. This essay was based on the observation of many illness patterns. In explaining the cause, the author appealed to current science and attributed the disease to obstruction of phlegm in the brain.

Many other diseases were associated with imbalance in the humours – too much or too little blood, too much or too little phlegm. Some were located in specific body parts. Treatments of bleeding, baths, fumigations, and diets were intended to restore the disrupted balance. External causes, such as trauma, noxious air, and unhealthy places, worked their harmful influence through the physical structures of the body. Like most other medical writings, these accounts conform to the organismic theory (disease affects individuals, is bad and discontinuous). From a cause-based perceptive and in contrast to earlier texts, their reliance on the theory of imbalance in the internal humours tends to make them physiological. Concepts similar to this imbalance, such as disharmony or conflict in the natural components of the body, can be found in the medical systems of ancient India and China.

Another writer famed for his classic descriptions was Aretaeus of Cappadocia, who lived around 100 A.D. His vivid accounts of the symptoms of diabetes and disorders of liver, kidney, and gut sometimes ornament modern texts. The extensive works of Galen in the second century A.D. also contain case histories, as well as essays on diseases, diagnosis, and therapeutics, and commentaries on earlier authors. Galen's pathology was eclectic, but again the five functions described in the opening to this chapter are easily found. Frequently his pathology was used to justify his success as a practitioner; few examples of unanticipated therapeutic failure are described. Galen anchored some explanations in anatomy, although he did not dissect human subjects (see chapter 2). But he also made reference to the four humours and the life force. Except in cases of trauma or harmful airs, his disease concepts, like those of Hippocrates, tended to be organismic and physiological.

Galen's ideas dominated pathology in Europe, just as they dominated physiology, until early modern times (see chapter 3). Medieval philosophy advocated complete submission to the will of God. Galenical remedies could be attempted for sickness, but cure was the product of divine will. Only the arrogant would attempt to refine diagnosis by distinguishing between diseases or by improving on Galen. Some historians, with Fielding Garrison, have accused Galenism of 'preventing the advancement of medical science' because of its vitalistic reasoning, theory of blood flow, and therapeutics (*Introduction to the History of Medicine*, 1929, 106). But it is unfair to blame Galen for his successors' lack of imagination. The longevity of his influence was neither his idea nor his fault; rather it was a manifestation of prevailing attitudes and practices.

Disease = Patterns of Suffering (Nosology)

Gradually medical authors began to distinguish between diseases on the basis of their symptoms in a practice called nosology (derived from the Greek words for 'disease' and 'theory about'). Hippocrates, Galen, and other ancient writers had described fevers with and without skin rash, and fevers with diurnal variations. In the ninth century A.D. a specific clinical distinction was made between the two febrile diseases with rashes, measles and smallpox, by the Persian physician-encyclopedist Rhazes (Abu-Bakr Mohammed Ibn Zakaria Al-Razi). Rhazes' twenty-volume compendium, *Continents*, was translated from Arabic into Latin in 1280. In the late fourteenth century, after Europe was ravaged by the bubonic plague – a disease that could not be found in Galen – scholars rediscovered Rhazes in looking for new ways of identifying disease. By 1476 Rhazes' *Continents* had been summarized in Padua, and twelve years later his treatise on plague was translated into Latin.

In the Renaissance, spiritualistic and vitalistic explanations of the natural world lost credibility. Hippocratic observation was glorified, while rigid Galenism waned, together with the interdictions on human dissection. Physiological experimentation was revived with iatromechanism and iatrochemistry (see chapter 3). Doctors developed techniques to integrate the new sciences of chemistry. For example, uroscopy (the examination of urine) became a new diagnostic tool added to examination of the pulse. Charts were constructed to allow physicians to associate the colour, odour, turbidity, sweetness, and other chemical properties of urine with a specific diagnosis.

But linking acid urine with illness rarely led to benefits. Medical practitioners were caught up in the realities of the bedside: people suffered from symptoms, such as pain and shortness of breath, not from acid urine. The new scientific endeavours could not yet be mapped onto the analysis of a sick person, and their effects on pathology were modest. Nevertheless, with the decline in Galenism and the rise of sensualist observation, doctors hesitated to invoke unknown causes for disease. Instead, they built a new system of diagnosis, deliberately labelled nosology, based on the careful observation of symptoms. It was a self-conscious effort to avoid theorizing. A flurry of classic disease descriptions followed.

The English physician Thomas Sydenham, writing in Latin, published his clinical observations about diseases, especially fevers, and their treatment. In the tradition of Rhazes, he separated scarlet fever from measles (1676), and he described chorea (1686), the movement disorder that follows scarlet fever and now bears his name. With his friend, the physician-philosopher John Locke, he emphasized the importance of observation and the dangers of theory. Sydenham's treatise on podagra, or gout (1683), has become a classic for its rich description of the manifestations of the disease, from which he himself suffered. Sydenham refered to the humours, but for him, the basis of diagnosis was well-developed characteristics of each disease. His diseases existed independent of the patient, as 'tyrants' or 'friends.'

In the century after Sydenham, nosology became an established form of pathology. Medical writers, who actually called themselves 'nosologists,' classified diseases into conceptual trees with branches for classes, orders, genera, and species. Symptoms and their sequence were used to categorize diseases as if they were entities, or 'beings,' like animals and plants. Authors devised original systems, each hoping to find the perfect reflection of natural order. Some classifications recognized several thousand species of disease. Among the nosologists were François Boissier de Sauvages and Philippe Pinel of France, William Cullen of Scotland, and Carolus Linnaeus of Sweden – the same man who classified animals and plants. Working mostly from books and only rarely at the bedside, medical students were obliged to memorize the 'correct' classification and characteristics of each disease, depending on their place of study. The disease theories that apply best to Rhazes' measles, Sydenham's gout, and the nosological classifications include the organismic theory – as usual – and the ontological theory.

Diseases with Personality

If [bleeding] be continued ... gout will take up its quarters even in a young subject, and its empire will be no government, but a tyranny.

– Thomas Sydenham on Gout (1683), in *The Works of Thomas Sydenham*, trans. R.G. Latham (London: New Sydenham Society, 1848), 2: 131

Pneumonia may well be called the friend of the aged. Taken off by it in an acute, short, not often painful illness, the old man escapes those 'cold gradations of decay' so distressing to himself and to his friends.

– William Osler, *Principles and Practice of Medicine* (1892; 3rd ed., Edinburgh: Young J. Pentland, 1898), 109

Nosological classifications are still used today in pathology and clinical medicine. In a manner reminiscent of the Hippocratic epigraph of this chapter, they simplify the mass of information gleaned from an accumulation of fleeting opportunities in clinical experience by giving it order and structure, to serve judgment in diagnosis and prognosis. In contrast with eighteenth-century nosology, most nosological systems now refer to anatomical or chemical changes. Only in psychiatry, where physical lesions are usually absent, do we continue to find a similar ordering of knowledge, based on observation of symptoms and behaviour (see chapter 12).

Pathology Moves into the Morgue

Disease = Altered Anatomy

Our present concepts of pathology are inseparable from anatomical change. Two centuries ago, however, the relevance of anatomy to bedside medicine was obscure, for three reasons: (1) changes inside the body were hidden until the patient was dead; (2) alterations visible at autopsy might result from death not disease; and (3) internal changes could not be repaired. Nevertheless, anatomists continued to dissect, establishing the boundaries of normal and abnormal structure (see chapter 2).

While clinicians were organizing disease by its symptoms, some anatomists began to compile abnormalities found in cadavers. Four treatises, in particular, are worthy of note. The book of the Italian physician Antonio Benivieni was published posthumously in 1507, nearly forty years before Vesalius's *Fabrica*. The Latin title, *De abditis nonnulis ac mirandis morborum et sanationum causis* (*On Some of the Causes Unknown and Surprising of Diseases and Treatments*), refered to the 'hidden' and 'wondrous' causes of disease that were revealed by autopsies in the 111 case histories. Benivieni was among the first to relate diseases to organic change.

In 1679 the Swiss physician Théophile Bonet (see figure 4.1) published another collection of abnormal anatomy, which contained more than 3,000 observations from his own practice and those of other writers since antiquity. He divided the work into four sections: head, thorax, abdomen, and systemic conditions such as fevers and wounds. Emphasizing the somewhat para-medical nature of his endeavour, he called his treatise *Sepulchretum anatomicum* (*Anatomical Graveyard*). Bonet's book was longer and more developed than that of Benivieni, but his title reflected the marginal status of anatomy in medicine.

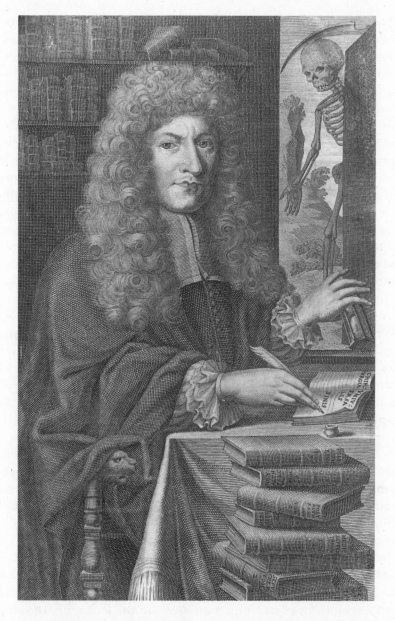

4.1   Théophile Bonet, as he chose to portray himself. Notice the grim reaper peeking through the door. *Sepulchretum anatomicum*, 1700, frontispiece

Nearly a century later, Giovanni Battista Morgagni of Padua published a prolix three-volume treatise, amplifying the work of his predecessor with his own experience. Unlike Bonet's title, Morgagni's
Sedibus et causis morborum per anatomen indagatis (*The Seats and Causes
of Diseases Investigated by Anatomy,* 1761) emphasized the importance
of autopsies to clinical medicine. He tried to make pathological anatomy more accessible to clinicians by including an index for diseases
and another for lesions; knowledge of one might lead a reader to
knowledge of the other. For his emphasis on autopsies, many historians cite Morgagni as a founder of modern pathology. A shorter
and more accessible work was published in 1793 by Matthew Bail-
lie, called *The Morbid Anatomy of Some of the Most Important Parts of the
Human Body.* Many doctors grew interested in pathological anatomy,
but they were baffled by its relevance to practice, since both diagnosis
and therapeutics were predicated on symptoms. Methods of examination before death revealed little about the internal organs. To have
a 'disease' in the eighteenth century, a person had to feel sick.

A synthesis between anatomy and clinical medicine took place in
the early nineteenth century with the advent of physical diagnosis
– an approach that incorporated the inventions of thoracic percussion by Leopold Auenbrugger of Vienna and auscultation by R.T.H.
Laennec of Paris. Symptoms of living patients could now be linked to
anatomical changes. In 1830 Jean Cruveilhier published the first volume of his lavishly illustrated treatise on pathological anatomy. New
trends in disease concepts had fostered this technology: if a disease
was anatomical then it could appear in a picture. Once established,
anatomical pathology generated a further shift in disease concepts –
from emphasis on how the patient felt, to emphasis on what lesion
could be found (see chapter 9). Reflecting the rise of anatomy in
pathology, disease names changed, for example, from phthisis (or
consumption) to tuberculosis.

In the early nineteenth century, doctors realized that not all patients
would display every symptom of any given disease: some might have
a few; others, all. In 1825 P.C.A. Louis of Paris analysed 2,000 cases
of tuberculosis by correlating mortality with the frequency of various
symptoms and the age and sex of sufferers. Well before the mathematical tools of probability and statistics had been fully elaborated,

he is said to have founded 'numerical medicine.' The technique was further systematized by his student L.D.J. Gavarret. Numerical medicine was pathology's response to the positivism that had permeated experimental physiology (see chapter 3). Its many successors include the 'evidence-based' medicine of the late twentieth century. The word 'natural,' meaning health, was gradually replaced by the mathematically loaded word 'normal' (see J.H. Warner, *Therapeutic Perspective*, Cambridge, MA: Harvard University Press, 1986, 89–91).

In this period, several more 'classic' descriptions of disease appeared, each reflecting the new scientific preoccupation with anatomy. Named for their discoverers, they were connected to the specific organic change that constituted their diagnosis; for example, Bright's disease of kidney (1827), Hodgkin's disease (1832) (see figure 4.2), Graves' disease (1835), and Addison's disease (1855). The anchoring of diseases to three-dimensional anatomical forms, which could be illustrated, may have triggered the current passion for images in medical communication.

Most anatomical pathology was done with the naked eye until the 1830s, when microscopes were improved. The idea of tissues had originated three decades earlier in the macroscopic observations of J.C. Smyth, P. Pinel, and Xavier Bichat; but improvements in microscopes reified it. Diseases could be identified and classified by their changes at the level of tissues. For example, the ancient concept of 'inflammation,' characterized by redness, swelling, heat, pain, and loss of function, took on new characteristics derived from microscopy. Czech-born Karl Rokitansky of Vienna wrote a German-language text of pathological anatomy (1842–6) and is said to have performed more than 30,000 autopsies in his career, but he was reluctant to use the microscope. Rudolf Virchow was convinced of its value; he described leukemia (1846), founded a journal of pathological anatomy (1847), and wrote a treatise on cellular pathology (1858), which is often called a 'cornerstone' of the discipline (see also chapter 8). Based on his study of tumours, Virchow brought anatomical cell theory to pathology; he concluded that the anatomy and physiology of a single cell was passed on to all its 'daughter' cells. He was also a liberal politician (see chapter 15).

Elegant technological innovations linked microscopic and sub-

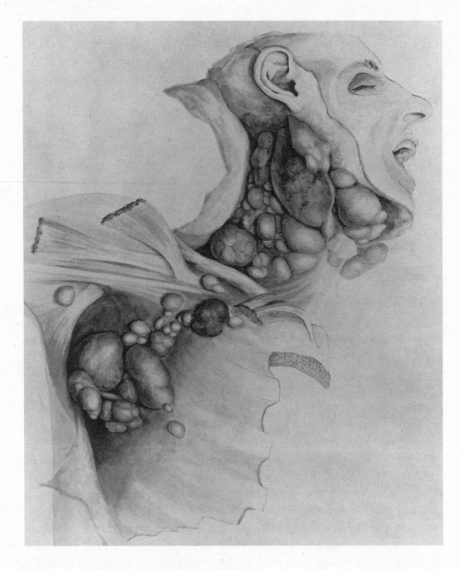

4.2   Hodgkin's disease. Watercolour by Robert Carswell, used to illustrate
the reading of Thomas Hodgkin's original paper, 1832. The enlarged lymph
glands were the anatomical definition of this disease. Medical School Library,
University College, London

microscopic changes in structure to illness. This method prevails in our present system of medical knowledge. To determine what disease a patient has, doctors seek changes, be they anatomical, chemical (such as high blood sugar), or physical (such as an elevated blood pressure). In contrast to the eighteenth century, a person no longer needs to feel sick to have a disease. Diagnosis is not about how the patient feels but what the doctor finds (see chapter 9).

Anatomical methods of describing and identifying disease correspond to the organismic theory; with respect to causes, they can be both external (ontological) and internal (physiological). Favouring the ontological view is the fact that the physical lesion – a three-dimensional entity – is equated with the disease. Conversely, and favouring the physiological view, lesions seemed to emerge from within the patient – and may somehow have depended on who the patient was. In the late nineteenth century, germ theory challenged that idea and set pathology on a new course.

Disease = Damaged Organs

Symptoms, then, are in reality nothing but the cry from suffering organs.

– J.M. Charcot, *Clinical Lectures on the Senile and Chronic Diseases* (1868; English ed., London: Sydenham Society, 1881), 4

Surgery does the ideal thing – it separates the patient from his disease. It puts the patient back to bed and the disease in a bottle.

– Logan Clendening, *Modern Methods of Treatment* (St Louis: Mosby, 1925), 17

Disease = Invasion by Living Organisms

An ontological view of disease was consolidated in the 1880s with the triumph of germ theory, resulting from the work of a French chemist, a British surgeon, and a German physician; they approached the problem simultaneously, each from a different angle. Despite their numerous predecessors, medicine had long hesitated to accept the idea that diseases were caused by germs (see chapter 7).

Chemist Louis Pasteur studied fermentation to explore (and refute) the notion of spontaneous generation of living organisms. He demonstrated the link between bacteria and diseases, and in some impressive public demonstrations he proved that inoculation could convey immunity to domestic animals. Doctors were sceptical of his work for a variety of reasons: germs could be found everywhere, even in the healthy. Furthermore, Pasteur was not a physician.

The surgeon Joseph Lister applied Pasteur's germ theory to the practice of wound dressing, using carbolic acid to deliberately 'kill germs' and seal wounds. His 1865 success with an open fracture of a young boy's leg was published in the *Lancet* in 1867. Acceptance of this antiseptic technique varied, but the news spread quickly, publicizing the practical consequences of germ theory (see also chapter 10).

In 1882 Robert Koch identified *mycobacterium tuberculosis* as the cause of pulmonary tuberculosis, relying on the development of staining and culture techniques. Tuberculosis was the single most important cause of death in the nineteenth century; Koch's discovery had tremendous impact on scientists and the general public. He also laid down rules for establishing that a specific bacterium is the cause of a specific disease. Finding the organism in every case was a necessary prerequisite, he said, but it was not sufficient evidence for believing that the organism caused the disease. It was only the first of four criteria, known as 'Koch's postulates.' To be the proven cause of a disease, the organism must (1) be found in every case; (2) be isolated and grown in pure culture; (3) produce the same disease when injected into animals; (4) be recovered in all experimental cases. Satisfaction of 'Koch's postulates' is still a standard part of etiological investigation. Although his most famous work had been completed more than two decades earlier, Koch was awarded the Nobel Prize in 1905.

The triumph of germ theory as an explanation for disease immediately ratified the search for effective vaccines to convey immunity and for drugs to kill the invading organisms. Initial research concentrated on vaccines.

Pasteur's most famous experiment concerned his efforts to create a vaccine for rabies. Since antiquity, rabies had been known to be a lethal disease communicated by the bite of an infected creature. Pasteur discovered that the virulence of infected nerve tissue waned on long exposure to air. Hoping to develop an attenuated vaccine, he injected dogs over several days with increasingly virulent material taken from rabies-infected rabbit nerve tissue. At his door on the evening of 4 July 1885 appeared three people: nine-year-old Joseph Meister, who had been viciously attacked by a rabid dog; the boy's unharmed mother; and the dog's owner, who had himself been bitten in rescuing the child and killing his animal. Sticks, stones, and straw in the dog's stomach were the diagnostic sign of rabies. The owner was thought to be out of danger (his skin had not been broken), but the physicians whom Pasteur consulted concluded that the boy would die. The vaccine should be given, they thought, even if it offered only a slight chance of recovery. In a series of injections reminiscent of Jenner's experiment (see chapter 7), Pasteur gave the child a range of solutions prepared from rabies-infected rabbit tissue that had been incubated for less and less time; the last injection contained fresh material. The child lived and grew to be a man, ending his days as the gatekeeper at the Pasteur Institute in Paris. Using Pasteur's notebooks, historian Gerald Geison has shown that at least two other 'private' patients had been injected with rabies vaccine before young Meister; one died.

Germ theory shifted the cause of disease away from internal organs to external invaders. The long-frustrated social hygiene movements could now marshal science to help their efforts to clean up the world in a joint campaign against a living 'enemy' (see chapter 5). What's more, germ theory spawned the new science of bacteriology, which more than any other form of inquiry brought pathology into the medical spotlight. Bacteriology established the microscope as a tool for doctors as well as scientists. The staining techniques needed to visualize germs could also be applied to tissues, advancing the relevance of anatomy to the clinic.

Laboratory medicine was instrumental in transforming hospitals from places to be avoided into places of science and cure (see chapter 9). Soon every hospital needed a laboratory, with someone to run it – usually a doctor specializing in pathology. The rise of pathology as a distinct specialty is intimately connected to this shift, which corresponds to the beginnings of widespread specialization in all branches of medicine. By the turn of the twentieth century, pathologists worked in hospitals and medical schools of Europe and America. They were stars of medical science; their career paths were remarkably similar, as they reaped honours for bringing new sciences to clinical medicine.

From 1878, William Henry Welch taught pathology in New York. By 1885 – just three years after Koch's discovery – he had been lured to Baltimore to head up pathology at the planned Johns Hopkins Hospital (opened 1889). Reflecting the new priorities for science in medicine, it is no accident that he, a leading pathologist, was chosen as the first dean of the fledgling medical school in 1893. Eight years later, Welch became the first president of the Board of Directors of the Rockefeller Institute for Medical Research, a post that 'propell[ed] the 51-year-old portly pathologist to an even higher realm – the rarefied world of philanthropy, trusteeship and foundation service' (A.B. Swingle, *Hopkins Medical News*, Fall 2002). The blend of science and clinical medicine at Johns Hopkins medical school was widely copied by medical educators for more than half a century. Pathology was key.

In Britain, the physician Almroth Wright became a bacteriologist when he was appointed professor of pathology for the Army Medical School in 1892. Ten years later, he founded a research department at St Mary's Hospital Medical School in London, where he investigated vaccination. Four years later, he was knighted.

In Germany, Emil von Behring began with studies in medicine, served as a military doctor, and from 1888 worked with Koch at his research institute in Berlin, where he developed antitoxins against tetanus and diphtheria. Later, he moved to Marburg as professor of hygiene in the medical school. In 1901 von Behring became the first Nobel laureate in medicine for his work on diphtheria. Also in Germany the young Jewish physician Paul Ehrlich had experimented with tissue stains for his MD thesis of 1878. Like von Behring, he worked with Koch to devise a method for staining the tuberculosis bacillus. By 1882, he had an academic position in the Berlin medical school, and in 1908 he too was awarded the Nobel Prize.

In France, Émile Roux used his work on Pasteur's rabies vaccine as the basis of his MD thesis in 1881. Two years later he helped to found the Pasteur Institute, where he spent most of his career in administration and research on infectious diseases. Between 1901 and 1932, Roux was nominated more than one hundred times in twenty-four different years for the Nobel Prize, making him one of the most admired scientists to miss the honour. His younger colleague, Charles Nicolle, returned as professor to Rouen medical school; in 1896, just three years after obtaining his MD degree, he became director of its bacteriological laboratory. Later, he moved to Tunis to direct a branch of the Pasteur Institute, where he made his 1909 discovery of the role of lice in spreading typhus. For this achievement two decades later, he became a Nobel laureate.

The Canadian-born physician William Osler was fascinated by the potential of laboratory science in diagnosis. His first appointment was as a pathologist at McGill University in 1874. After a sojourn in Philadelphia, Osler joined Welch as a founding professor of clinical medicine at the influential Johns Hopkins medical school in Baltimore. His *Principles and Practice of Medicine* (1892) blended pathology with lucid case descriptions, making it the most durable and influential textbook of its time. He ended his career as the Regius Professor of Medicine at Oxford. He is still venerated in many circles including the American Osler Society, which continues to meet annually in his honour. Osler's protégée Maude Abbott organized McGill's superb museum of pathological specimens, and her classification of congenital abnormalities of the heart was an essential prerequisite for open-heart surgery. In the same tradition, the Scottish-Canadian pathologist William Boyd published the first of his many pathology texts in 1925. Admired for its use of science, his writing was also hailed for its riveting prose.

William Boyd's Textbook of 1925

On bronchiectasis:
'Stinking pools of pus' accumulate to cause 'exceedingly foul breath which makes a social outcast of the unfortunate victim so that he tends to live a life alone, apart, helpless and hopeless.'

On villous papilloma of the bladder viewed with the cystoscope:
The 'delicate many fingered growth ... unfolds its fragile processes when the bladder is filled with water until it looks like a piece of seaweed floating in a marine pool.'

– William Boyd, *A Textbook of Pathology* (1925; 8th ed.,
Philadelphia: Lea and Febiger, 1970), 698, 945

Typifying the international scope of these contributions was the career of Félix d'Hérelle. Originally from Montreal, he studied bacteriophage, the viruses whose nucleic acid became the prototype for molecular genetics. This interest took him to five continents; like Roux, he was nominated twenty-eight times between 1926 and 1937 without ever winning a Nobel.

Most people working in hospital laboratories and education did not enjoy such fame; sometimes, they were overworked and underappreciated. Once the importance of pathology to clinical medicine was firmly accepted, they organized for standards in training and practice and recognition as a distinct specialty. Just as for physiology (see chapter 3), although slightly later, this professionalization process involved societies, journals, departments, and conferences. Because pathology was a medical speciality it eventually involved separate certification examinations (see table 4.1).

The public imagination was captured by the brilliant promise of laboratory medicine in saving lives and solving crimes. The dramatic stories of researchers were celebrated by bacteriologist Paul de Kruif in his 1926 book *Microbe Hunters*, which inspired several generations of future medical scientists and itself has become the object of his-

Table 4.1 Some organizations formed by pathologists

Year	Country	Organization
1906	UK	Pathological Society of Great Britain and Ireland
1916	Germany	Deutsche Gesellschaft für Pathologie
1922	U.S.	American Society of Clinical Pathologists
1927	UK	Association of Clinical Pathologists
1936	U.S.	American Board of Pathology
1942	France	Société Française de Biologie Médicale
1947	U.S.	College of American Pathologists
1947	World	International Society of Clinical Pathology (becomes World Association, 1972)
1949	Canada	Canadian Association of Pathologists
1952	Japan	Japan Society of Clinical Pathology

torical study. De Kruif had worked at the Rockefeller Institute. Using popular caricatures, historian Bert Hansen has shown how the image of the doctor went from a fop in a frock coat to a scientist in a lab coat; he related it to sensation over a particular event. In December 1885, less than a year after the case of young Meister, Americans were riveted to newspaper reports of four little boys from Newark bitten by a dog and sent to Paris to be vaccinated by Pasteur.

The science of pathology and bacteriology emerged in fiction where it was (and remains) warmly embraced by the public. Sherlock Holmes, the 1887 creation of physician-author Arthur Conan Doyle, was based on the real surgeon Joseph Bell; his repertoire included the latest scientific discoveries. The immensely popular *Arrowsmith* (1925) tells the travails and triumphs of a physician scientist; its author, Sinclair Lewis, had dedicated the book to his friend de Kruif. He was awarded Pulitzer (declined) and Nobel prizes. Scottish physician-writer, A.J. Cronin created similar heroes in his novel *The Citadel* (1937). Pathologists continue to play supporting and starring roles in crime fiction, film, and television. Recent examples include women: Kay Scarpetta created by Patricia Cornwell, Samantha Ryan of BBC's *Silent Witness*, and Temperance Brennan, who, like her creator, Kathy Reichs, is a forensic anthropologist and the inspiration for the television series *Bones*. Many other successful crime writers had also worked in health care or forensics, including Agatha Christie and P.D. James.

The heady success of pathology was not without its opponents even in the early twentieth century. By 1906, germ theory had become so popular that it was mocked by George Bernard Shaw. Critics argued that germs could not explain everything: some people were more susceptible to infection than others; therefore, infection with germs must have something to do with the host as well as the invader, something that anatomical methods had not yet demonstrated.

The Overworked Germ of Overwork

RIDGEON: It's nothing. I was a little giddy just now. Overwork I suppose ...

B.B. [Sir Ralph Bloomfield Bonington]: Overwork! There's no such thing. I do the work of ten men. Am I giddy? No. NO. If you're not well, you have a disease. It may be a slight one, but it's a disease. And what is a disease? The lodgment in the system of a pathogenic germ, and the multiplication of that germ. What is the remedy? A very simple one. Find the germ and kill it.

SIR PATRICK: Suppose there's no germ.

B.B.: Impossible ... there must be a germ: else how could the patient be ill? ... [severely] There is nothing that cannot be explained by science.

– G.B. Shaw, *The Doctor's Dilemma* (1906; reprint, Harmondsworth: Penguin, 1957), 102, 112 [Ridgeon was a thinly veiled version of Almroth Wright.]

Heredity Strikes Back

Disease = Molecules

The concept of heredity is ancient. That some people have distinct physical and psychological traits had been conveyed in words like 'temperament.' So too, certain diseases had long been thought to 'run in families.' But hereditarian explanations began to seem antiquated after the arrival of germ theory. As bacteriology dragged pathology into hospitals and medical schools, work on heredity continued in the hands of other scientists in botany, entomology, and agriculture.

An international priority dispute in 1900 led to the rediscovery of the laws of heredity that had been published more than thirty years earlier by the Austrian botanist and cleric Gregor Mendel. Mendel's work with peas was so perfect that some historians now believe that he fudged his results; nevertheless, the sorting and inheritance of traits along dominant and recessive lines made sense. Two years later, in 1902, Archibald Edward Garrod of England worked out the inheritance of alcaptonuria, making it the first human disease shown to follow Mendelian laws. Suddenly this holistic observation gave substance to the physiological views of disease that had been eclipsed by ontological germ theory. It matters who you are to explain what you get.

Further improvements in microscopes were prompted by the success of bacteriology, meaning that tissues and cells could also be seen more clearly. In the late nineteenth century, scientists had observed chromosomes; the effect of colchicine on mitosis was reported in 1889, making experiments possible. The early history of genetics was played out in the United States and arose from the margins of descriptive anatomy and cell biology. Embryologist Thomas Hunt Morgan was not a doctor; his 1890 PhD was in comparative zoology. Appointed professor in experimental zoology at Columbia University in 1904, he began working on the fruit fly (*Drosophilia melanogaster*). With colchicine, chromosome patterns could be studied under the light microscope. Soon Morgan hypothesized that the hereditary units resided on the chromosomes; they were called 'genes,' a word coined in 1909. By 1910, Morgan had worked out the principles of sex-linked transmission and went on to analyse crossing over in cell division. The concept of X-linkage was applied to certain conditions that had long been known to occur only in boys, such as muscular dystrophy and hemophilia. However, since no one yet understood what exactly was a gene and how it might work, little could be done with this new way of expressing the obvious. Morgan's many achievements were recognized with a Nobel Prize in 1933, delayed perhaps because of the excitements over bacteriology.

Once it became possible to visualize, measure, and experiment with chromosomes, heredity seemed to catch up to become a special field of science. Still it was conducted outside of medical centres, often relying on methods of physics and chemistry. The discoveries crept closer and closer to clinical relevance; and still they were American. For example, in 1927, Hermann J. Müller showed that fruit fly chromosomes could be damaged by X-rays – a discovery that blurred the sharp rivalry between inside and outside causes. Around the same time, Barbara McClintock, working with maize, studied how chromosomes change in reproduction; in the 1940s, she found that some genes misbehave by hopping from one chromosomal place to another in a process called transposition. Her conclusions were considered heretical for a long time. Also in the 1940s, George Beadle and Edward Tatum brought genetics closer to clinical relevance with their 'one gene, one enzyme' hypothesis. Unlike the bacteriologists, none of these researchers had been physicians. All would eventually win the Nobel Prize in medicine, but some had to wait many years.

In the meantime, the popular eugenics movement co-opted the science of genetics (see chapter 13). Most geneticists, however, beginning with Morgan, eventually came to suspect the pernicious applications of their field in justifying discriminatory measures on the basis of race, class, and political philosophy.

It was the discovery of the structure of DNA in 1952 that pushed genetics into the spotlight, giving it the kind of front-page attention that bacteriology had enjoyed a half-century earlier. Researchers expected that genes would turn out to be proteins. Canadian-born Oswald Avery directed attention to the nucleic acid DNA in 1944. But how could this molecule convey the complicated information needed to build an organism? By 1950 biochemist Erwin Chargaff, an Austrian Jewish immigrant to New York, had made observations that would be crucial to unravelling the mystery: in the four amino acids of DNA, the number of guanine units is equal to the number of cytosine units; similarly, adenine equals thymidine. Working at Cambridge, James Watson and Francis Crick used this information and the X-ray crystallography photographs taken by others to discover the double helix structure. It established their fame and brought genetics to the doors of clinical medicine.

Table 4.2
Some clinical problems linked to chromosome abnormalities

Name of syndrome	Abnormality	Clinical description	Chromosomal or enzyme description
Down	extra 21st	1866	1959
Klinefelter	XXY (male)	1942	1956
Turner	0X (female)	1930–8	1959
Hurler	recessive gene	1919	1959
CM leukemia*	Philadelphia chr.	1845	1960
Fragile X			1968

* The translocation from chromosome 9 to 22 was described in 1973.

Multiple-symptom constellations could now be reduced to a chromosomal abnormality or even a single molecular substitution in DNA, detected by missing or altered enzymes. By 1959, people who were odd from birth were given closer attention, grouped into clinical patterns that were quickly connected to chromosomal or enzyme changes. Some conditions had been known for decades; other rarer forms were actively sought. Indeed, on occasion the chromosomal description uncovered the clinical disease. Jérôme Lejeune, who described 21-trisomy in 1959, pointed out the racist implications in the term 'mongolism' that had been chosen by his predecessor J. Langdon Down. All too often the eponym identified someone who was not the original discoverer, or someone whose opinions were no longer respected. Names of clinical discoverers stuck to those syndromes described earlier (see table 4.2); by the 1960s eponyms waned in favour of cities and chromosomal patterns. For example, Lejeune also discovered Fragile X syndrome; yet no disease bears his name.

Alterations of many inherited and acquired disorders have now been defined at the phenotypic, chromosomal, and nucleic acid levels – for example, Tay-Sachs disease (assay of hexosaminidase A, 1970), sickle-cell anemia (locus on small arm of chromosome 11 for beta-globin chain synthesis, 1980); muscular dystrophy (gene mapping, 1987), and cystic fibrosis (gene mapping, 1989). The discovery in the mid-1950s of the human histocompatibility complex (HLA antigens) helped to explain inherited predisposition to certain diseases and contributed to tissue-typing for organ donation between related and unrelated donors; indeed, HLA typing can be seen as the modern rendition of the ancient concept of individual 'temperament.' Sometimes the methods of genetics served to justify clinical realities that had been disputed: one example is the form of congenital muscular dystrophy recognized by Yokio Fukuyama of Japan (see his abstract *Brain and Nerve* 60, no. 1 (2008): 43–51). Just as bacteriology dominated the early Nobel Prizes, genetics dominated a century later.

With the precision of molecular identification, pathology has grown beyond medicine and the law to become a highly respected instrument for studying the past. Re-examination of Egyptian mummies has become a new specialty, while discoveries of bony remains and frozen corpses result in great public and scientific interest. Recent finds given wide attention include bodies from the Franklin expedition (from 1981 on), Ötzi the 5,000-year-old alpine iceman (1991), and the opening of 1918 influenza graves in the Spitzbergen permafrost (1998). Not only can paleopathology explain the characteristics, diseases, and death of individuals from long ago, it can demonstrate the links and origins of all people today.

The Medical Model of Today and Its Problems

Returning to the causal views of disease, we can now find elements of both external (ontological) and internal (physiological) causes in the current medical model. The former are seen in diseases caused by viruses or bacteria, modified physiologically by the accompanying immune status of the host. The latter are seen in genetic or autoimmune disorders, modified ontologically by concepts such as post-viral autoimmunity for conditions such as diabetes and multiple sclerosis. Nevertheless, disease descriptions in medical textbooks conform overwhelmingly to an organismic view of disease – something undesirable and hopefully discontinuous that affects individuals.

Extrapolations of these theoretical perspectives can be dangerous. For example, rigid adherence to the ontological view of disease as the product of demonized external invaders sometimes led society to recoil from people who appeared to be at risk. In nineteenth-century Canada, immigrants thought to be susceptible to cholera were forcibly confined in unhygienic sheds, where those who had not previously been infected soon sickened and died. Similarly, in more recent times, homosexuals and Haitians have been equated with AIDS. The advent of SARS in 2003 triggered xenophobic reactions against people from southeast Asia. Controls are proposed against groups at risk as if their members were equivalent to the disease or its cause (see chapter 7).

Similarly, extrapolation of physiological views of disease allows observers to blame patients for their illnesses. For example, some disease descriptions incorporated prejudicial notions of race, gender, and class: 'Jewish' diseases, 'negro' diseases, women's diseases, and diseases of poverty. Historian Robert Aronowitz suggests that the concept of risk factors developed since the 1960s has helped to mitigate the stark differences and disadvantages of these two causal views: the risk factors predisposing to a disease are expressed statistically and in combination with each other, rather than as consequences instrinsic to certain traits of existence.

Being ideas, diseases are built of words and metaphors. Sometimes deliberately, sometimes unintentionally, metaphors convey social attitudes as they try to express dispassionate science. Consequently, disease, like bodies, can be 'socially constructed' (see also chapters 2 and 7). As literary critic Susan Sontag has shown, stereotypes may be triggered by the presence of the illness itself in a certain group.

Not only do social attitudes change, science can also turn out to be 'wrong.' Pathology is vulnerable to its distortions, abuses, and errors. For example, phrenology was the study of character, intelligence, and disease by reading the shape of the head (see figure 4.3). All too easily discredited now, phrenology was indeed scientific when clinical anatomy was on the rise and doctors were intent on finding external clues to hidden changes of the internal organs. Many distinguished physicians had been students of phrenology and willed their brains for its use.

On phrenology and numerous other topics, medical authorities pronounced with great confidence opinions that later were found to be wrong. The flagrant errors of the past persisted because they seemed to fit the observed data, offered explanation, and corresponded to contemporary science. Critics of modern medicine point

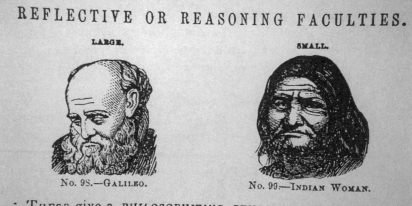

REFLECTIVE OR REASONING FACULTIES.

LARGE.

SMALL.

No. 98.—GALILEO.

No. 99.—INDIAN WOMAN.

THESE give a PHILOSOPHIZING, PENETRATING, INVESTIGAT-
ING, ORIGINATING cast of mind ; ascertain CAUSES and abstract
RELATIONS ; CONTRIVE, INVENT, ORIGINATE ideas, etc. Adapted
to the first principles, or laws of things.

4.3   Phrenological comparison illustrating the relative reasoning power
(and head shape) of Galileo and an Indian woman. From O.S. and L.N.
Fowler, *Self-Instructor in Phrenology and Physiology*, 1859, 159

to the past errors as a sign of danger in the medical present. Surely
some of what we think is right now will eventually be wrong, but we
cannot know which part.

Critics also complain that in the medical model suffering is less
important than the objective lesions demonstrated by doctors: doctors have too much power in making diagnoses. These complaints
have philosophical implications. For example, people with 'chronic
fatigue syndrome' experience many symptoms, but the credibility
of their disorder is low compared with that of symptomless conditions such as carcinoma in situ, hypertension, or HIV seropositivity.
Sometimes the situation leads to ironic if not absurd contrasts: the
disturbing rise in reported hepatitis C took place on a background
of the virtual disappearance of clinical forms of transfusion hepatitis
(see Duffin 2005). With the rise in treatable risk factors, some of the
greatest drug expenditures are for 'diseases' with no symptoms at all:
hypertension, hyperlipidemia, and mild diabetes (see chapter 5).

Those who turn to alternative or complementary medicines yearn for a holistic integration of body and self, for a return to subjectivity. But holism is increasingly beyond the means of a medicine predicated on the demonstration of the smallest material change. The popular neurologist-writer Oliver Sacks also calls for a re-evaluation of medical knowledge. Citing the inadequacies of disease definitions that are confined to physics or chemistry, he describes the metaphysical aspects of illness and the strength of human adaptation in terms of organization and design. 'Nearly all my patients,' he says, 'whatever their problems, reach out to life – and not only despite their conditions, but often because of them, and even with their aid' (*An Anthropologist on Mars*, Knopf, 1995, xviii). In other words, the subjective should be part of a disease, just as it is part of being ill, and just as it was in the distant past. If we find a way to include the subjective in our concepts of disease, maybe we will also discover purpose and meaning in illness.

Narrative medicine, or storytelling, is one response to this need to put personal suffering back into pathology. It provides a corrective to the shortcomings of doctor-centred diagnosis and care, although most of its practitioners would scarcely imagine that it is a form of pathology. Stories are told by patients or their caregivers, to be read by strangers, other patients, and their families. An early example of the genre is the 'autopathography' of Norman Cousins, *Anatomy of an Illness* (1979), describing how he pampered and laughed himself out of his own ailment. The method extends also to poetry, art, film, and the reading of literary classics. Artists and scholars of literature now teach medical students and work with sick people. How does it work? If a man is convinced that his cancer arose because he was cruel to his mother, his doctor should recognize the notion, even if she does not believe it herself. If a woman with arthritis views her pain as an opportunity for spiritual growth, she may not tolerate her medications well.

What began as a trickle of articles by ethicists in the late 1980s has mushroomed since the year 2000. Research – even evidence-based research – on narration is discussed in conferences and journals. To serve these interests the online Literature, Arts, and Medicine Database has been growing steadily since 1993 under the editorial direction of physiologist Felice Aull at New York University. It is used by sick people, their caregivers, and students all over the world. A program was launched at Columbia University under the direction of Rita Charon in 1996. 'Narration' became a Medical Subject Heading (MeSH) in 2002. The history of this movement has yet to be written.

Finally, the unquestioned acceptance of an organismic view of disease in the medical model may be at odds with the political values of our time; it makes difficulties both for chronic diseases and for public health (see chapter 15). If, for the purpose of argument, we contemplate the opposite, a population-based view of disease, we find a world in which disease is constant and cannot be eradicated – indeed, probably should not be eradicated – a world in which some disease might actually be beneficial. This 'nonorganismic,' or population-based, theory has also been called the ecological theory of disease. Traces of it have surfaced in the past, but it is rarely to be found in medical texts. Medieval accounts of illness by writers such as Hildegard of Bingen emphasized the moral strength derived from a period of suffering. Closer to our own time, Social Darwinism or Malthusian concepts of 'survival of the fittest' also correspond to those ideals. For example, reference is often made to the supposed malaria protection provided by sickle hemoglobin, which favours persistence of the sickle allele in various populations.

But we do not need to examine the past for examples of a nonorganismic view. Current issues of health-care funding juxtapose hard fiscal realities against medical ideals and the rights of individuals to pursue a cure. Governments may decide that the elderly beyond a certain age are not entitled to expensive procedures such as dialysis and coronary bypass, or that premature infants under a certain gestational age do not warrant intensive care. They may also decide where and how physicians are to practise, or what groups are to be served by hospitals. This population view would maintain, together with Oliver Sacks, that disease may not actually be 'good,' but in creating the greatest good for the greatest number, some disease, at least, is 'tolerable' (see chapter 6).

Pathology is a sophisticated science that defines material change in reliable ways. It has been reduced, however, from a holistic study of suffering to a laboratory-based inquiry of what is wrong. Notwithstanding our efforts to incorporate quality, culture, and identity into our understanding of disease, the answer to the question 'what is wrong?'– which is the diagnosis – almost always lies in the smallest identifiable lesion within the body, the least material change.

Suggestions for Further Reading

At the bibliography website http://histmed.ca.

CHAPTER FIVE

First Do No Harm:
History of Treatment, Pharmacology,
and Pharmaceuticals*

If the whole materia medica as used, could be sunk in the bottom of the sea, it would be all the better for mankind and all the worse for the fishes.

– Oliver Wendell Holmes (1883)

In June 1991 the body of American President Zachary Taylor was exhumed for a medico-legal examination. He had been dead since 1850 – officially of diarrhea – but a question of poisoning had been raised. The president may not have been murdered, the papers claimed, but he had been killed by his physicians.

Stories like this one irritate me. The writers presume that the patient was not seriously ill until he accepted treatment, and that the illness did not contribute to his demise. Without denying the dangers of past therapy, I find these tales disturbing, because they hit close to hematologic home. Chemotherapy makes people vomit and lose their hair; it also reduces their immunity – and, by the way, it shrinks tumours. One of my teachers used to call it 'poison with anti-cancer side effects.' We hope that safer and more effective treatments will be found in the future. In the meantime, however, we give these potentially lethal drugs – not to kill our patients but to help them live longer and better. Are we deluding ourselves?

*Learning objectives for this chapter are found on p. 451.

The Latest Frontier

The history of therapeutics is the latest frontier of medical history partly because it is so embarrassing. Until recently, ridicule was the goal of the few who wrote about past medicines. Current practices are assumed to be rational and scientific, while those of predecessors are not; what we do now is flawless, and what they did back then could not possibly have worked. Many recent examples of this literature abound; none appear in the bibliography for this chapter. History conducted through such a prejudicial lens (called 'presentism' by historians; see chapter 16) will be limited and insensitive, even if it is lively and well written. Only recently have historians begun to examine why certain drugs now thought dangerous were once endorsed by orthodox medicine. Others study the parallel folk medicines of self-help – a much more difficult task, lacking sources that can easily be identified.

Most therapies were discovered by empirical means – observation, accident, and trial and error. Eating or doing something was followed by improvement. But the empirical methods do not prevent 'reasoning' from helping to transform observation into medical dogma. And they rely on at least two prior conditions: agreement on what constitutes the disease (i.e., the need) and an opportunity to observe. For pharmacology, these conditions comprise the Pastorian 'preparation of the mind' before a treatment is discovered (see chapter 3). A rationale for why the treatment was presumed to work will always have been applied – in many cases, *after* the drug's benefits were noticed – and it will be subject to historical vogue in science.

Change in a disease concept can alter the rationale without necessarily changing the treatment. By the same token, a drug's mechanism of action can shift without refuting its benefits. For example, in the 1970s hydrochlorothiazide was thought to lower blood pressure through its diuretic and saliuretic effect; now it is thought to have some additional effect on the smooth muscle of blood vessels. A similar revision can be applied to digitalis, as we will see below.

Undesirable side effects can also lead to new applications. For example, minoxidil was introduced in the mid-1970s as a powerful antihypertensive, with the depressing side effect of hirsutism; now it is prescribed for external use as a treatment for baldness. Similarly, the adrenergic drug methylphenidate (Ritalin) was originally used as a stimulant, but its paradoxically calming side effect on children with hyperactivity (now called 'attention deficit disorder') became its principal application.

Defunct medical practices were neither irrational nor unscientific in their heyday; the rationale was reconciled with prevailing science and concepts of disease. For example, when medicine looked for acids or bases in urine, remedies were selected to alter urinary acidity toward health; when fevers were associated with too much blood, bloodletting made sense. When syphilis first appeared as an import from the New World, the wood product guaiacum was thought to 'work' for two reasons: first, like the ailment, it came from America; second, the naturally occurring, spontaneous remissions in the disease could be attributed to whatever intervention had preceded them. Similarly, the colour red was a therapy for smallpox since at least the tenth century in Japan and Europe: red clothes, red rooms, red food, and red light – erythrotherapy. This idea persisted into the twentieth century with the work of the 1903 Nobel laureate Niels R. Finsen.

Therapeutic rationale depends on the time and place. All medical systems appeal to reasoning, including the past of orthodox medicine and the present of 'unorthodox,' or 'alternative,' medicine. In homeopathy, invented in the late eighteenth century by Samuel Hahnemann, the dominant assumption is that 'like cures like' – often expressed in Latin as *similia similibus curantur*. The best remedy will be the one which, if taken in large doses, produces symptoms similar to the disease; treatment then consists of giving that remedy in tiny, 'homeopathic doses.'

Therapeutic rationale also changes with perceptions of disease. For example, when peptic ulcer was associated with personality, stress, hyperacidity, and disordered motility, the correct treatments dealt with those problems. But in the late 1970s, histamine-2 antagonists dramatically altered prescribing practices for ulcer. By the early 1990s, a microbial explanation came to the fore, and management of the now-infectious condition changed accordingly.

Therapeutic rationale may vary by patient, and perceptions of people can also alter through time. In the medical journals of the 1950s and 1960s, tranquillizers promised to help women cope with the strain of housework. The idea that increased opportunities for outside employment might offer a better solution was not a therapeutic consideration. Since then, tranquillizer remedies have not been discarded, but their target population has altered in conjunction with cultural norms of health and behaviour.

Finally, some medically sanctioned treatments once hailed as miracle cures turned out to be useless or harmful. In the last century, increasing awareness of this possibility led to legislation designed to protect professionals and their patients from unjustified claims and unforeseen side effects. Pharmaceutical literature changed accordingly, and the 'small print' increased with time. Advertisements from a century ago contain few such warnings about composition, side effects, drug interactions, and contraindications. The less-than-noble therapeutic past has itself become a mover in the history of pharmacology. Nevertheless wild swings in acceptable treatments still occur. Since the first edition of this book, several top remedies have vanished, as we will see below. They were shown to have unacceptable side effects on the heart and other organs.

Mysticism, Religion, and Magic: Do They Work?

Since prehistoric times, doctors have been making recommendations for therapeutic intervention. Ancient remedies 'worked,' and some still work, including magic, prayer, and divine supplication. Sick people are among the pilgrims who flock to shrines such as Lourdes in France, Fatima in Portugal, Santiago de Compostella in Spain, and the Oratoire St-Joseph, Cap-de-la-Madeleine, and Ste-Anne-de-Beaupré in Quebec. Sites of divine healing enjoy a charisma akin to that of medical meccas such as the Mayo Clinic. In our time, however, physicians leave the prescribing of pilgrimages to other professionals.

The spiritualistic or vitalistic aspect of treatment has been reified in the concept of 'placebo' (from Latin 'I shall please'). The term 'placebo' long signified the administration of harmless but inert compounds; however, in the mid-twentieth century, placebo was found to be effective in virtually every form of intervention and for any kind of disease. The last decade has witnessed an explosion of interest in its nature, uses, and history.

An Experiment: Shifting Therapeutic Claims

Go to the library (not the Web!) and examine drug advertisements in the medical journals of the past (the online archives often omit advertising). You will find:

- drugs that are no longer used because they are now considered dangerous;
- drugs that have been replaced by others with completely different actions, because our idea of the disease has changed (e.g., anxiolytics and antispasmodics for ulcers);
- drugs for problems no longer considered diseases (e.g., agents to promote weight gain);
- drugs to help women cope with housework and school meetings;
- advertisements that seem tasteless, humourless, or corny because aesthetic standards have changed too.

The older the journal, the more curiosities will be encountered; however, even recent publications contain advertisements for products that are now considered inefficacious or harmful.

Finally, imagine how advertisements for present practice might appear to observers in fifty or one hundred years from now.

Greco-Roman Treatments and Medical Botany

Greco-Roman diseases arose from an imbalance in the humours (see chapter 3); therefore, treatment consisted of trying to re-establish the balance. Modification of diet and lifestyle were intended to alter the relative proportions of the elemental substances. After spiritual therapies, they are probably the oldest forms of medicine.

The Hippocratic treatises of the fifth century B.C. refer to many non-drug remedies, such as bloodletting, special diets, baths, exercise or rest, and applications of heat or cold. In addition, more than 300 medications are cited, most of plant origin; they could be administered either externally or internally by mouth, rectum, vagina, and other orifices. Hippocratic doctors tended to be conservative in their treatment philosophy. They believed in the healing power of nature (*vis medicatrix naturae*), which governed the body's response to illness. Medicine was to help the body heal itself; it was not supposed to hurt, but the Hippocratics readily acknowledged that, sometimes, it could. 'To help, or at least to do no harm' (*Epidemics* I, 11) is a saying often written in Latin as *primum non nocere* (first, do no harm).

'Expectant' treatment – patiently waiting for nature's cure – has wandered in and out of fashion since the fifth century B.C. In their eagerness to glorify Hippocrates, some historians may have projected more caution onto their Greek predecessors than the texts would justify. At the time of writing, expectant medicine is no longer in vogue despite an energetic public lobby for its rediscovery. Folk medicines, herbal remedies, and natural products now compete for market share with the purveyors of gleaming capsules. Because medical practice tends to follow demand, orthodoxy may eventually bend toward *la médecine douce* (gentle medicine); some physicians are expanding their practice to include these areas, but most medical schools do not require instruction in them. Certainly, since the year 2000, pharmacies have embraced the so-called natural trend with rapidly expanding sections for these over-the-counter remedies that would not be recommended by doctors, mostly because doctors know little or nothing about them.

The Greek word for drug, *pharmakon*, from which pharmacology is derived, means a drug, a remedy, and a poison. In the earliest classifications, drugs were either toxins or antidotes; the antidotes were medicinal. In the first century B.C., King Mithridates VI of Pontus in Asia Minor feared being murdered by the Romans, with whom he was often at war. He is thought to have experimentally immunized himself against poisons by drinking the blood of ducks fed on toxic substances. A universal antidote bore his name. Ironically, the king was later unable to commit suicide with poison and had to ask a servant to polish him off with a sword.

Another ancient antidote was theriac, which was developed to counteract animal poisons. The word 'theriac' is derived from the Greek word *therion* (wild beast) and reflects the composition of the remedy as well as its purpose. Depending on which of the many recipes was followed, theriac contained up to seventy ingredients, including the flesh of vipers. Both theriac and mithridates were used to treat infectious diseases, conceived of as 'pests,' or poisons. These remedies enjoyed almost mystical stature into the nineteenth century, and medical museums display magnificent faience jars for their keeping. The nineteenth-century physiologist Claude Bernard worked in a pharmacy in his youth, where he saw theriac made by mixing the dregs of all the other preparations in a vat.

Galen, of the second century A.D., was a successful therapist. Among his many medications were vegetable derivatives, which came to be known as galenicals, or simples. His treatments could be aggressive, but he knew of placebo and that his patients' confidence in his reputation could help him to effect cures. He was ready to take credit for the healing accomplished by nature or by stealth.

A Galenic Therapeutic Strategy: Winning Confidence

I completely won the admiration of the philosopher Glaucon by the diagnosis which I made in the case of one of his friends ... Observing on the window sill a vessel containing a mixture of hyssop and honey, I made up my mind that the patient, who was himself a physician, believed that the malady from which he was suffering was a pleurisy ... Placing my hand on the patient's right side ... I remarked: 'This is the spot where the disease is located.' He ... replied with a look which plainly expressed admiration mingled with astonishment.

– Galen, *De locis affectis*, cited in L. Clendening,
Source Book of Medical History (New York: Dover, 1960), 45–7

Galen's pharmacopoeia embraced the therapies of his predecessor, Dioscorides, a first-century Greek surgeon who served the army

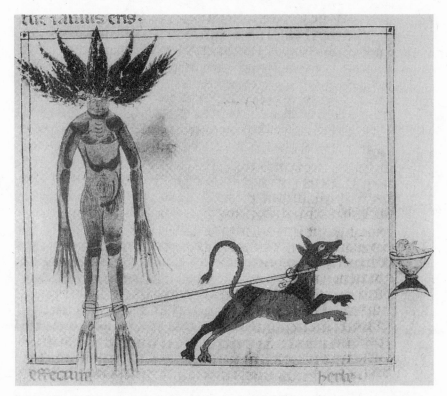

5.1   *Mandragora* (mandrake root) from a mid-thirteenth-century manuscript copy of a herbal by Apuleius. Wellcome Institute Library, London, WMS 573

of the Roman Emperor Nero. Dioscorides' medical botany described more than 600 plants, animals, and their derivatives. He classified his remedies by their physical qualities: oils, animals, cereals, herbs, roots, and wines. Wine made with *mandragora* (mandrake root) was a love potion and anesthetic (see figure 5.1). Mandrake's anthropoid appearance may have had something to do with its legendary powers. Humans daring to pull it from the ground would be killed by its screams; a dog should be tied to the root and tempted to 'harvest' it with a nearby dish of meat.

Dioscorides' botany remained the most influential book on *materia medica* (medical substances) for 1,400 years. Most other medical botanies were simply commentaries on his work. The first medical book printed by the German inventor Johannes Gutenberg was the 1457

Laxierkalender, a collection of laxative remedies. Some herbals were written first in Greek, translated into Arabic, then Latin, and finally a modern language. Often the texts are garbled with missing passages. None of the original Greek illustrations have survived. Illustrations in later manuscripts or books are highly stylized or mismatched; sometimes they describe plants that are difficult to identify or no longer exist, as in the illustrated commentary of Pietro Andrea Matthioli of 1554. Research on the ancient writings of Dioscorides and other botanists continues; its success relies on accurate translation and knowledge of manuscript sources as well as the plants.

Advent of Metals

Copper had been mentioned in the Hippocratic treatises, but it was not until the late fifteenth century that metals were widely used as medical therapy. By then, the Greco-Roman element 'earth' was thought to have expanded to include three new elements: mercury, salt, and sulphur. Among the proponents of medical metals was Theophrastus Bombastus von Hohenheim, who called himself Paracelsus. Born in 1493 in the German-speaking Swiss mining town of Einsedeln, he deplored the fact that minerals were not used in pharmacy. Influenced by alchemists, he thought that plants and minerals contained specific healing properties called *arcana*. For every disease, he maintained, a specific remedy must exist, and he proposed that diseases be classified by the drugs that cured them, a notion that has currency today in the concept of the therapeutic trial. Paracelsus expounded his ideas with elaborate demonstrations, including public burnings of the works of Galen and Avicenna. Such behaviour did little to help him find and keep employment, and he wandered over Europe for much of his career.

To today's student and many earlier observers, Paracelsus's writings seem confused and incoherent. For his bombastic style, he has been portrayed as a ridiculous villain whose legacy is easily dismissed. Recently, however, scholars in history, medicine, and even public administration have reconsidered his work to find that his impact may have been greater than previously thought, if only because he dared to challenge the established authority of ancient writers.

New substances, including mercury, sulphur, and antimony, became the wonder drugs of the late Renaissance. In the early sixteenth century, Girolamo Fracastoro recommended mercury to treat the 'new' European epidemic of syphilis. Mercury causes gastrointestinal disturbances, gum swelling, salivation, and neurological toxicity, but it does appear to have been an effective treatment for syphilis.

Similarly, antimony compounds produce nausea, vomiting, purging, and cardiovascular collapse. This toxicity led to a ban on antimony at several medical faculties, including Heidelberg and Paris. In the form of tartar emetic, however, the drug was said to cure almost everything, and the ban was overturned by popular demand after it was credited with saving the French king, Louis XIV, from typhoid fever in 1657. In the nineteenth century, high-dose tartar emetic was used for pneumonia; clinical statistics testified to its efficacy, but toxicity led to its disappearance once again. One of my own research projects, with Dr Pierre René of Montreal's Royal Victoria Hospital, demonstrated that – its toxicity notwithstanding – tartar emetic has bactericidal properties.

Apothecaries and the Persistence of Plants

Botany was a standard subject in medical education until about 1900. Medical schools and hospitals maintained botanical gardens, not only for teaching but also for a reliable supply of remedies. A few of these gardens remain, such as the Chelsea Physic garden in London; many others have been recreated. But doctors were not the experts; an apothecary tradition in Europe was well established as a distinct guild. Training was by apprenticeship, and a wide variety of standards and forms of practice arose – a situation referred to as 'pluralism.' Inheriting an apothecary practice was one of the earliest professional opportunities for women. Gradually the role of the English apothecary shifted to become the basis of general practice (see chapter 14). The Worshipful Society of Apothecaries of London has roots going back to the twelfth century. Still in existence, it operates an excellent website and runs many fascinating courses, including a prestigious course in medical history and training in conflict and catastrophe medicine.

Reflecting the intimate relationship between medicine and growing plants, the first Europeans to cultivate land in New France are said to have been the family of the apothecary-settler, Louis Hébert of Paris, who arrived in 1617. Some eighty years later, the first herbarium of North American plants was collected by the French physician and surgeon Michel Sarrazin also of Quebec; he corresponded with scientists in France and is said to have collected over 800 specimens of native North American flora, among them the pitcher plant (*Sarracenia purpurea*). The identities of the first apothecaries of colonial America are unknown. Wise women and autodidacts served this function, as did politicians and preachers; many early doctors, especially those in rural areas, were obliged to prepare their own remedies. The earliest apothecary stores were attached to medical practices as dispensaries: the 1698 account book of Bartholomew Browne of Salem, Massachusetts, attests to this activity. By 1721, Boston is said to have had fourteen apothecaries, and the Irish immigrant, Christopher Marshall, opened his Philadelphia shop in 1729. During the Revolutionary War, the military position of Apothecary General for the rebels was filled by the twenty-one-year-old Scot, Andrew Craigie. The first college of pharmacy in the United States was established in Philadelphia in 1821.

Many drugs still in use today were originally derived from plants, although most are now synthesized in laboratories for commercial distribution. Some have been around for a long time. Senna has been known as a laxative since at least 1550 B.C.; castor oil comes from the garden plant ricinus, which also was known to the Egyptians; foxglove has provided digitalis since at least the eighteenth century; and an aspirin-like substance is found in the bark of willow trees and yellow birch. The benefits of some vegetable remedies are rediscovered with much fanfare, as was the case with the gastrointestinal effects of bran, promoted by Denis P. Burkitt in 1973. Similarly, the cholesterol-lowering value of oat bran was widely publicized in the 1980s. Modern treatments originally derived from plants include the antileukemia drug vincristine, found in the Madagascar periwinkle; the podophyllotoxins (VP-16 and etopiside), derived from the root of the mayapple; and the breast cancer agent taxol, first extracted from ancient yew trees of Japan and the Pacific Northwest.

Effective remedies extracted from complex plants challenge scientists to imagine other miracle cures lurking in the bushes. In the early twentieth century, Parke Davis became one of the first drug companies to sponsor a systematic search of the jungle for new remedies. The 1960s fascination with the psychedelic plants known to aboriginal peoples also brought ethnobotany to the attention of scientists. More recently, the destruction of the rain forest has led to a certain panic over the potential extinction of three-quarters of the world's plant species, with a presumed loss of thousands of potential remedies, some of which may be known to indigenous peoples. The *Journal of Ethnopharmacology*, founded in 1979, provides a forum for investigators. Several projects, both botanical and anthropological, are under way to survey, identify, and analyse the medical potential of plants, some of which are already used by the peoples of Amazonia.

Botanist John Thor Arnason of the University of Ottawa identified and studied the pharmacological properties of plant products known to the native peoples of North America. Like the classicists who study antiquity, ethnobotanists need language skills to interpret myriad dialects and oral traditions; much information has already been lost. For example, early accounts of European settlement tell how the 1535–6 winter encampment of Jacques Cartier at Stadacona (Quebec) was healed of 'great disease,' probably scurvy, by a so-called white cedar (or spruce) tea given them by the natives. By the winter of 1605–6, when Samuel de Champlain founded the habitation at Port-Royal (Annapolis Royal, Nova Scotia), the remedy could no longer be identified, although Champlain knew of Cartier's experience. Evergreen needles contain vitamin C, but dialect discrepancies over the precise plant name mean that scientists have been unable to trace the exact cure.

Classification and Therapeutic Change

The earliest classifications sorted drugs into poisons and antidotes. Other classifications were based on their physical properties (Dioscorides) and, later, their physiological effects. For example, poppy juice (containing opium) and nightshade (containing atropine) were both classified as sleep-inducing narcotics, although the latter is no longer thought of in that context. Willow bark, which contains salicylic acid, was an 'astringent' that dried secretions, explaining its effect on gout. Substances that produced vomiting were emetics. Those that caused diarrhea were laxatives, cathartics, or purges, depending on their ferocity. Sudorifics made patients sweat. Stimulants woke them up. Diuretics made them urinate. The classification followed the description of the physiological effects, whether or not the effects were the reason for administering the drug. To a certain extent, we still view drugs in this way, but now we tend to explain the side effects through a chemical rationale.

For example, digitalis was first thought to be a diuretic because it reduced peripheral swelling and increased urinary flow. It is now a heart-strengthening drug or cardiotonic, but still it reduces edema and increases urinary output. In other words, the rationale has changed, but the benefits are constant. In his treatise of 1785, William Withering brought digitalis into medical orthodoxy, described its harmful effects, and reported his experiments on poor patients. He had learned of foxglove leaf, he said, from a secret remedy belonging to 'an old woman in Shropshire, who sometimes made cures after the more regular practitioners had failed.' Sadly, the identity of this woman is unknown, although some say that her name was Hutton. Medical history holds many other unknown progenitors, while experiments conducted on disadvantaged people without consent continued well into the twentieth century (see chapters 6, 7, 11 and 13).

During the nineteenth century, the pharmacopoeias of Europe and North America contained drugs that are now considered poisons: mercury in the form of calomel; antimony in the form of tartar emetic; jalap, a powerful cathartic; strychnine to stimulate appetite and bowel action; opium and laudanum for pain and sleep; alcohol as a stimulant. Combined with restrictive diets, vicious enemas or clysters, and various means of bleeding, such as phlebotomy, leeches, and cupping, this style of interventionist therapy has been called drastic, or heroic. Not everyone took it lying down – hence, the famous artistic and literary lampoons of Molière, Thomas Rowlandson, James Gilray, Honoré Daumier, and G.B. Shaw. The word 'heroic,' which normally signifies admiration, became a pejorative term in medicine. Originating from the vigorous last-ditch attempts to save lives, it now implies overdrugging, overdosing, and overreacting.

Wonder Drug, 1665

SGANARELLE: What, sir, you are a heathen about medicine
as well? ... You mean you don't believe in senna or cassia
or emetic wine? ... You must have a very unbelieving soul.
But look what a reputation emetic wine has got in the last
years. Its wonders have won over the most sceptical. Why,
only three weeks ago, I saw a wonderful proof myself. ... A
man was at the point of death for six whole days. They didn't
know what to do for him. Nothing had any effect. Then suddenly they decided to give him a dose of emetic wine.
DON JUAN: And he recovered?
SGANARELLE: No. He died. ... Could anything be more effective?

– Molière, *Don Juan*, Act 3 (1665), from *Don Juan and Other Plays by Molière*, trans.
Ian Maclean and George Graveley (Oxford: Oxford University Press, 1998), 60

Medical therapeutics has undergone greater change in the last two
hundred years than in the preceding two thousand. Why? A number
of reasons can be offered. No doubt, the fashion of period and place
had an influence. For example, in postrevolutionary France, things
associated with the old order were rejected because they were old.
Reflecting this ideal, the physiologist François Magendie hoped that
physicians would abandon the complex derivatives of the past in
favour of new, chemically pure drugs. In eight editions of the for-
mulary for the Hôtel-Dieu hospital in Paris between 1821 and 1834,
he recommended purified chemicals over the older 'simples' (the
Galenic plant-based precursors), morphine over opium, quinine
over cinchona bark. He referred to his animal tests of new alkaloids,
such as codeine and bromide. Some scientists favoured therapeutic
nihilism, but the degree to which it was actually practised is difficult
to determine.

Three other reasons may account for the decline in drastic remedies. First was the rise of surgery following the advent of anesthesia and antisepsis. Why give a nasty pill forever if an operation will
cure the problem in an instant? Second, the wide acceptance of germ

theory in the 1880s (see chapter 4) and the discovery of hormones soon after caused doctors to turn from modifying disease symptoms to finding a set of 'magic bullets' to eliminate the causes of disease. Third, pressures from homeopathy and other medical competition may have pushed medicine toward less drastic therapy. Using a computer-assisted analysis of prescription records from two urban hospitals, John Harley Warner (*Therapeutic Perspective*, 1997) elucidated a change in doctors' prescriptions between 1820 and 1885: side-effect-ridden 'heroics' were replaced by more gentle therapies. Among other factors, Warner related the change to issues of professional identity between doctors (allopaths) and unorthodox practitioners whose remedies were less harmful and more attractive to patients. Other historians suggest that resistance to homeopathy prompted the professional organization of American physicians (see chapter 6).

Magic Bullets: Antibiotics, Hormones, and Twentieth-Century Optimism

When microorganisms became accepted as a cause of disease, research focused initially on producing vaccines to heighten natural immunity (see chapter 4); only secondarily were agents sought to attack bacteria. Cinchona (or Jesuit bark) had been used to prevent and treat malaria since the seventeenth century, long before the *Plasmodium* organism had been visualized; its 'rationale' was as a 'tonic' that heightened resistance to the noxious atmospheres thought to cause malaria. Discovery of the parasite in 1880 by the future Nobel laureate Charles Laveran provided an entirely new rationale for the still effective quinine. The conscious quest for agents that kill germ invaders yet leave a living, healthy patient has been called 'the search for the magic bullet.'

The first two magic bullets were developed by Paul Ehrlich: the dye, trypan red, for experimental trypanosomiasis (1903); and the arsenic-containing Salvarsan, for human syphilis (1910). Ehrlich worked with dyes and stains that had a special affinity for bacteria, hoping that they would selectively carry a toxin into the invading cell. His 1908 Nobel Prize was awarded for theoretical work on immunity, although his work on drugs is better known.

Sulpha drugs also formed part of the magic bullet agenda. Gerhard Domagk, working for the Bayer laboratories in Elberfeld, Germany, developed the first sulpha drug, Prontosil. Having proved that it was effective against streptococcal infections in rats, Domagk's first human trial was conducted on his own daughter, who suddenly developed septicemia in December 1933. She recovered. Domagk was awarded the Nobel Prize in 1939, but he was arrested and jailed by the Gestapo for having attracted undue foreign approbation. He did not receive his award until 1947, when the prize money was no longer available. Few present-day physicians have heard of Domagk, possibly because of the wartime hostilities with Germany and possibly because he worked for a big pharmaceutical firm.

The most famous magic bullet is penicillin. Schoolchildren are taught the story of Alexander Fleming, who, in culturing bacteria, rejected plates that had been infected with mould – until he was struck by the significance. But historians have shown that Fleming's 1928 'discovery' that penicillium mould kills bacteria had been published earlier by others (notably, Bartolomeo Gosio of Rome in 1896 and E. Duchesnes of Lyons in 1897). Montreal mycologist Jules Brunel also reported that elderly Québécois had long used moulds on jam as therapy for respiratory ailments. Fleming recognized the potential of his findings but did not pursue applications, nor did he cite his predecessors. The Oxford researchers, Howard W. Florey and Ernst Chain, extracted, purified, and manufactured penicillin, which was released in 1939 a decade after Fleming's observation. Fleming, Florey, and Chain shared the Nobel Prize in 1945.

Interferon is not really a magic bullet, because it does not kill germs directly so much as it helps the body to do so by stimulating the immune system. It is a cytokine that occurs naturally in response to foreign proteins. As a result it is used for treatment of viral infections, cancer, and autoimmune diseases, as it encourages the body to destroy or control invasions of viruses, malignant cells, or irrational antibodies that attack the self. Discovered by Japanese scientists in the 1950s, it was scarce until 1980, when the techniques of recombinant DNA enabled manufacture on a large scale, making it one of the first drugs to result from genetic engineering. The many different types now available are applied to infectious and non-infectious diseases, including hepatitis C and multiple sclerosis.

Hormones and vitamins do not kill invading organisms, but they

too act as magic bullets when they specifically target and replace deficiencies. (On vitamins, see chapter 13.) The isolation and elaboration of several hormones early in the twentieth century contributed
to a rising medical optimism (see chapter 3). Frederick G. Banting,
a practitioner in London, Ontario, became convinced from his reading that the cause of diabetes mellitus was in the pancreas. In the
summer of 1921 he borrowed laboratory space from J.J.R. Macleod
at the University of Toronto to work with medical student Charles
Best on experimentally induced diabetes in dogs. The rapid isolation
and purification of the hormone was the elegant work of biochemist
J.B. Collip. Within a short time, insulin was the first hormone to be
developed as specific replacement therapy for this widespread and
previously fatal disease. The 1923 Nobel committee overlooked Best
and Collip and gave the prize to Banting and Macleod, who shared it
with the other two.

Hormones were soon applied to the treatment of tumours, fuel-
ling the growing quest for substances that could not only replace
deficiencies but cure all disease. Several hormone discoveries and
treatments followed in succession. P.S. Hench and E.C. Kendall of
the Mayo Clinic found the hormone of the adrenal cortex in 1949;
in keeping with the buoyant mood of the time, their Nobel Prize
was awarded the following year. Soon after their achievement had
been announced, an awestruck clinician rushed up to historian E.H.
Ackerknecht to tell him that he was a lucky man: all diseases would
soon be wiped out and the only professor left in the medical faculty
would be the historian (Ackerknecht, *Therapeutics*, 1973, 2). One of
the byproducts of this overwhelming enthusiasm would be an effect
on history itself – toward further ridicule of the past.

Clinical Trials

Historical comparisons with untreated human groups had long been
made to introduce new treatments. Deliberate clinical testing began
in the early nineteenth century in parallel with the development of
statistical methods (see chapter 4). For example, P.C.A. Louis applied
his numerical medicine to cast doubt on the value of bleeding. Animal trials, much used by Magendie and Bernard, continued to precede trials on humans.

In response to the many pharmacological discoveries of the early twentieth century, committees were formed to develop standards to ensure that results could be ascribed only to the drug and not to other extraneous factors (e.g., British MRC Therapeutics Trial Committee 1931). The active recruiting of concurrent, untreated 'controls' was a conscious development of the twentieth century. They began with self or alternate controls (ca 1900); randomized controls came later (ca 1940). The practice of 'blinding' observers as well as subjects increased after 1940 as a means of dealing with the powerful placebo effect. Standardization meant that drugs were carefully tested on 'the seventy-kilogram man'; effects on women, pregnant women, and racial minorities were often ignored. The zeal to investigate trod on patients' rights, sometimes with disastrous results; the postwar Nuremberg Code was devised to address these abuses and clarify the process of informed consent (see chapter 15). The first randomized controlled trial (RCT) is often said to have been the Medical Research Council (MRC) study of streptomycin in tuberculosis (*British Medical Journal* 2 [1948]: 769–88); however other contenders for this honour have been identified, including a 1944 MRC-funded trial on patulin for the common cold. Throughout the 1950s many clinical trials were used in cancer medicine.

Randomized controlled trials and the evidence-based medicine (EBM) movement are indelibly associated with Scottish epidemiologist Archie L. Cochrane. He claimed his 'first, worst, and most successful' trial was a 1941 study on nutritional value of yeast and vitamins conducted on himself and twenty other starving prisoners of war. After the war, he did field research in Wales for the Medical Research Council. In his influential book of 1972 (*Effectiveness and Efficiency*), he complained that, despite many years of RCTs, most treatments were prescribed without good evidence of benefit. In his name, an international program was founded in 1993: the Cochrane Collaboration endeavours to collate all available RCT information in various areas of practice through systematic reviews.

'Evidence-based medicine' is a term coined in 1991 by Gordon Guyatt of McMaster University, Canada. He pioneered the movement with colleague David Sackett; they conducted research into improving methodologies and Sackett later directed a special centre at Oxford University. Another leader in this field was Iain Chalmers, who began to direct the Perinatal Epidemiology Unit of the United Kingdom in 1978 (see chapter 11). He became the founding director of the Cochrane Collaboration and was knighted in 2000.

The persuasive arguments of EBM proponents resulted in widespread acceptance of these principles for advancing and changing therapeutic practice as well as medical education. Keating and Cambrosio (2007) argue that it has created a new form of practice. Its history has yet to be written. But most medical historians are allergic to the term: they claim that it relies on static diagnostic categories and tends to imply (albeit unintentionally) that our predecessors did not consider evidence at all. Medline is now rife with articles showing that the great but forgotten 'so-and-so' wielded EBM principles first and long ago. As P.K. Rangachari aptly put it, EBM is 'old French wine with a new Canadian label' (*J Royal Soc Med* 90 [1997]: 280–4). Social critics of medicine argue that the turn to EBM forces individuals to conform to group norms. EBM proponents protest that these criticisms unfairly address unintended consequences or unrealistic applications of the method.

Recent Scepticism: Is There No Magic Bullet?

The mid-twentieth-century optimism was premature, if understandable. Aside from their many side effects, magic bullets created magic microbes. We now have drug-resistant malaria and gonorrhea, while multi-drug-resistant staphylococcus (MRSA) stalks the literature and the wards, colonizing unsuspecting patients, especially in chronic care facilities. And we worry about penicillin-resistant syphilis. Dreadful nosocomial infections lurk in the antibiotic-ridden ferment of hospitals, where few but resistant strains can survive. In his *Medical Nemesis* (1975), Ivan Illich suggested that the medical establishment had become a serious threat to health. More recently, the blunt title of Allan Brandt's history of venereal disease, *No Magic Bullet*, expressed the postmodern disillusionment with the goal of universal disease eradication.

Antibiotics have certainly saved individual lives, but did they really prolong life expectancy? Few historians were prepared to assess the possibility that the new drugs, so effective in individual cases, might not be good for the collective. People live longer now than they did two hundred years ago, but how much of that enhanced longevity is actually due to medicine? For example, we now know that mortality from the leading killer, tuberculosis, began to decline *before* the advent of vaccination and antituberculous drugs. In other words, hygiene, diet, wealth, and lifestyle probably counted as much for the decline, if not more. The rise of tuberculosis in parts of North America during the 1990s coincided with decline in wealth, living conditions, and nutrition. A spate of novel infections beginning in the late 1990s only enhanced the scepticism (see chapter 7).

Thalidomide

The story of thalidomide provides a powerful example of innovation gone awry; it shook confidence in medicine on a global scale. A highly effective sedative developed in the late 1950s, thalidomide was applied often to morning sickness of pregnancy. Used in Germany from 1957 and in England from 1958, it was linked to birth defects in late 1961 by Australian William McBride and German geneticist Widukind Lenz after nearly a year of studying what seemed to be an epidemic rise in gross limb abnormalities in infants (phocomelia). Its removal in Canada came five months later in April 1962; the first affected Canadians were born in Saskatoon in February and June 1962 (*CMAJ* 87 [1962], 412, 670). Because the drug was teratogenic in the earliest weeks of pregnancy, the full scope of the tragedy was not known until nine months later. A total of 10,000 children in at least twenty-five countries were affected: 5,000 in Germany, 540 in Britain, 300 in Japan, 125 in Canada, 107 in Sweden. Probably many more pregnancies ended in miscarriage. The tragedy was averted in the United States because the drug had not yet been fully licensed, owing to the hesitation of physician-scientist Frances Oldham Kelsey of the Food and Drug Administration (FDA). In 1962, President Kennedy presented her with the award for distinguished Federal Civilian service. In 2005, she retired at age 90 from the FDA, a much lauded national hero.

Affected people were of normal intelligence and eager to work despite their missing limbs and other disabilities. The German drug

company, Grünenthal, was sued, but an out-of-court settlement resulted in the company contributing 100M DM, matched by the government, into a trust fund for pensions. A similar trust begain in Great
Britain in 1973. In Canada, affected people received no compensa-
tion until September 1992, when they were thirty years old. Because
the drug had been properly licensed, the government was held liable,
not the pharmaceutical industry and not the medical practitioners
who had prescribed it. Ironically, and some would argue inappropriately, thalidomide has now been reintroduced for the management of various skin conditions, including graft-versus-host disease,
an iatrogenic disorder. The memory of the tragedy meant that these
newer uses met with vigorous opposition.

Thalidomide is an extreme example of therapeutic disaster; even
its victims understand that their deformities were unintended. But it
should not be forgotten. Thalidomide reminds us that good intentions do not prevent medicine from being harmful; it helps to account
for the complicated licensing procedures that are so often criticized
for slowing innovation. Animal rights activists point out that animal
testing has greatly increased since the tragedy; yet they argue that it
is often futile as a tool for studying humans: for example, the original
pregnant animal tests for thalidomide had been negative. The thalidomide story also renews and explains the public's continued mistrust of the medical establishment. The negative image guarantees a
market for the dissenting literature and for products of the largely
unregulated folk-medicine and health-food industry, an industry
whose net worth is difficult to determine, but in the United States
alone, the annual market is said to exceed $60 billion.

Rational Derivatives

Magic bullets were extracted from the living tissues of animals, plants,
and moulds, and they could also be synthesized in the laboratory.
They were designed to repair the biological causes of infections and
deficiencies. But in the early twentieth century, many other diseases
were defined in a chemical or molecular sense. Attempts to 'design'
rational remedies are based on an understanding of the precise biochemical error producing the disease. For example, in Parkinson's

disease, chemicals that appear to be deficient in the brain become the medicines administered by doctors. Other examples abound: histamine antagonists to reduce gastric acid secretion; beta-blockers to prevent transmission of certain nervous impulses; calcium channel blockers for ischemic heart disease. In the majority of these cases, the 'designer drug' emerged out of trials as the most effective and least toxic of a series of related compounds created in a laboratory to solve a chemical problem.

The 1988 Nobel Prize was awarded to James Black, Gertrude B. Elion, and George H. Hitchings for the development of '*rational methods for designing*' treatments; most of the drugs that they 'discovered' or developed are still widely used: cimetidine, propanolol, 6-mercapto-purine, 6-thioguanine, allopurinol, and trimethoprim. In each case, the drug was a chemical device invented to solve a chemical problem.

By the year 2000, the human genome project showed how many diseases could be defined by molecules; therefore, virtually any genetically defined problem could become a call for a rational derivative. Relying on the Nobel-winning technology of hybridoma research, 'genetic engineering,' so much discussed in the twentieth century, finally began to cash out. First used in 1977, the word 'drugable' reflects the pharmaceutical potential of molecular discovery (see figure 5.2). The best but not the only examples of drugable products are the '-mabs' – monoclonal antibodies targeted directly against enzymes and tumour antigens: imatinib for chronic leukemia; rituximab for lymphoma; trastuzumab for breast cancer; dozens of others are in the pipeline. These wonder drugs offer hope to millions, but they are very expensive to make and to use. (On biotechnology see chaper 9.)

The Pharmaceutical Industry

Since the late 1800s, when specific chemical agents were isolated and characterized, the need for standardization and synthesis of natural substances favoured the development of a drug industry. For more than a century, drug companies have engaged in and supported research with funds and laboratories. Not only does the industry have

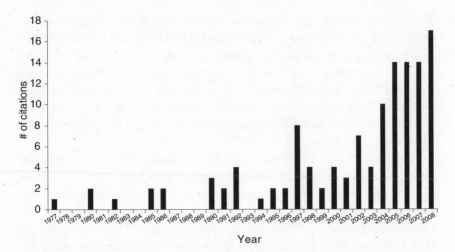

Year

5.2   The word 'drugable' (also 'drug-able') in medical literature, 1977–2008 (N=126). Keyword search on Medline, May 2009

power over the sales and distribution of remedies, it controls more than 70 per cent of the funds spent on drug research even when that research is done in universities. Privately funded research is often extremely productive. Like Domagk of sulpha fame, the 1988 Nobel laureates were employees of major pharmaceutical firms.

Medical and public reaction to drug companies is ambivalent. Their discoveries are welcome, and for expensive new treatments their financial input is essential. But their big profits and their research grants are sources of discomfort. Critics worry that drug-funded research is ethically compromised or that accepting sponsorship is a form of advertising; scholars show that it skews publication. They also point to the financial gain from selling drugs, claiming that the industry is not motivated to cure disease; chronic illness is good for business. These worries are heightened by cases like that of Toronto's Dr Nancy Olivieri, whose 1996 expression of concern over the side effects of a trial drug resulted in withdrawal of industry support for the trial and serious personal and professional harassment from her academic colleagues.

Drug patents have a long history extending back to the early modern period when they reflected royal approbation. Since the late eighteenth century, patent protections meant that the contents of remedies could remain secret for a period of time, usually seventeen years. Historically speaking, the term is often used to refer to nostrums and 'quack' remedies, but all drugs were eligible for patents, and all newly developed medications still seek them. The complex history of patents is written in precedents from case law and legislation in various countries, where swings between private protection of investments and public distrust of monopolies result in modifications and changes. Furthermore, wide cultural variation exists in different developed nations about the appropriateness of taking pills: Japan and France lead the world in taking medicines.

In the 1970s various procedures were implemented to allow Canadian pharmacists to replace expensive brand-name drugs with the least expensive substitute, often a copy with the same composition manufactured by a 'generic' company that had not invested in developing the drug. These policies were unpopular with the research industry because they ignored its heavy investment in developing products. The situation created problems with international trading partners. For example, in 1987 and again in 1993, Canada's patent laws were to satisfy the demands of the General Agreement on Tariffs and Trade (GATT). Similar changes took place in other countries. The new laws guaranteed patent owners up to twenty years of exclusive sales of their product (seventeen years in the United States). In return, the pharmaceutical industry was obliged to increase its spending on research and development (R&D). It has complied, and private funding of academic research has increased, but it continues to lobby against drug substitution policies as cost-control measures.

But because of, or in spite of the changes, drug prices rose. In countries with universal health insurance, the higher costs take a larger slice out of the tax dollar, since drug spending for seniors and welfare recipients are covered benefits. These governments were motivated to regulate costs. Therefore around the mid-1990s, as laws changed to afford longer patent protection, national regulatory bodies for controlling the prices of patent drugs were established in Canada, France, Germany, Italy, Sweden, the United Kingdom, and elsewhere. Their methods vary. In Canada the agency can intervene to ensure that prices rise no higher than the consumer price index.

The United States does not regulate drug prices. Also around 1993, some countries, lead by Britain, established bodies to establish and monitor 'codes of practice' concerning ethics and safety in the promoting and selling of drugs. In developing countries, the protected drugs are so expensive that they are unavailable, and international efforts focus on new regulations to allow generic substitutes or charitable donations.

Without regulation, prices in the United States rose much higher than in other countries. Critics argued that the sick were being forced to pay for the heavier advertising in direct-to-consumer practices that are illegal elsewhere; the sick must also bear the higher financial burden imposed by the for-profit health insurance industry and a litigious culture that spawns expensive lawsuits. In 2003, a grassroots movement of Americans organized for action: comprising mostly seniors living in border states such as Maine and Michigan, they travelled to Canada in busloads, or they ordered medications by mail. Internet suppliers leapt to the fore and Canadian physicians were pressured by 'friends of friends' to prescribe for people whom they had never met. The legality of the matter and the quality of Canadian medications were called into question by the U.S. FDA, although most of the products sought were identical to those sold (and approved) in the United States. In 2007, some clarity was established when legislation allowed American pharmacies to import drugs; however, interpretations have been variable and the U.S. Senate rejected a bill in late 2009.

Sensitive to the criticism of making money during a time of fiscal restraint and feeling unfairly blamed for the high costs of innovations, pharmaceutical manufacturers began to defend themselves in the early 1990s through their professional associations. In aggressive campaigns for public information, they argued that research into newer and better drugs for the management of illness helps to control health-care costs by keeping people out of hospital; it also supports academic inquiry and provides jobs. The contributions to research meant that by 2003, according to *JAMA* (289, 454–65), at least a quarter of medical scientists in North America had financial affiliations with industry and two-thirds of universities held equity in companies – a growing problem of conflict of interest. In 2005 the approximately fifty member companies of the Canadian pharmaceutical organization donated $86 million to charity and invested almost C$1.2 billion in R&D. In 2006, the equivalent group in Britain gave £3.9 billion to R&D, while in the United States the figure was US$43 billion. With the 2003 amendments to the agreement governing intellectual property (TRIPS), the World Trade Organization has attempted to make low-cost remedies available to poor countries while continuing to provide patent protection in rich nations. Canada's first shipment of generic anti-HIV drugs went to Rwanda in September 2008.

The Industry View and Some Questions

British doctors are still reluctant to prescribe new medicines – clinicians in other countries are far more likely to prescribe medicines that have come on to the market in the past five years.

— Association of the British Pharmaceutical Industry (ABPI),
http://www.abpi.org.uk/ (accessed 3 November 2008)

According to the same website, eight of the ten top-selling drugs in Britain were launched within the preceding decade (average time since launch 7.9 years). Of the fifty top-selling drugs in Britain only two had been on the market for twenty or more years (L-thyroxine and Zoladex).

Is the relative reluctance of British doctors to prescribe newer drugs a bad thing in your opinion? In the opinion of the ABPI? Why?

Why have most best-selling drugs been on the market for less than twenty years?

What is the purpose of the ABPI?

The pharmaceutical industry also exercises considerable, though not exclusive, control over drug information. Doctors are usually unable or ill-equipped to examine the research literature. As a result, they tend to learn about new drugs from roving representatives,

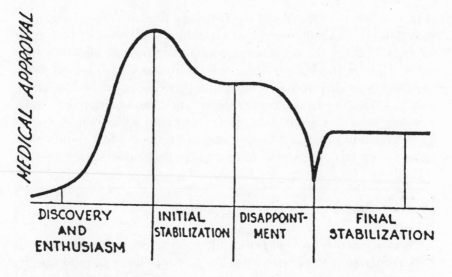

5.3   Graph depicting the phases in a drug's use. From Ernest Jawetz, *Annual Review of Medicine* 5 (1954): 2

advertisements in medical journals, and conferences, all vulnerable to industry influence. Continuing Medical Education initiatives of medical schools and professional bodies are working to improve the situation by keeping the onus for disseminating news of innovations and dangers in the hands of supposedly impartial practitioners. Rare scholars, such as Joel Lexchin and Jeremy Greene, try to sort out the relationships of doctors and industry now and in the past.

The Life Cycle of Innovations in Treatment

By 1954 Ernest Jawetz had shown that medical approval follows a pattern. At first, the use of a new remedy rises quickly in a period of optimism; then some untoward side effect is noted, and the approval drops rapidly to a low based on mistrust and fear; finally, use stabilizes at a moderate level – swings that have been called 'from panacea to poison to pedestrian' (see figure 5.3). The Jawetz model certainly fits the life cycle of chloramphenicol, which was developed in 1948 as an effective antibiotic. By 1967, it was found to cause aplastic anemia in one of every 30,000 recipients. Sales fell dramatically, and its manufacturer, Parke Davis, was forced to merge with Warner Lambert. Since then, chloramphenicol use has risen slowly to a stable but lower level.

Jawetz's curve has been applied to the natural history of other remedies, including thalidomide and digitalis; the latter suffered a long period of unpopularity. For digitalis, the margin between therapeutic and toxic is narrow; levels high enough to be of benefit are close to those causing side effects. Only when dosage could be stabilized was medical approval stabilized too (Estes 1979).

Legislation and careful drug testing are intended to level off peaks and troughs, but the Jawetz curve is unlikely ever to become a straight line. Increasingly careful drug testing may eliminate the precipitous drops due to unexpected side effects, but gradual decline in a drug's use will always occur as one remedy is replaced by safer and more effective products, or as the disease in question becomes something else (see chapter 4). Dips in the curve are generated not only by the recognized side effects but also by what disease happens to be in fashion and who comprises the target population.

The most used or most sold drugs have changed markedly in the last two centuries (see table 5.1). But information for recent years is difficult to gather, and it is even more difficult to draw meaningful comparisons in time and space. Some is provided in terms of retail sales; some in terms of frequency of use (compare the differences in table 5.1 in columns 1997 and 2004). A top-selling drug means that it generates the most money – it does not mean that it is prescribed most often. Once a patent expires, generic companies can begin to sell cheaper versions of the same drug. As a result, the R&D pharmaceuticals are constantly looking for new 'follow on' drugs to answer to the same problems. Some critics argue that newer products have only slight differences from the substances that they replace, and that they might not be better.

At the time of writing, the list of best-selling drugs in Canada, Britain, and the United States is dominated by agents for the treatment of the risk factors (rather than symptoms) of heart disease, hypertension, and high cholesterol, and for asthma, heartburn, mental disorders, and arthritis – all chronic problems, many the product of diet and lifestyle, conditions that can be treated unto death. The list is yet another sign of an aging society in which neither patients nor practitioners are particularly enamoured of the concept of dis-

Table 5.1
Top drugs/treatments used or sold in various practices, 1795–2007

1795[a]	1850s[b]	1880s[b]	1931[c]	1995[d]	2007[e]
opium	quinine	cupping	codeine	diltiazem (Cardizem)	atorvastatin (Lipitor)
blisters	opium	opium	acetylsalicylic acid	omeprazole Mg (Losec)	fluticasone (Seretide)
senna	venesection	tartar emetic	sod. bicarbonate	nifedipine (Adalat)	clopidogrel (Plavix)
aloes	tartar emetic	chloroform	acetphenetidin	fluoxetine HCl (Prozac)	olanzapine (Zyprexa)
tartar	calomel (mercury)	discontinue order	elix. pepsin comp.	lovastatin (Mevacor)	etanercept (Enbrel)
cinchona	blisters	bromide/ergot	sodium bromide	beclomethasone (Beclovent)	budesonide / formoterol (Symbicort)
licorice	ipecac	aconite	glycerin	enalapril (Vasotec)	tiotropium (Spiriva)
enemata	cupping	chloral hydrate	sodium salicylate	simvastatin (Zocor)	trastuzumab (Herceptin)
mercurials	iron	enemata	nux vomica	ciprofloxacin (Cipro)	venlafaxine (Effexor)
jalap	jalap	milk	ammonium cl.	sertraline (Zoloft)	simvastatin (Zocor)

SOURCES:

[a]Based on a practitioner's prescriptions: J.W. Estes, 'Drug Use at the Infirmary, the Example of Dr. Andrew Duncan, Sr,' in Guenter B. Risse, *Hospital Life in Enlightenment Scotland: Care and Teaching at the Royal Infirmary of Edinburgh* (Cambridge: Cambridge University Press 1986), 351–84

[b]Based on a practitioner's prescriptions: J. Duffin, *Langstaff: A Nineteenth-Century Medical Life* (Toronto: University of Toronto Press, 1993), 75

[c]Based on survey of >120,000 pharmacy prescriptions in four states. E.N. Gathercoal, *The Prescription Ingredient Survey* (American Pharmaceutical Association, 1933), 22

[d]Based on national sales of prescription drugs: Pharmaceutical Manufacturers Association of Canada, *Annual Review* (Ottawa: PMAC, 1996–7), 23

[e]Assocation of the British Pharmaceutical Industry, Facts and Statistics, 2007 http://www.abpi.org/uk/statistics/intro.asp, accessed December 2009

ease prevention. The target diseases depend on place: for example, comparatively more asthma products are top-sellers in Britain; more heartburn remedies are top-sellers in the United States. Is this because of differences in the disease incidence, or is it because of geographic differences in rates of diagnosis and in willingness to take medication?

Over-the-counter remedies are not always included in these reports, although user surveys suggest that they are probably the most frequently used medications of all. Similarly because they generate less income, generic versions of older, off-patent remedies occupy lower places on the best-seller lists; but that list does not reflect frequency of use; nor does it comment on effectiveness.

The pharmaceutical industry also participates in the creation of disease to create larger markets for its products. The launch of Viagra was accompanied by an advertising campaign that was packaged as 'raising awareness.' But it also raised the status of the condition, changing its name from the weakling 'impotence' to the manly 'ED' (erectile dysfunction), and implying that one did not have to have a real disease to benefit from the pill. 'E.D. is more common than you think.' Similarly the 1986 launch of Prozac, patented in 1977, was accompanied by a vigorous campaign, again packaged as 'raising awareness,' that, at its peak, resulted in the drug being taken for shyness and nervousness and netted the company $3 billion in the year 2000; being alive was a Prozac-deficient state. At its official website Eli Lilly now boasts that Prozac is 'the most widely prescribed antidepressant medication in history' and has been prescribed to 'over 54 million people worldwide.' However, this statement belies the serious problems that the company suffered in early 2002 when it finally lost its fight to extend the patent. (For more on SSRI drugs like Prozac, see chapter 12.)

The clock starts ticking on a patent as soon as it is filed; drug development can take another ten years before it can be sold. The generic version of fluoxetine sold for approximately 10 per cent of the Prozac price. Lilly lost 90 per cent of its Prozac market in a year; its net worth collapsed $35 billion in a single day. Although fluoxetine is not among the best-selling drugs when measured by sales, its generic versions are used by millions of people every day. This example shows how a successful company uses the Jawetz curve and the duration of patents; it must plan to replace its new drugs even as they are launched, meaning that the search for something better is also driven by a parallel search for something different – a search that preoccupies economic and intellectual resources in finding another version of the same thing at the expense of finding solutions to rare diseases or putting useful remedies into the hands of poor people and poor countries.

More spectacular shifts in drug popularity were to come. In July 2002, *JAMA* published a clinical trial that showed hormone replacement therapy was associated with a higher risk of heart disease and cancer. Overnight, the widespread practice of giving prophylactic estrogen to all menopausal women virtually disappeared with the predicted economic consequences. In September 2004, another clinical trial implicated a 'coxib' drug, designed to treat arthritis, with causing heart disease. Merck, the company making a related drug (but not the one studied) withdrew its product (Vioxx) from the market; overnight, its stock collapsed; personal injury lawsuits mushroomed and are still being fought. Many earlier trials had attested to the benefits of these remedies.

Swings in drug fortunes can go the other way. Trastuzumab (Herceptin) is one of the elegant drugs designed from molecular medicine to treat a specific antigenic type of aggressive breast cancer (see chapter 8). When a clinical trial in 2005 showed that it was beneficial at the early stage, women took to the streets, generated petitions, lobbied their governments, and demanded the drug be made available to all who qualify, despite the $50K cost for a single patient. At the time of writing, whether adjuvant Herceptin is 'the right thing to do' depends on nationality, private insurance, or personal wealth.

As pharmacology as becomes more and more precise, the wild swings in fortune and practice seem no less extreme. Achieving the promise of clinical trials must lie ahead, because it cannot be found in the past.

Suggestions for Further Reading

At the bibliography website http://histmed.ca.

CHAPTER SIX

On Becoming and Being a Doctor: Education, Licensing, Payment, and Bioethics*

That any sane nation, having observed that you could provide for the supply of bread by giving bakers a pecuniary interest in baking for you, should go on to give a surgeon a pecuniary interest in cutting off your leg, is enough to make one despair of political humanity.

– G.B. Shaw, *The Doctor's Dilemma* (1911), 1

The Doctor–Patient Contract

Doctors can be doctors only when someone else agrees. A contract has always existed between physician and patient, although it was not always recorded in writing. This contract assumes that doctors' expert knowledge will fill patient expectations. When these expectations are met, patients grant doctors the privileges of authority and professional control: autonomy over examination, licensing, and discipline. Privileges continue as long as the contract is filled to the satisfaction of both parties. When doctors fail to meet expectations, problems arise and solutions are determined by rules.

The history of the profession is a history of this contract and how it has been negotiated and changed. Simply meeting its terms does not necessarily guarantee adulation or even respect. The profession has passed through periods of ascendancy and decline. Becoming and

*Learning objectives for this chapter are found on pp. 451–2.

being a doctor is intimately connected to these changes, and at its heart is the socially condoned connection to the patient.

On Fildes's Doctor: An Image

The 1891 painting by Sir Luke Fildes, called *The Doctor* (see figure 6.1), is a magnificent example of nineteenth-century strength and pathos. The caring physician sits beside a suffering child, whose distraught parents hover in the background. He comforts with his presence, even if he appears to offer little in the way of medicine.

Few would dispute the values symbolized by Fildes: patience, tenderness, wisdom, even courage, as the physician exposes himself to disease. The bearded man is distinguished and wise; he has come to the patient's home without special equipment, and he gives all the time that the family needs. The parents are displaced by his authority. Indeed, they willingly cede their place. An accord is implicit in the shared culture of the family and the doctor. It is probable (though not evident in the painting) that he has treated the child with mercury, antimony, bloodletting, or other measures considered dangerous today. Whether she lives or dies, the parents will owe him money; whether or not he accepts their payment is another matter, but he certainly has the account in his ledger at home. Failure to save the child's life will bring sorrow to the family, but it is unlikely to bring a subpoena for malpractice.

A Fleeting History of Medical Education

The first step in the contract is obtaining the status of expert, becoming a doctor. The education of doctors began as clustered apprenticeships around knowledgeable physicians, loosely termed 'schools' by modern observers. Egyptian scrolls from ca 3000 B.C. and Mesopotamian tablets from the seventh century B.C. attest to communication of knowledge. The Aegean island of Cos is said to have been the leg-

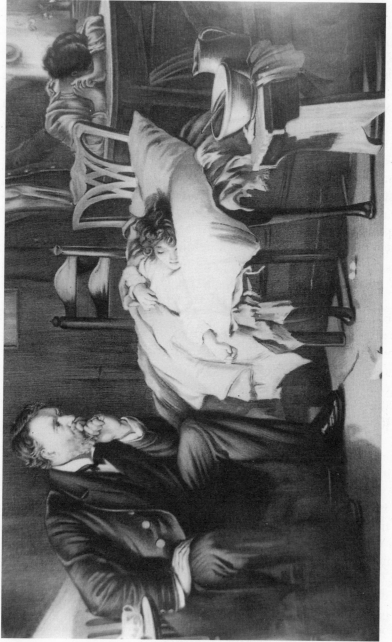

6.1   *The Doctor*, by Luke Fildes, 1891 (detail). Colour engraving based on original in the Tate Gallery, London. Gift of Dr J.W. Kerr, Faculty of Health Sciences, Queen's University

endary home of Hippocrates. Ancient medical 'schools' of the Mediterranean were also located in Cnidus and Alexandria. From at least the fifth century A.D. schools in Persia centred around hospitals, such as the one in Gundishapur (Jondishapour) in present-day southwest Iran; they combined their own traditions with Greek and Roman wisdom – a process that continued following Arab invasions and Islamic rule. Most of the ancient Greek and Latin medical texts were preserved by scholars in the middle east, North Africa, and Spain.

In the era of medieval universities, these texts were recovered. The earliest European medical school was founded by the tenth century at the southern Italian city of Salerno; this region, it is said, had the benefit of four traditions: Greek, Roman, Islamic, and Jewish. Despite many ups and downs, the Salerno school survived until around 1800, when it was closed by the conquering Napoleon Bonaparte. By 2006, a new faculty was being revived. Montpellier in southern France boasts the oldest continuously operating medical school in the Western world; its founders were probably Jewish physicians who migrated from Spain in the twelfth century. Its botanical garden dates from the late sixteenth century.

Until the eighteenth century, formal medical education, associated with universities, was separate from that of surgeons, who had their own guilds in which apprenticeship and practical training were emphasized over books (see chapter 10). Hospitals might now be a logical place to find medical students, but they were run as hospices by religious caregivers; the intrusion of educators was unwelcome and largely unimagined (see chapter 9). Until they chose to practise, doctors trained as scholars, philosophers, and natural scientists. In Britain, four schools claim early origins: Oxford (thirteenth century), Aberdeen (1495), Cambridge (1540), and Glasgow (1637).

In the late eighteenth century, political and social changes meant that hospitals increasingly belonged to municipalities rather than religious orders. Rising appreciation of anatomy and the physical examination also meant that 'hands-on' learning was valued for both doctors and surgeons; their traditions could profitably merge (see chapter 2). These changes swept Europe. Older schools were revamped – for example seeking more space, Montpellier took over a Benedictine monastery which it still occupies; and new schools

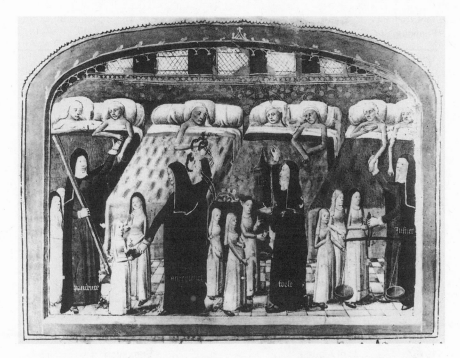

6.2   A medieval hospital scene. Care was the objective of religious sites of
healing; cure, a gift of God. From the fifteenth-century French manuscript
by Jehan Henry, 'Livre de vie active.' Musée de l'Assistance Publique, Paris

arose around clinics and hospitals in Leiden, Jena, Vienna, Edinburgh, London, Berlin, Rome, and many other cities. Some were
free-standing institutions, others associated with colleges and universities; all looked to hospitals for teaching opportunities. British
medical schools, especially, were associated with hospitals and still
are, although, since 1990, a number merged with each other and
with universities.

In North America, the earliest European physicians had trained
somewhere else. The idea of creating schools in the colonies did not
materialize until almost two centuries after first settlement. The first
medical school for colonial America opened at Philadelphia in 1765;
and for Canada, at Montreal in 1822. In the boom of the early nineteenth century, many other schools opened, some privately owned,

Table 6.1
Founding of Canadian medical schools and their predecessors

1822–9	Montreal Medical Institution (became McGill U)	Montreal
1824–6	Rolph and Duncombe	St Thomas
1829	McGill U	Montreal
1843–91	Toronto School (merged with U of T)	Toronto
1843–53	King's College (at U of T)	Toronto
1843–90	École de Montréal (merged with Laval)	Montreal
1850–?	Upper Canada / Trinity College	Toronto
1852	U Laval	Quebec City
1854	Queen's U	Kingston
1854–74	Victoria U, Cobourg	Toronto
1866–90	Victoria U, Cobourg (merged with École)	Montreal
1868	Dalhousie U	Halifax
1870-1903	Trinity (merged with U of T)	Toronto
1871–1905	Bishop's (merged with McGill)	Montreal/Lennoxville
1878–1920	Laval succursale (became U de M)	Montreal
1882	U of Western Ontario (renamed Schulich School, 2004)	London
1883	U of Manitoba	Winnipeg
1883–95	Women's Medical College	Kingston
1883–1906	Woman's Medical College	Toronto
1891	U of Toronto	Toronto
1913	U of Alberta	Edmonton
1920	U de Montréal	Montreal
1926–44	U of Saskatchewan (premed only)	Saskatoon
1944	U of Saskatchewan (full program)	Saskatoon
1945	U of Ottawa	Ottawa
1950	U of British Columbia	Vancouver
1966	U de Sherbrooke	Sherbrooke
1967	U of Calgary	Calgary
1969	McMaster U	Hamilton
1969	Memorial U	St John's
2005	Northern Ontario School of Medicine Lakehead U and Laurentian U	Thunder Bay Sudbury

others associated with colleges (see table 6.1). Standards were variable and a large number did not survive. Figure 6.3 shows that the demand for new doctors varies through time.

Following the late nineteenth-century advent of germ theory and bacteriology (see chapter 4), laboratory science became crucial for future doctors. The school of medicine at Johns Hopkins University in Baltimore was founded to exemplify these values. From its incep-

Founding of Medical Schools in the United States and United Kingdom, 1725–2009

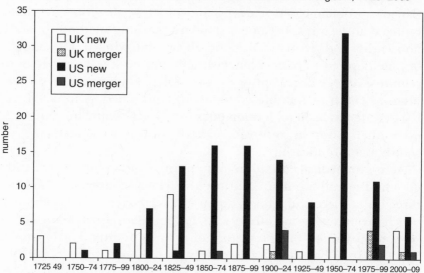

6.3   Founding of British and American medical schools by quarter century. Excludes the four UK schools with earlier origins (Oxford, Aberdeen, Cambridge, and Glasgow), and schools that disappeared without successors. Founding dates of the schools involved in mergers are retained. A merger creates a new school but diminishes the total number. Source: Historical information at the websites of extant 27 schools in UK and 130 schools in U.S., 2008–9.

tion in 1893, medical training was divided into two years of basic science and two of clinical medicine. This became the ideal. It was spread and maintained in North America and with some modification even beyond for more than seven decades, owing to the impact of the highly influential survey of Abraham Flexner in 1910. The more schools resembled Johns Hopkins, the better they fared in his judgment; some were forced to close altogether.

Between 1920 and 1960 few new medical schools appeared in the English-speaking world. The result was that the graduate-per-capita ratio slowly declined. Surveys again showed that more doctors were needed. Another boom in creating medical schools took place from the late 1960s in Britain, Canada, the United States and many other countries of Europe. Following the lead of McMaster University in Canada, problem-based learning and other small group methods, rather than lectures, became a standard teaching method. In addition, earlier and greater clinical training was introduced. The amount of time devoted to basic science shrank, but most schools began to require a college degree prior to entry; science subjects were prerequisites. Length of training consequently shortened. A trend of the last decade has been to develop links with isolated satellite centres or even other countries to provide experience in remote medicine – a return to apprenticeship.

Access to medical education for minorities and women was restricted until the mid-twentieth century. Medicine is conservative and the directors of successful schools espoused their own cultural traditions, which meant excluding others who did not share them. Many books have been written on the history of restricted entry. For example, Todd L. Savitt has written extensively on the endeavours of African Americans. Following emancipation, they were educated at segregated schools opened by missionaries, including Howard University, Meharry College, and Shaw University. By the late 1880s, some of those graduates founded their own proprietary schools because blacks were still excluded from many northern schools. Women too found opportunities in segregated schools, after a handful of individual successes in male schools (see chapter 11). Even after admission became possible, discrimination persisted: racial and religious minorities, including Jews, and women were subjected to limiting quotas that fluctuated with social pressure. These restrictions persisted until at least the 1970s. Affirmative action programs to enhance access have had limited roles with medical schools. With no shortage of applicants, conservative forces prefer to rely on high achievement in leading colleges, as if undergraduate grades should correlate with good doctoring. At the time of writing, the biggest barrier to medical education for intellectually endowed and motivated students is financial.

Becoming a doctor is only one step of several socially determined elements in the doctor–patient contract. The degree does not grant a licence to practise.

Controlling Practice: Guilds, Professional Bodies, and Licensing

Simply claiming to be a physician is not enough. Doctors have always been subjected to sanctions when they failed to live up to expectations. In antiquity, penalties for medical failure within state laws could be severe: ranging from amputation of both hands as recommended by the Code of Hammurabi (ca 1700 B.C.) to crucifixion as recommended by Alexander the Great (Plutarch, *Life of Alexander*, ch. 72; Arrian, *Anabasis*, 7, 14). The less drastic penalties of our own time include fines, revocation of the licence to practice, public humiliation, and jail. Professional authority is still a privilege, not a right.

Credentials

For most of the past, physicians and barber-surgeons competed with a wide variety of other healers, including wise women, quacks, charlatans, and the adepts of alternative theories. The history of medical professionalization is the shift from pluralistic health care to a monopoly of a powerful orthodoxy.

The trend to monopoly was advanced by claims for the power of medical knowledge. During the dominance of Christianity, the perfect practitioner was one who combined knowledge of disease with deference to God's will. Nevertheless, by the middle of the fourteenth century, most European jurisdictions required some form of a licence, to be obtained through examination by a guild, a public authority, or a university (see table 6.2).

From the sixteenth century, with the so-called scientific revolution, religion and medicine were formally separated and the independent power of doctors began to grow. European doctors scientificized illness in new ways and touted their superior abilities as healers. They were aware that some colleagues might not be safe and that others might limit their earnings; to minimize the damage done to patients and reputations by unworthy doctors, they demanded the right to decide who was acceptable and who was not. In Italy 'Protomedicato' committees granted licences to practise from the mid-sixteenth century. After considerable petitioning, charters of autonomy were

Table 6.2
Some early milestones in the medical professionalization of Europe

Date	Authority	Licence requirement or limitation
Mid-12th C	Roger II of Sicily	Public examinations of practitioners
1215	Fourth Lateran Council	Clergy forbidden to cauterize or incise
1219	Bologna	Examination by archdeacon
1231	Frederick II of Sicily	Salerno masters have right to examine
13th C	Montpellier	Barber-surgeon guild
1260	Collège St Côme	Paris surgeons' guild
1418	Montpellier	Barber-surgeon guild examinations
1423	London	Brief merger of surgeons and physicians
1505	Edinburgh	Barber-surgeon guild
1518	London	Royal College of Physicians
1540	England	Company of Barber Surgeons
1599	Glasgow	Royal College of Physicians & Surgeons
1617	London	Apothecaries separate from physicians
1654	Dublin	Royal College of Physicians
1681	Edinburgh	College of Physicians
1699	Louis XIV of France	Dentists examined by surgeons

granted to physicians and to guilds of barber-surgeons, first by cities, then by nations. Being a professional was not only about education and college degrees; it was defined by membership in a body of practitioners who held the privilege of examining, licensing, and disciplining their own – independent of government.

In Canada, medical practice has been regulated by regional licensing bodies since the seventeenth century. Before any Canadian medical schools were founded, a degree from elite institutions in Europe was sufficient for a licence. American and other graduates were subject to examinations. In the early nineteenth century, with the founding of the first Canadian schools, examination eventually became compulsory for all. Licences are granted by states and provinces. But a number of twentieth-century modifications make the credentials portable on a national scale. For example, since 1911, the licence of the Medical Council of Canada (founded 1906) has been portable across all provinces. Special examinations are required of foreign medical graduates who come to the United States or Canada (called ECFMG, first held in 1958).

Medical power and prestige increased further with the advent of specialties in the late nineteenth century. In Britain, where the royal colleges for surgery and medicine already dated back hundreds of years, each new specialty developed its own 'college.' Eventually a loose merger formed in 1974, the Academy of Medical Royal Colleges, but each specialty college maintains its own offices and staff. Australia's system is similar. The first autonomous specialty board appeared in the United States in 1924. By 1933 plans were afoot to share facilities for several specialties and make the standards nationwide. Twenty-four boards, representing many more subspecialties, operate within the American Board of Medical Specialties. Similarly, in Canada, the Royal College of Physicians and Surgeons was founded in 1929 to train, examine, and license specialists in medicine, surgery, and laboratory science; twenty-eight specialties with sixty-one disciplines are certified, but offices are centralized in Ottawa. Both North American organizations looked to Europe, especially England, France, and Denmark in the early years.

The Mace of the Royal College of Physicians and Surgeons of Canada

A gift of the Royal College of Surgeons of England in 1964, the mace symbolizes the 'corporate power' of the college and is carried by the executive member-at-large during academic processions. The original was stolen in 1992, but a replacement was quickly commissioned and completed in 1993. Canadian specialists take their power and its symbols very seriously.

Professional Associations

Beyond the credentials of licensing and certification, membership in professional associations allowed practitioners to participate in negotiating the rules that governed them. The goals of the professional societies were and still are to protect and advance standards of medical knowledge through meetings, publication, and licensing; they were also to lobby for the interests of doctors. It is no accident that they were formed at a time when new medical schools were being created in Europe and North America.

The British Medical Association was founded in July 1832 at a meeting of fifty doctors in Worcester. Its role has always been to promote medical science and serve the interests and honour of the profession. In nineteenth-century America, doctors resented the financial threat and personal success (as much as they mistrusted the knowledge) of their 'unorthodox' colleagues, the homeopathics, eclectics, Thomsonians, and midwives. The American Medical Association (AMA) was founded in 1847 partly as a professional lobby to protect the market share of doctors against homeopathists. The Canadian Medical Association emerged from a variety of provincial and municipal precursors, some of which still exist, with the goals of disseminating knowledge and protecting the interests of physicians; its constitution was ratified in 1907. All three associations publish influential journals founded soon after their creation: the *British Medical Journal* (*BMJ*, 1840), the *Journal of the American Medical Association* (*JAMA*, 1883; replaced *Transactions*, 1848–82), and the *Canadian Medical Association Journal* (*CMAJ*, 1911). Not only do these publications bring relevant science and news to doctors, they are a fabulous source of professional opinion for historians.

Patient Expectations: Rising, Falling, and the Double Bind

On the patient side of the contract, expectations have changed dramatically since medical writing began some 3,500 years ago, and most changes are recent. In antiquity, being a successful doctor meant being able to predict the outcome of an illness. Alleviation of suffering was also important, but knowledge of the condition and its prognosis for death or healing constituted medical triumph. Most patients accepted the potential limitations of treatment, and the physician was just one among many different advisers, including soothsayers, oracles, and priests.

In the early modern period, society may have acknowledged the advantages of the new scientific learning, but expectations of what a physician could actually accomplish changed little. Some were amused by the credibility gap. Playwrights such as Shakespeare and Molière, and caricaturists such as Rowlandson, Cruikshank, and

Daumier, poked fun at pompous doctors – expensive, ineffective, and incomprehensible purveyors of drastics that killed as readily as they cured (see figures 6.4 and 6.5).

Patient expectations of medicine began to rise in the mid-nineteenth century with the major discoveries of anesthesia and antisepsis. Anesthesia has been cited as the most important technology in shaping the modern contract: diseases once accepted as fatal or chronic could suddenly be painlessly repaired (see chapter 10). Patients 'now expected a "technical fix" for every pain,' but by acquiescing to medical expertise, they lost individual autonomy over their well-being (Pernick 1985, 233). The advent of antibiotics in the 1930s and 1940s had a similar effect, as did each major discovery in medical science (see chapter 5). Now that a cure was *sometimes* possible, it quickly became an imperative. The fact that everyone dies sometime faded from medical and cultural view.

Between 1850 and 1950, the medical profession could point to a succession of surgical and medical giants, hailed as national institutions within their homelands. The great books of these great men sustained Fildes's country doctor through his bedside vigils year after year. Knowledge was static and safe. In the early twentieth century, simply *being* a doctor was automatically a reason to be accorded admiration and respect.

The marked rise in patient expectations turned hope for health into demand. People now want and expect to be cured. They insist on 'the best,' even if it means immediate heart surgery or intrauterine correction of fetal defects. Newspapers report on families who have lost loved ones while waiting for procedures to be done, as if no one ever dies on the table and the procedures are fail-safe.

But in the late twentieth century patient expectations altered yet again. Without relinquishing the expectation of cure, large sections of the population began to doubt medicine's ability to provide it. True, some continue to venerate the medical profession, but it is no longer a given. Practitioners are not necessarily trusted; nor do they possess the same control over practice that they once enjoyed. While miracle cures continue to be expected, parallel expectations of medical professionals have declined to 'low': doctors are sometimes said

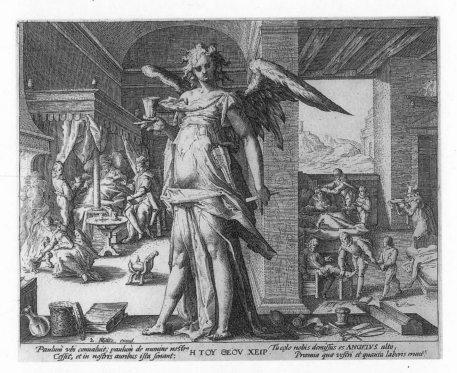

Paulum vbi conualuit; paulum de numine noſtro H TOY ΘΕΟV ΧΕΙΡ. Tu colo nobis demiſſus es ANGELVS alto,
Ceſſit, et in noſtris auribus iſta ſonant: Præmia qua veſtri et quanta laboris erunt?

6.4 and 6.5   The physician as angel (above) and as devil (opposite). Both anonymous Dutch, 1587, after Hendrik Goltzius. These are the second and fourth images in an allegory of the medical profession from the patient's perspective. The doctor changes from a god hearing a prayer for help, to an angel dispensing medicine, to an ordinary man who hurts as he tries to help, and finally to a devil seeking payment. Philadelphia Museum of Art

to be dangerous, unsympathetic, and cruel. The result is a double bind that further challenges the doctor–patient contract.

Many reasons contributed to the decline in respect. First, it is now widely known that medical knowledge has sometimes been 'wrong.' Errors of the last century may be no more frequent nor damaging than those in earlier times; however, now they are more conspicuous. Procedures touted as panaceas have waned or been abandoned; examples include tonsillectomy, and surgery for visceroptosis (see chapter 10). Some practices were hounded into quackery: the once-respectable Brinkley procedure, begun in the 1890s, purported to

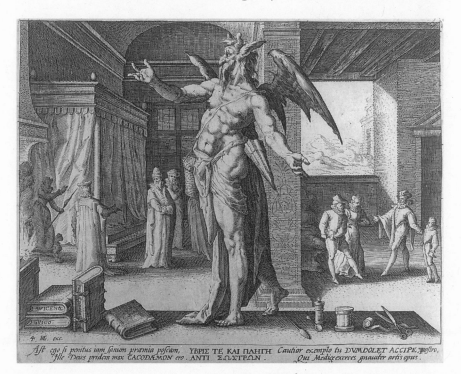

Aſt ego ſi penitus iam ſanum præmia poſcam,   YBPIΣ TE KAI ΠΛΗΓΗ   *Cautior exemplo tu DVMDOLET ACCIPE, noſtro,*
Ille Deus pridem max CACODÆMON ero. ANTI   Σ.Ω.ΣΤΡ.ΩΝ.   Qui Medicæ exerces gnauiter artis opus.

rejuvenate by 'transplanting' monkey or goat gonads; by 1930, the
editor of *JAMA* brought charges against John R. Brinkley of Kansas,
despite patient testimonials in his defence. Most drugs have undesirable side effects, but some have resulted in serious harm that is widely
publicized – for example, thalidomide, chloramphenicol, phenace-
tin, arthritis remedies, and hormone replacement (see chapter 5).
The same is true for objects such as intrauterine devices and breast
implants. And like medicine, science too has been 'wrong.' Science
brought the atom bomb, Love Canal, ozone depletion, Chernobyl,
air pollution, genetically modified organisms, and global warming.
Inspired by environmental ethics, patients say that they don't want
to poison their systems with drugs. Doctors who administer dangerous treatments have generally been protected from blame. In most
cases, it is the drug companies, manufacturers, and, occasionally, governments who bear the legal responsibility. Will doctors continue to
make unfortunate decisions? Yes. Will they always enjoy relative insu-

---

A Less Respectful View

Mistrust of authority is also reflected in the writings of current historians, whose works on 'great doctors' seldom fail to address shortcomings that previously might have been passed over as virtues or quirks. Galen, we are told, fled Rome during a plague. Similarly, Thomas Sydenham fled London during an epidemic. William Withering first tested digitalis on the poor. Edward Jenner's courageous demonstration of vaccination would not meet present-day standards of ethics, nor would that of Louis Pasteur. William Osler perpetrated practical jokes. William Halsted used cocaine. Alexander Fleming was given more credit for penicillin than he deserved. Norman Bethune drank and womanized. Frederick Banting hit his wife.

---

lation from blame? Will they readily acknowledge their errors? We do not know. But the informed public is wary of doctors, because they are gatekeepers of scientific products.

Second, the *nature* of medical knowledge is changing as much as its content. Some claim that 'knowledge is increasing,' but the increase is in information – not knowledge. Medline provides references to the medical literature; its precursor, the *Index Medicus*, appeared as printed books. In 1879 it was a single volume, five centimetres thick. That slim size shrinks in comparison with the more than thirty-fold expansion that was required to hold the nineteen fat volumes of the 1997 edition. With the switch to digital resources, the burgeoning of information is difficult to 'see' in the same way, but the relative quantity continues to explode. How can any doctor profess to 'know' the tens of thousands of medical periodicals filled with so-called new knowledge? Ideas that are true at the beginning of a medical educa-tion are sometimes false by the end. Faced with a labyrinth of con-flicting information, how do doctors learn when to reject what they have been taught in favour of something new? In having so much more information about different things, do today's doctors really *know* more than the man painted by Fildes? Is it better knowledge? And has it come with no cost? An informed public worries that the doctor cannot possibly know everything.

Third, medical heroes may continue to hold authority in some countries, but they are no longer fashionable in North America. In France, a 1990s campaign put the faces of the country's famous oncologists on billboards, exhorting the citizens to give generously. This project would not do well where doctors are relatively unknown and mistrusted; the pleas of patients are more effective. Mistrust of heroes is not confined to medicine. Our age has become suspicious of class distinctions, authority, and anything labelled scientific.

Given a willingness to look on the dark side, historians, journalists, and the public can find lots to complain about in the medical past. Being human, doctors sometimes make costly mistakes. They also used their knowledge deliberately for harm in the service of political and cultural ideology. In experimentation, the rights of disadvantaged people were on many occasions cast aside. What is different now is a far greater public awareness of the accidents and the crimes of the past. For example, the Tuskegee study of *untreated* syphilis in African-American men continued until the 1970s, long after effective treatments were known. Participants thought that they were being given good care and contributing to scientific knowledge. Not until May 1997, after a number of historians exposed the tragedy, did the survivors receive a formal apology from President Bill Clinton for the U.S. government's role in that project. Many relate awareness of that flagrant abuse as a reason for mistrust of medicine in the present. Sobering recent histories dissect the actions of Nazi doctors, who somehow managed to reconcile racial extermination with their Hippocratic oath to 'do no harm' (see chapter 15). Recently doctors are severely criticized for accepting the perks provided by the pharmaceutical industry, and high-profile dismissals add to the distrust. For example, Charles Nemeroff stepped down from his position at Emory University in 2008 over his vast, undeclared profits from the pharmaceutical industry. Past and present abuses of medical power and privilege constitute a reason for the public's lack of respect and low expectations for medicine today.

Injured? Need a Lawyer? Call 1–800–XXX-XXXX

– Billboard on many eastern U.S. interstate highways, 2008

Fourth, Western culture now endorses blame. Medical professionals live with the threat of malpractice lawsuits resulting from dou-
ble-bind of the conflicted patient expectations. When every person
expects a cure, a society that equally mistrusts medical science and
authority will never be short of people to blame for shortcomings.
Doctors have been sued for failing to cure an incurable disease, as if
someone must be held responsible for natural decay.

Malpractice insurance fees in the United States have risen to
unprecedented levels. A form of cooperative protection functions in
Canada; the single service makes it possible for historians to quickly
grasp the effects on a national scale. In Canada, contingency fees
are illegal and malpractice suits less frequent; nevertheless, the effect
of a litigious society is visible. Premiums have been rising steadily in
parallel with spiralling costs. For example, in 1976 Canadian Medical Protective Association disbursements in damages and legal fees
were about $4.5 million; by 1981 they had more than doubled to just
over $10 million; in 1991, they were in excess of $60 million; and by
1995 they had doubled again to $120 million; by 2007 they were $393
million, an eighty-seven-fold increase in thirty years. Over the same
period, the rise in the Canadian consumer price index was approximately fourfold.

Recognizing these problems has prompted the rise in bioethics
(see below) and resulted in a 'patient-centred' focus in medical training. For example, in the 1990s, Ontario initiated a 'demand-side'
approach in a program called Educating Future Physicians (EFPO);
it defined twelve complementary and sometimes conflicting roles for
doctors. These in turn influenced national bodies for accreditation;
now called 'CanMEDS Roles of Physician Competency,' they are used
in accreditation processes in several countries. Young doctors are
reminded to find out what the patient wants.

Finally, the difficulties of paying well-off doctors does not enhance
public sympathy, especially when rich doctors go on strike.

Table 6.3
Founding of health-care systems

Year	Country	Legislation
1883	Germany	Compulsory health insurance for workers in wage category
1888	Austria	"
1891	Hungary	"
1893	France	Free medical care for the poor
1911	Britain	National Health Insurance Act
1916	Saskatchewan	Municipal doctors' scheme (salaries)
1947	Saskatchewan	Hospital services insurance
1948	Britain	National Health Service
1962	Saskatchewan	Medical services insurance
1968	Canada	National medicare program launched
1984	Canada	Canada Health Act

Paying the Doctor: Health-Care Systems

Illness can easily ruin patients and their families. The problem of paying the doctor found various solutions over the years, each reflecting the political and cultural ideals of place and time. In many countries, a third party has entered the doctor–patient contract. The contract duet has become a trio.

Beginning in the 1700s, charity clinics were (and are) served by prominent doctors, while wealthy patients paid according to approved fee schedules, modified to fit the medic's reputation. Benevolent societies were organized to care for the sick, sometimes in workhouses that closely resembled jails. Many people simply went without medical care. With the rise in technology and expectations of success, the 'need' for physician services was all the more pressing. Philanthropists sought ways to provide for the poor, and entrepreneurs perceived a window of opportunity. Health insurance schemes grew in the late nineteenth and early twentieth centuries, many run by doctors. Their purpose is to reimburse expenses and pay health-care personnel.

Illness also makes demands on employers and governments. Eventually inequities in access to medical care became a problem for governments rather than private charities, and a variety of national health programs emerged (see table 6.3). Some covered all costs, while others covered only hospital and/or doctor care and excluded dentistry, drugs, physiotherapy, and other forms of health care. At first, special consideration was given to people with certain devastating diseases, such as tuberculosis or cancer; later, systems were extended to all citizens in a country, healthy or not.

The purpose of these systems – be they private or public – is threefold: first, to remove the onus for payment from the sick or the poor; second, to ensure that services are remunerated; and third, to prevent disease. The first two goals are often met; the third, however, is not. 'Health-care system' is a euphemism for managing and paying the wages of disease. The systems range from health-insurance programs (in which the citizen pays a premium, the doctor receives a fee for service, and the government is the broker) to state-medicine programs (in which the doctor is salaried, and health care is funded from taxes and provided 'free').

The first compulsory national health-insurance plan appeared in Germany in 1883 under the direction of the statesman Otto von Bismarck. Workers whose earnings fell within a specified range were obliged to pay premiums for coverage of health-related services, including dental, hospital, and medical care. Those whose wages fell below the range were not covered and obliged to seek charity. People who earned more than the range were recommended to private coverage.

Nationalized health plans have been demonized as the thin edge of a communist wedge; however, Bismarck's aim was the exact opposite: he reasoned that providing health care for workers within a capitalist system would thwart the growing labour movement by eliminating one of its chief complaints. The German system received wide attention because the country's well-funded laboratories were a leading destination for physicians (see chapter 3).

The National Health Insurance Act of Britain was passed in 1911 under the leadership of the future prime minister David Lloyd George. It did not cover hospital expenses, except for tuberculosis patients, and it forced employers to pay premiums for workers; the unemployed were excluded. The Russian Revolution created a decentralized system of clinics in which paramedical professionals, called feldshers, played a prominent role and fees for service were abolished. France had enacted free medical care for the poor in 1893; insurance companies and employer-paid benefits covered a variety of situations for others until after the Second World War; then influenced by Britain, France extended coverage slowly but surely, to the elderly, pregnant women, children, and eventually the entire population by 1999. These sweeping changes to the method and amount of doctor payments in other countries heightened suspicions in the United States.

Fear of Health Care: The Radio Debate on State Medicine, 12 November 1935

A publicly funded medical service 'would socialize if not communize one phase of American life ... We shall become a nation of automatons, moving, breathing, living, suffering and dying at the will of politicians and political masters.'

– Morris Fishbein, editor of *JAMA*.
American Medical Association Bulletin, November 1935, reprint, 7

In 1948, further reforms were implemented in Britain prompted by the 1943 report of the distinguished economist William Henry Beveridge. Health care was to be only one item in a comprehensive program of welfare 'from the cradle to the grave.' Beveridge intended state services to complement but not stifle individual initiative. British doctors who participated were paid a salary and limited to certain sites of practice. Negotiations resulted in compromises, and a parallel private system quickly became the sanctuary of elite physicians who served the wealthy – the 'Harley Street set.'

Most European countries, as well as Australia, New Zealand, and other developed nations now have health-care systems administered by the state. These countries enjoy better health. Wealthy jurisdictions without nationwide medical care must face some depressing statistics. Following its own revolution in 1959, Cuba also adopted a system of salaried doctors and capitation, charging them with responsibilities for health maintenance and reporting; although doctors' earnings are small, the health statistics of that country are admirable.

In the United States, social programs cover the poorest in the population and the elderly. Many earlier attempts to introduce health-care legislation on a national scale in the United States have met with failure, most recently under the Clinton administration. At the time of writing, fierce opposition in Congress to President Barack Obama's plans for health-care legislation comes from members of both political parties. Now at least 46 million citizens have no insurance at all. The majority of those who died in a 1990 measles epidemic in Texas were unvaccinated African-American or Hispanic children living in poverty. Creative solutions were found to allow the middle class to buy into 'managed-care' programs with various restrictions: the health maintenance organizations. Health-care coverage and fear of its loss become factors in job choice. Some states, such as Massachusetts, now require that all residents acquire private health insurance with subsidies for those living in poverty. The private insurance industry constitutes one of the largest lobbies against a universal health care system; thousands of jobs in the middle-management sector are paid for by the premiums and by higher costs of services in order to generate profits. The tragic situation of *insured* Americans was the subject of filmmaker Michael Moore's acclaimed and demonized documentary *Sicko* (2007).

In such a system, the public and the medical profession have relatively more difficulty dealing with the 'social determinants' of illness: poverty, illiteracy, lifestyle, pollution, and war. Efforts to address these issues have been left to less effective, remote bureaucracies, such as the United Nations and the World Health Organization, or to the efforts of extra-professional groupings of highly motivated individuals (see chapter 15). A group of American historians has formed a lobby, the Sigerist Circle, that uses history as a weapon in the struggle toward universal health care.

Canada's health care system has been an object of scrutiny by many nations. During the Second World War, the country embarked on economic measures to prevent another disaster like the Great Depression of the 1930s. All political parties endorsed the concept of state funding of health care. Canadian doctors were interested in the decentralized systems of their Russian ally. Following the provincial election in 1944 of the Co-operative Commonwealth Federation government of Baptist preacher Tommy C. Douglas, Saskatchewan became the first North American jurisdiction to enact hospital and medical insurance. The plan began with province-wide hospital coverage and a pilot project of full medical services in the town of Swift Current. A handful of doctors participated, but most others opposed the changes until they realized that they were earning more than they had in the past (see chapter 15).

In 1962 Saskatchewan extended medical coverage to the entire province, and doctors went on strike for twenty-three days. In 1964 a royal commission, chaired by judge Emmett Hall, recommended a national system modelled on the Saskatchewan plan. The initial legislation was passed in 1966, the program was launched in 1968, and the Canada Health Act was signed into law in 1984; provinces were brought on side with promises of transfer payments.

Despite criticism from many practitioners and some Americans, the Canadian health-care system compares favourably with others in the Western world in terms of life expectancy, infant mortality, and smoking cessation. However, Canada has fewer doctors, nurses, and MRI machines than average, and its system is the second most expensive (next to the United States). The system has changed the doctor–patient contract. Access to care is also called a 'right.' But doctors are less autonomous than in the past. Even when they fill most expectations, keep up to date, and do not make mistakes, control no longer belongs entirely to them, but to the third party who pays. Fees are negotiated with governments and shaped by fiscal pressures. Patients, however, are content; it is the most popular social program in the country, endorsed by all political parties, and strengthened through later royal commissions.

Services are rationed through waiting times, a problem receiving active research attention. Audits of practice billings are conducted; however, after Ontario physician Anthony Hsu committed suicide in 2003 following a critical review of his practice, these audits were judged to be too severe and prejudicial. And in 2005, the Supreme Court confused matters with a ruling that restrictions on private health clinics (illegal according to the Canada Health Act) were

Table 6.4
Doctors' strikes or threatened strikes – a partial list

Countries
Australia, 1984, 1993, 2001 (Tasmania), 2002 (threat), 2008
Bangladesh, 2007
Bulgaria, 1922–3
Britain, 1911 (threat)
Congo, 2008
Czech Republic, 1995, 2007
Denmark, 1981
Dominican Republic, 2000, 2009
El Salvador, 1998, 2002
Finland, 1984, 2001
France, 1995, 1996, 2002, 2005, 2008
Germany, 1904 (Leipzig), 1982 (West), 1996 (threat), 1999, 2005–6
Greece, 2000
Haiti, 2005
Hungary, 1914, 1998 (threat)
India, 1987, 1992, 1995, 1998, 1999, 2001, 2004, 2005, 2006, 2007, 2008, 2009
Iraq, 2005
Ireland, 2002 (residents), 2003 (public health), 2008 (residents)
Israel, 1983 (118 days), 2000 (127 days), 2005
Italy, 2004
Korea, Republic of (South), 2000
Malta, 2009
Nepal, 2006, 2008
New Zealand, 1992 (residents), 2006 (residents)
Nigeria, 2004, 2009
Pakistan, 2002, 2008
Peru, 2008
Poland, 2007
Portugal, 1998-99
Russia, 1905, 1917–18, 1992 (threats), 2005
Serbia, 2003
South Africa, 2009
Spain, 1995
Sri Lanka, 1999, 2001, 2009
Switzerland, 2009
Tanzania, 2005
United States, 1969 (Charleston, SC), 1975 (New York City; California hospitals), 1990
    (California housestaff), 2003 (West Virginia and Philadelphia), 2004 (Maryland)
West Bank and Gaza, 1999, 2008
Zimbabwe, 1998, 2001, 2002, 2003, 2007, 2009

Canada
Alberta, 1998 (threat)
British Columbia, 1983 (threat), 1992, 1998 (threat), 1999, 2000 (Prince George), 2002
    (threat)

Table 6.4
Doctors' strikes or threatened strikes – a partial list *(concluded)*

Manitoba, 1932–4 (Winnipeg), 1990
New Brunswick, 2001
Newfoundland, 1982 (threat), 2002
Nova Scotia, April 1984 (threat)
Ontario, June 1982 (1 day), June 1986 (25 days), 1996
Quebec, 1991 (threat), 1998 (threat)
Saskatchewan, 1962

---

against the Charter of Rights and Freedoms. And like other countries, Canada soon saw more of that peculiarly twentieth-century phenomenon, the doctors' strike (see table 6.4).

Doctors' Strikes

Strikes in most countries are for better physician wages; they are most prevalent where the doctor can pretend that it is not the patient but the third-party payer who is the opponent. In the United States, they are much less frequent and have been by salaried residents or by other doctors who object to their high malpractice fees. Doctor strikes do not work, and they result in more hostility toward the profession, a further lowering of expectations.

Striking doctors display few of the qualities that earned the social standing of their predecessors. They appear to act against their patients as well as the system, and they abrogate public responsibility by refusing to participate in a society's occasional need for financial restructuring. Striking doctors lose public esteem, and their gains in financial concessions come at a moral cost. The unemployed and people on low incomes may tolerate the huge salaries of sports 'heroes,' but they do not sympathize with the strikes of imperfect physicians – medical 'villains' – whose earnings continue to be well above the national average.

The twenty-five-day doctors' strike in Ontario in June 1986 was over the right to bill the patient for the remaining small percentage of the fee not covered under the system – a right that had been outlawed two years earlier by the Canada Health Act. The doctors' goal of 'full billing' was labelled 'extra billing' by legislators and the media. The government won the issue, instigating a global rollback of fees – a legislated charitable donation. In a leading ethics journal, Eric Meslin characterized the strike as a double failure for the profession: it lost its case, and, having reneged on a moral duty to provide health care, it lost sympathy and credibility. Epidemiologists discovered that the death rate actually decreased during the strike, and policymakers added this statistic to other arguments for limiting physician practice. (Similar statements were made about the Israeli strike of 2000 – fewer doctors may be good for your health.)

Despite the rhetoric of medical lobby groups, striking doctors can never convince a thinking public that their motivation is patient well-being. Instead, they appear to be preoccupied with their own incomes, especially those of their senior members rather than those of younger doctors or fellow professionals in nursing, midwifery, and rehabilitation. For example, on several occasions some medical associations proposed disincentives against new graduates. Similarly, Canadian doctors long resisted the notion of mandatory retirement at age sixty-five – a concept that once applied to most citizens and other government-funded workers; it was abolished in a nationwide human rights process between 2006 and 2009.

How Much Money and How Many Doctors?

Questions have been asked about physician incomes, patient entitlements, and the allocation of costly instruments and procedures. In the early 1990s, economists recognized that the more doctors there are, the more they will cost. Canada and Britain limited the number of medical school and residency positions and added new controls on physician numbers and earnings. Different methods were used within the same country. For example, Quebec capped the income of general practitioners in the early 1980s. Later in the same decade, British Columbia tried to deny billing rights to newcomers. In Alberta, however, the number of doctors increased by 20 per cent in the early 1990s, while the population remained stable. The Alberta government then made drastic cutbacks in services and hospital funding and refused to prosecute the illegal private clinics that were wielding expensive technologies – taking wealthy people out of the government-funded system. Ontario decreased the number of medical school spaces and residency positions in the same year, severely stressing access to postgraduate training for some time.

Now it is said that the pendulum has swung too far and physician shortages prevail in many parts of the developed world, including large cities; the shortages are especially severe for family doctors (see chapter 14). Many blame women who have entered the profession in large numbers but refuse to work the long hours of their predecessors – as if the long hours were a good thing. Women and their male allies point out that long hours are not good for anyone, including patients. Schools have been allowed to increase in numbers and expand their enrolments. International medical graduates (IMGs) are being admitted to training with unprecedented enthusiasm. This trend has drawn sharp criticism of poaching from countries, such as South Africa and India, where needs are much greater.

Economists and policymakers also point to the tremendous savings that would result from concentrating our efforts on the prevention of heart disease, stroke, and lung disease rather than waiting to deal with their consequences. Others cite the global inequities of spending millions of dollars to prolong the lives of elderly, sedentary, and well-heeled people while thousands of children die every year from malnutrition and simple infections (see chapter 15). These population-based arguments have little resonance for the caregivers and families of individuals who are already sick. The discrepancy underscores a fundamental problem in trying to alter the medical model of disease in the context of democracy (see chapter 4). Suffering individuals cannot accept that procedures available for some may not be available to all. The traditional contractual obligation to the individual must be reconciled with providing optimal care for the majority at minimum cost.

With a third-party payer, be it public or private, doctors complain about loss of autonomy and control. Some hold press conferences with bereaved families to protest delays for surgery. Others move from nations with restrictions to the United States hoping for bigger incomes and greater freedom. They express nostalgia for the respect enjoyed by their less-effective nineteenth-century predecessors. But the past was not as rosy as it may seem. Practitioners worked long hours for relatively low wages, and they knew by name and face the identity of their charity cases. The weeping parents in the background of the Fildes painting could be indebted to the doctor for the rest of their lives. Some respect derived from his generosity. True, legislated limits on physician earnings and control over sites of practice are a form of charity, but they lack the personal appeal of the one-on-one benevolence of the past. Hard-working doctors do not readily accept the concept of anonymous, enforced charity; patients scarcely perceive it.

The Rise of Bioethics and Palliative Care

The good behaviour of doctors has been an element of the doctor–patient contract since writing began. In the Code of Hammurabi and the Oath of Hippocrates rules were laid down to protect vulnerable people from exploitation of any kind. Decorum at the bedside was part of this tradition. Some treatises from the Middle Ages and into the eighteenth century contained explicit instructions for how to act, dress, and behave in moments of uncertainty and in matters of payment. One of the founders of modern medical ethics was Thomas Percival, whose 1794 code served as a template for the American Medical Association at its founding in 1847. These codes serve to remind doctors of the negotiated nature of their contract.

But medical ethics as we know it today has a short history. Relying on the code emerging from the Nuremberg doctors' trial (see chapter 15), it was newly professionalized as a particular branch of moral philosophy in the 1960s. The ethics courses of medical schools, if they had existed at all, turned to PhD philosophers as well as interested doctors. (Tellingly, this turn to humanities expertise occurred in medical history too and at around the same time.) To distinguish this brand of philosophy from other older forms, the word 'bioethics' was coined around 1972.

The recent rise in bioethics is further reflected in the founding of chairs and departments and in the increase in journals for scholarly research. Although it had several less formal precursors, the prestigious *Journal of Medicine and Philosophy* began in 1976. Since then, a hive of scholarly activity resulted in a number of journals that

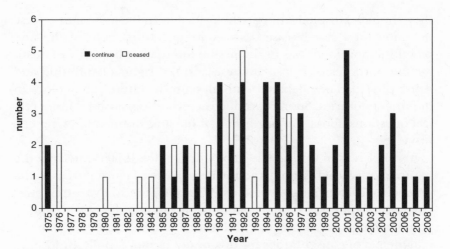

6.6   Medical Ethics Journals, 1975–2008. Source: Holdings of the National Library of Medicine, N=64 titles containing 'medical' or 'clinical ethics' or 'bioethics.'

appeared or disappeared through failure or merger (see figure 6.6). Following intense activity from 1985 to 2005, the enthusiasm may have stabilized.

Several discrete forces contributed to the rise of bioethics. Some are intimately connected to the changes in the doctor–patient contract described above. For example, given that expectations went from care to cure, all doctors will more frequently (and inevitably) fail to meet expectations. Does failure mean that they are bad doctors? Ethics promised to help in coping with such distressing situations. Similarly, with the frequent examples of medical error, the occasional pain of doctors' strikes, and the resultant erosion of respect, doctors need to be aware of (and protected from) the climate of suspicion that surrounds their acts. A certain amount of this education entails an understanding of the law as well as moral obligation. Indeed, further pressure for bioethics comes from the results of the litigious nature of modern society.

The innovations of technology also created a demand for ethicists. New possibilities of keeping people alive, creating or preventing conception, and determining inheritance caused doctors to remember that just because they *can* do something does not mean that they should. Hospital ethicists help to determine the right course of action on a case-by-case basis. Among the first tasks of the new bioethics movement was to define the moment and quality of death for the purposes of transplantation and the rights of suffering and dying people. They debated euthanasia with differing outcomes in different countries. Soon reproductive technologies raised more ethical questions about the beginning of life and ownership of genetic property.

Another reason for the rise in bioethics since 1990 came from the nature of medical research and the prevalence of clinical trials in the practice of evidence-based medicine (see chapter 5). Every trial must have ethics approval – every committee needs an ethicist who understands enough medicine and philosophy in order to determine the parameters of consent. Jobs for doctorates in moral philosophy have never been so plentiful.

Bringing this story full circle, the rise in ethics forced doctors to listen more carefully to complaints of people. Surveys conducted during the 1950s revealed that physicians understood little about pain relief; they also showed that dying under medical care could be horrifying for both patients and their families. The ancient role was all too easily neglected with new technologies and the irrational expectation of cure. Doctors often feared death more than their patients; and when they could not alleviate suffering, they avoided contact.

> 'Go and read medicine. It's the doctors who desert the dying and there's so much to be learned about pain. If you don't do it properly you'll only be frustrated, and they won't listen to you.' (Advice against a nursing career.)
>
> – Norman Barrett, surgeon (ca 1948), cited by
> C. Saunders, *J. Royal Soc. Med.* 94 (2001): 430–2

The hospice movement of the 1960s and the rise of palliative care as a distinct specialty meant that doctors, patients, and the public at large were forced to relearn how to comfort and serve the dying. Often motivated by religious faith, leaders in this field included some radically unconventional women: Elizabeth Kubler-Ross of Arizona, Cicely Saunders of London, and Mother Teresa of Calcutta. Journals in palliative care began to appear about a decade after those in bioethics.

A Word about Alternative Medicines

This history has been told as a tale of a monopoly arising from pluralism. But the monopoly was never total, and to a certain extent it is beginning to wane in conjunction with the same forces that generated the bioethics movement. This book addresses the history of medicine as taught in orthodox schools of today, but it is important to recognize that no system develops in a vacuum. Many other practices have arisen, each with adherents and satisfied patients, the effects of which are felt in regular medicine. And as Roberta Bivins has observed, no medicine can be 'alternative' until another dominates.

Founded in Europe, homeopathy was popular in the nineteenth century (see chapter 5); it played a significant role in North American medical education and professionalization and is still prominent in Europe, especially France. Other systems appeared in America, reflecting the cultural openness and opportunity of that society. Sometimes they emerged as 'natural medicines' in direct reaction to the horrendous side effects of 'allopathic' medicine. All alternative schools were generally more open to minority students and women.

The most successful of these systems were regulated rather than defeated. They achieved survival and credibility by adapting to the rules of medical education, examination, and licensing. They have since spread to the rest of the world.

Osteopathy was founded in 1874 by a man from Missouri, Andrew Taylor Still, the physician son of a doctor. His search for a new method of healing was prompted by the loss of three of his children to meningitis. It relies heavily on palpation of the tissues of the body, and treatment aims to relieve pain and restore balance. Regulated in the United States since the 1930s, twenty-five colleges of osteopathy operate in the United States, eight in the United Kingdom, and one in Canada, with satellites in four cities from Halifax to Vancouver.

Chiropractic was created or 'discovered' by the Canadian-born

Daniel David Palmer of Iowa, who had been fascinated by magnetism in health; he treated his first patient with a spinal adjustment in 1895. He was prosecuted for practising without a licence. His system concentrates on an understanding of neuromuscular control, especially of the spine, and treatment is through manipulation. There are eighteen American colleges of chiropractic, three in Britain, and two in Canada. A bust in honour of Palmer adorns the lakefront of his home town of Port Perry, Ontario.

Naturopathy is more recent. A blend of homeopathy, botanical medicine, and Asian wisdom, naturopathy claims to be as old as healing itself, but its handful of schools did not begin until the mid-1950s, not all are accredited, and its practice is still confined to a small but growing number of states and provinces. So far the United Kingdom offers only a two-year diploma, available only to those holding other credentials.

Colleges for osteopathy and chiropractic exist in many other countries and on every continent. With greater emphasis on freedom of choice and patient-centred care, demand for these therapies is expanding: several new schools have appeared since 2000. In short, pluralism persists despite medical hostility.

Back to the Doctor

Is the message conveyed by Fildes's moving picture still valid in our own time? Now the doctor may not share the cultural, religious, or racial origins of the patient. The family is apt to have brought the child to the unfamiliar setting of a brightly lit emergency room, bustling with sparkling white coats, electronic gadgets, and strange sounds, where the doctors, almost half of whom will be women, have no time to sit and ponder. Furthermore, the family will not wish to be displaced from the bedside in unquestioning acquiescence with the doctor's opinion.

True, many schools educate their students in the importance of honing communications skills, reviving the house call, and providing reassurance for those confronted with the terrors of a modern hospital. But as much as doctors and patients alike may wish to emulate this empathy, patient expectations continue to go well beyond those of the stricken family in Fildes's painting of a century ago. We seem to be unable to provide the curative technology without sacrificing much of what is perceived to be valuable in Fildes's picture.

A Thought Experiment

A dean at Queen's University once dreamed of giving every new student a copy of the Fildes picture, 'because,' he said, 'that's what medicine is really all about.' If students could keep that image foremost in their minds, they might remember the attributes that earned the respect enjoyed by their professional predecessors.

Another colleague, in the Community Health and Epidemiology Department, agreed and recommended that the picture should have an empty thought-bubble above the doctor's head; students could imagine what he might be thinking. Some suggestions showed a marked preference for the present:

'I wish I could get an X-ray.'

'Why did I leave my tracheostomy set at home?'

'Will the family pay my bill?'

'If only we had clean water.'

In a postwar attempt to block the public health insurance initiatives that were launched in the United States, the American Medical Association distributed copies of Fildes's painting to every physician in the country under the headings 'Keep Politics Out of This Picture' and 'Do You Want Your Own Doctor or a Job Holder?' In 1947, the image also appeared on a U.S. postage stamp. And on 19 October 1950, in the newspaper *Journal American*, 'our doctor' sat with 'Mr and Mrs America' defending their child from 'the fever of socialism.' The campaign worked. But neither the Americans, who succeeded in keeping out the so-called threat of socialized medicine, nor their Canadian neighbours, who 'failed,' can claim to have preserved the ambience so movingly portrayed by Fildes.

Suggestions for Further Reading

At the bibliography website http://histmed.ca.

CHAPTER SEVEN

Plagues and Peoples: Epidemic Diseases in History*

Behold, a pale horse and its rider's name was Death, and Hades followed him; and they were given power over a fourth of the earth, to kill with sword and with famine and with pestilence.

– Revelation 6:8

Epidemics have destroyed populations and significantly altered economic, social, intellectual, and political aspects of life. With apologies to W.H. McNeill, whose 1976 title I borrow, this chapter will explore themes common to epidemics, emphasizing their impact on human life.

The Plague of Athens (ca 430 B.C.): What Was It, and Does It Matter?

Panic and breakdown of social order typify human reactions to epidemic illness. The Greek historian Thucydides, in his *History of the Peloponnesian War* (Bk 2, 47–54) told how a lethal contagious disease afflicted the Athenians while Spartans lay siege to their city. The symptoms included fever, painful skin rash, and great thirst. No treatment was effective. Physicians, who were quickly exposed to many cases, died first; even birds and animals disappeared. Among the

*Learning objectives for this chapter are found on pp. 452–3.

dead was Pericles, the ruler of Athens and builder of the Parthenon. Thucydides too had been sick, but he reported that the few survivors were considered immune. Opinion on the origin of the disease was divided. One rumour held that it came from Africa, but some thought it was new, stemming from starvation and the strife of war. Still others said that Spartans had poisoned the wells. Religious people were convinced that it was divine punishment for unrevealed sins; however, oracles and priests were no better than doctors at relieving the suffering.

Thucydides' account is the sole surviving record of this disaster. The absence of other testimony raises many questions, including the possibility that the historian simply invented his tale. Doctors, however, have long been intrigued by the plague of Athens, finding the vivid description credible – even irresistible. They have sought to discover the precise retrospective diagnosis; contenders include smallpox, typhus, and anthrax. And whenever a new infectious disease is described, it seems that sooner or later someone connects it to the plague of Athens. Recent studies apply modern techniques to postulate toxic shock syndrome, legionnaires' disease, AIDS, measles, and Ebola fever as the 'real' diagnosis. But most would-be diagnosticians fail to account for the bioecological reality of rapidly mutating germs. The improbability (if not impossibility) of applying a modern diagnosis to the plague of Athens is a 'Heisenberg uncertainty principle' in medical history. The riddle will likely continue to defy solution.

This ancient disease may not be reduced to our own terms, but Thucydides' story has come to exemplify the timeless extracorporeal side effects of any epidemic. During the plague, social structure decayed, crime was rampant, and codes of behaviour were abandoned. Family members shunned their ailing relatives and often neglected the dead; bodies were thrown on pyres built for others – a sacrilege as well as a crime. The epidemic passed, but Athens lost that war and did not regain its former power.

The Great Dying, or Black Death: Bubonic Plague (1348 and After)

The most famous epidemic in Western history was the fourteenth-century bubonic plague of Europe. Known at the time as the 'great dying,' its gothic and durable name, Black Death, was bestowed in 1832 by the German physician-historian J.F.C. Hecker. Earlier outbreaks of plague had occurred, including a sizeable epidemic during the reign of the Byzantine Emperor Justinian in the sixth century A.D.; however, none matched the scope and horror of the fourteenth-century scourge. According to witnesses, European plague travelled from Asia in ships and seemed to begin with the arrival of Genoese vessels at the Sicilian port of Messina in October 1347. From there, the disease marched rapidly north, fanning across Europe to reach Moscow by 1351. The symptoms were fever, swollen and oozing nodes (buboes), dehydration, and death.

Social practices were overturned in the manner described by Thucydides. People abandoned their urban homes to wander in the country; sick family members were left to die. Corpses were shunned, and officials tried to establish controls and forced criminals to heap bodies into mass graves. In this atmosphere, the Florentine writer Giovanni Boccaccio, whose father had died of plague, wrote the *Decameron* – one hundred risqué and diverting stories told by a group of young men and women sheltering from the epidemic. Boccaccio's introduction is a famous record of the first wave of plague. But plague remained in Europe and returned in successive waves for centuries; major epidemics ravaged Italy in 1630 and 1656, England in 1665, and southern France in 1720.

In the fourteenth century, many hypotheses for the cause of plague were expounded, each of which subtended control measures. A new form of medical literature, the 'plague tractate,' arose to express these ideas. According to the surgeon Guy de Chauliac, the Paris faculty of medicine attributed plague to atmospheric alterations resulting from a rare conjunction of planets in the constellation Aquarius in March 1345. Others saw it as divine punishment for the corruption of priests; this argument gained credibility with the successive waves of plague during the Great Schism (1378–1417), when the church split over rival popes – one in Rome, the other in Avignon. Still others blamed minorities, strangers, and travellers. The desperate search for cures brought confrontations between folk healers and academic physicians.

Whatever its remote origin, plague was perceived to be contagious. Many doctors fled; those who stayed used a variety of remedies, all viewed with scepticism. Physicians sometimes wore 'protective covering,' consisting of a gown, gloves, and a mask with mica goggles and a beaklike snout to contain healthful, fragrant herbs. Since travellers were potential carriers of the disease, states enacted laws of quarantine (from the Italian *quaranta*, meaning 'forty'), the first of which can be traced to the town of Ragusa (now Dubrovnik) in 1377 and to Venice in the early fifteenth century. The number related to Christ's self-denial marked by the forty-day period of Lent. Ships were required to wait forty days before unloading cargo or releasing passengers. Some cities passed harsher rules to restrict travel and freedoms. If plague appeared in a dwelling, all occupants might be confined there under 'house arrest' until they died or the disease passed. The wealthy tried to avoid these rules.

Foreign travellers were not the only people blamed for plague; minorities who lived in the midst of the illness (and suffered from it too) were also suspected of having provoked it. Village idiots, vagrants, beggars, 'witch' women, and Jews were tortured for confessions, driven away, or burned alive (see figure 7.1). The semi-religious flagellants atoned by zealous mortification of their own (and others') flesh; they enjoyed a surge in popularity that threatened organized religion. Other responses included the 'infectious' tarantism, or dancing mania. These practices are now seen to resemble forms of mass hysteria, fed by hopes for protection, salvation, absolution, and control.

One-quarter to one-third of the population of Europe is thought to have died in the first wave of plague, and many more succumbed in further outbreaks that occurred over the centuries. Once isolation became standard practice, special 'pest-houses' were built to house if not care for the sick. The devastation extended beyond the immediate human carnage. Grain was left to rot in the fields, seed was scarce, and years of famine ensued with other attendant illnesses. It has been argued that the lack of peasant labourers contributed to the collapse of the feudal system and the rise of an urban middle class. For their inability to cope with plague, clerics and medics alike lost credibility. Education, which had previously been dominated by the church, became anticlerical – or at least a-clerical. In medicine, the authority of Galen was challenged, because his copious writings do

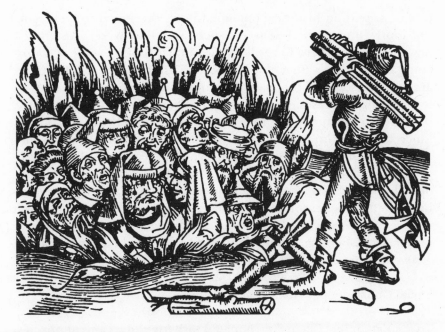

7.1   Woodcut depicting the burning of Jews in response to plague. From Hartmann Schedel, *The Nuremberg Chronicle* (*Buch der Chroniken*), 1493, facsimile. New York: Landmark Press, 1979

not describe the disease. The effects of plague even extended to the artistic portrayal of naked and dead bodies. In her essay 'The Black Death and the Silver Lining,' historian Faye Getz has shown how later students of plague emphasized the positive outcomes, as if the catastrophe had somehow 'caused' the Renaissance; she speculates on why these writers looked for good in so much bad.

We now understand that plague is spread by direct inoculation of *Yersinia pestis*, a bacterium that infects the flea, *Xenopsylla cheopis*, which will parasitize humans but only when its usual host, the black rat, has become scarce. Under certain conditions, plague can become pneumonic (involving the lung); then it is spread by droplets from human to human. But this etiological framework was unknown until the 1890s and the work of A.J.E. Yersin on the bacillus and of P.L. Simond on the flea.

By the end of the twentieth century, doubts were raised about the role of *Y. pestis* in historical epidemics long presumed to be plague. Previously unexploited sources, such as religious records, raised new questions: Where were all the dead rats? Why do some accounts emphasize rashes rather than buboes? Historians took sides. They argued that some of the many 'plague' epidemics represented clusters of other diseases, perhaps typhus or anthrax. Since 2003 DNA probes have been applied to paleopathological remains to confirm 'once and for all' the role of particular strains of *Y. pestis* in the plagues of Justinian and the fourteenth century. But the jury is still out. Partisan readers of literature cast doubt upon DNA evidence derived from dental pulp of a few skeletons of uncertain age. Plague has recently been cited as the reason for the uneven prevalence of certain genetic variants, such as hemochromatosis, which may have offered relative protection. Of course, none of this was known by the Europeans who were confronted with the great dying.

Social Construction: Definition and Examples

To the extent that plague was equated with foreigners and minorities, it was 'socially constructed' (see chapter 4). The social position of sufferers entered into the medical concept of the disease. Treatment, therefore, included the persecution or elimination of dangerous strangers and practices. Social construction has not been confined to plague.

Syphilis

Social construction is amply demonstrated in syphilis. The origins of this disease are controversial. A virulent outbreak, apparently without precedent, afflicted the French armies and their Spanish mercenaries during a siege of Naples in the mid-1490s. As a result, the prevailing view is that syphilis was transported to Europe from the Americas more than five hundred years ago by the crew of Christopher Columbus. Syphilis was called the 'great pox,' but it has also been called the 'French disease' by the Italians, the 'English disease' and the 'Spanish disease' by the French, and the 'Neapolitan disease' by the Spaniards.

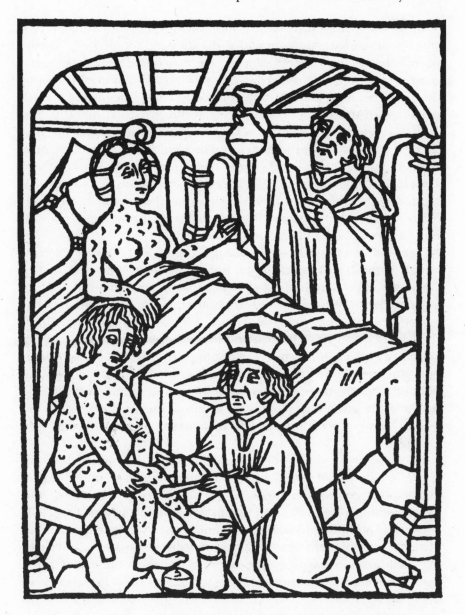

7.2   People being treated for the 'French disease.' From B. Steber, *A malafranzos*, 1498, facsimile by K. Sudhoff and C. Singer, 1925, 263

In the early sixteenth century, the Italian physician Girolamo Fracastoro suggested that contagious diseases were caused by 'seeds' transmitted by people and objects. He concluded that these seeds must be alive, a *contagium vivum*, able to divide and multiply; without this property, he reasoned, they would diminish to negligible quantities through transmission. Fracastoro also understood that this new French disease was spread by sexual contact: he knew that the first lesions appeared on the genitalia, and he cautioned his readers not to 'succumb to the attractions of love.' The name 'syphilis' is taken from his allegorical poem of 1530 in which the cause was 'sin': the shepherd, Syphilus [*sic*], worshipped a king instead of a god; the angered deity punished him with the disease. Probably through euphemism, the great pox came to bear the shepherd's name.

The skin manifestations of fifteenth-century syphilis were excruciatingly painful, and infection led rapidly to death. Fracastoro advocated mercury ointments and fumigations, applied until toxicity appeared in the form of sweating, salivation, and sore gums. Mercury probably was of some benefit, and it persisted as therapy until the twentieth century. Because spontaneous remissions occur in the course of syphilis, any remedy might appear to be effective. Numerous other methods were recommended, including guaiacum, the bark of a North American tree, which inspired confidence because it shared the presumed geographic origin of the infection. Later, the arsenic compound Salvarsan was formulated by Paul Ehrlich (see chapter 5).

Recognition of the modes of transmission of syphilis led to an alteration in sexual practices, the disappearance of public baths, and explicit connections between love and death (see figure 7.3). Many measures were directed against presumed carriers, especially prostitutes and foreigners. In nineteenth-century France, J.A. Auzias-Turenne attempted to treat infants born with the disease by 'vaccinating' wet nurses with syphilis-infected material; the women contracted the disease either from the vaccine or the babies. Later in Germany in 1898, the dermatologist Albert Neisser, who had identified the germ of gonorrhea, also attempted to vaccinate against syphilis by injecting serum from infected people into young prostitutes, all under age twenty; the experiment did not work, and some of the young women

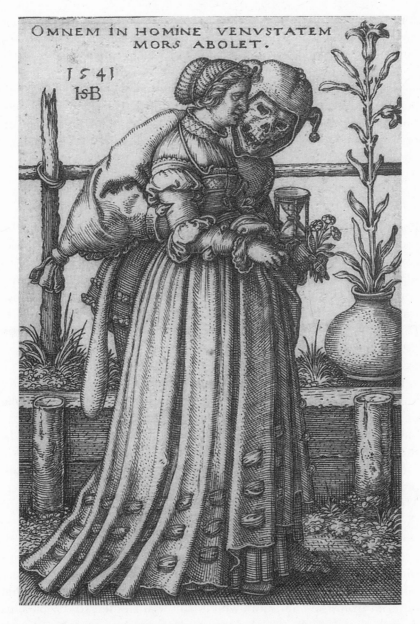

OMNEM IN HOMINE VENVSTATEM
MORS ABOLET.

1541
HsB

7.3   *Young Woman Accompanied by Death as a Jester* by Hans Beham, 1541. A post-syphilis *memento mori*. National Gallery of Canada

contracted syphilis. Because he had not obtained consent, he was
sued, fined, and reprimanded. His discoveries and research make
him an ideal subject for the Heroes and Villains game (see chapter
1).

Syphilis continues to be sensitive to the 'magic bullet,' penicillin,
but the disease has not been eradicated, nor has it been controlled.
The medical model treats infection inside the organism; however,
prevention and eradication rely on the more difficult task of interfer-
ing with behaviour.

Leprosy

Public health standards for water and waste management are the
product and legacy of earlier epidemics. Quarantine, for example,
continues to have currency, especially for localized outbreaks and
island jurisdictions such as the United Kingdom, Australia, Hawaii,
and Newfoundland. Influenced by contemporary ideas about disease
transmission, legislative measures can incorporate social prejudice.
Sometimes these historically determined controls seem to make little biological sense, and they are better explained by social, cultural,
psychological, and religious practices.

Leprosy, for example, is less infective than the responses to it would
imply. As we know it, the disease is only mildly contagious. Regulations probably had more to do with protecting the healthy rich from
having to confront the dreadful mutilations of the disfigured poor. In
the Old Testament of the Bible, leprosy denoted physical and moral
impurity and punishment for sin. Sufferers were forced to live in colonies and wear special clothes or bells to announce their presence.
The Order of Lazarus, founded in the twelfth century and named for
the man whom Christ raised from the dead, built special hospices to
isolate and care for sufferers. The 'lazaretto' catered to people with
problems other than leprosy or plague, but it became synonymous
with 'leprosarium' and 'pest-house.' Some historians maintain that
biblical and medieval leprosy comprised a variety of disorders that
differed from the condition, which is now attributed to the bacillus
described in 1871 by G.H.A. Hansen. Nevertheless, the old controls
persisted. Centres for leprosy (now Hansen's disease) still operate

in both rich and poor countries, including the United States, where a tiny colony continues on the Hawaiian island of Molokai. Since 2000, a museum is maintained at Carville, Louisiana, where a facility served for a hundred years. In Canada a colony was established in New Brunswick in the mid-nineteenth century. The care of Africans with leprosy was a mission of Cardinal Paul-Émile Léger of Montreal. In 1991, global elimination (less than 1 in 10,000 population) was targeted for 2000; the treatable disease has been eliminated from more than 120 countries, but it still persists in a few countries in Africa, Asia, and Latin America. Eradication is not feasible.

Epidemics and Numerical Medicine: Cholera and Typhus

With the advent of positivism in the early nineteenth century, numerical medicine soon influenced concepts of epidemic diseases (see chapters 3 and 4). The British reformers William Farr and Edwin Chadwick applied statistics to population health and uncovered powerful correlations between poverty, class, and disease. Their observations created a tension among middle-class reformers: some held the poor responsible, while others tried to help them. But the blaming approach was more popular, especially with bureaucrats who balanced budgets and with physicians who focused on disease rather than prevention. For example, the German physician and statesman Rudolf Virchow argued for education, employment, and social programs to promote health in a population ravaged by cholera and typhus, but he lost his job in the 1849 backlash against reform.

Public health measures are informed by scientific research and predicated on the impulse to help the sick and protect the well. Sometimes, however, they have been both discriminatory and ineffective, causing more disease than they prevented (see chapter 15). The nineteenth-century experience with cholera and typhus illustrates these points.

In the early 1830s, cholera swept across Europe from the Baltic in the second of seven great pandemics. British military action, colonial trade, and Russian wars all contributed to its spread beyond the usual endemic focus in India. Characterized by massive diarrhea, cholera can lead to death, sometimes within hours (see figure 7.4). The pre-

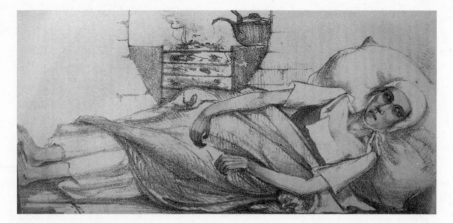

7.4   Blue stage of spasmodic cholera. This sketch of a girl who had recently died was published to educate physicians on how to recognize the new scourge. Her face, hands, and feet were hand-tinted in a blue-white wash. *Lancet*, 4 February 1832, opp. 669

cise global mortality for 1832 is impossible to determine but reliable figures include 20,000 deaths in Paris alone, 100,000 in all of France, 6,500 in London, 6,000 in Canada, and 150,000 across the United States.

Cholera came to North America on ships in 1832. Sick newcomers were confined to sheds without fresh water or sewage facilities. Healthy immigrants were herded into the same buildings to be 'quarantined' side by side with those who were already sick. Management of the sheds was a charity, funded by rich and middle-class citizens who were motivated by sympathy and a desire to keep the sickness at bay. The vast mortality endorsed the view that the dirty poor were the most susceptible. Successive waves of cholera were handled in the same way.

Cholera's link to drinking water was not established until twenty-two years after its epidemic debut in Europe. In 1854 the English doctor John Snow carefully tracked the location of victims to identify London's Broad Street pump as the source of an outbreak. Many doctors remained unconvinced, and competing biological hypotheses held sway for some time. Cholera seemed to be a disease of immigrants, the poor, and the dirty. Images portraying the link between foreigners and death were common (see figure 7.5).

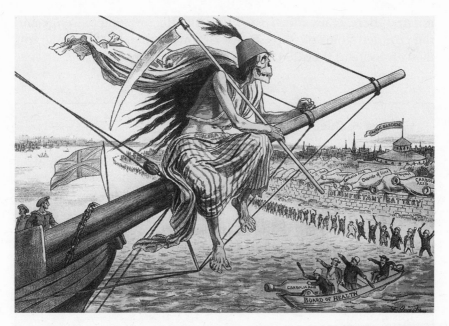

7.5   Cholera on the bowsprit, by Graetz. *Puck* magazine, 18 July 1883. 'The kind of "assisted emigrant" we can not afford to admit.' Disease is personified by the death's-head immigrant in Turkish garb. Bert Hansen Collection, New York.

Robert Koch eventually identified the *Vibrio cholerae* in 1884. This hardy bacterium can live in cool water; contamination cycles are maintained when sewage comes into contact with drinking water during floods, earthquakes, and war. Pandemics persisted well into our own time. At the time of writing, the World Health Organization (WHO, founded in 1948) is monitoring outbreaks in Guinea Bissau and Iraq.

Typhus, which is characterized by fever and rash, is now considered to be caused by the louse-borne agent *Rickettsia prowazeckii*. It had been endemic in Europe since antiquity, and severe epidemics occurred at various intervals, related to environmental conditions. An eighteenth-century outbreak in Nova Scotia decimated French troops, local Mi'kmaq natives, and the settlers in Halifax. From 1816 to 1819, typhus affected 700,000 of the 6 million living in Ireland. With the social instability and political revolutions of the late 1840s, it flared there again and crossed the Atlantic, ravaging passengers in the crowded holds of ships. In 1847–8, more than 9,000 immigrants died en route as they fled the Irish potato famine.

Cholera at Quebec, 1832

The dreadful cholera was depopulating Quebec and Montreal when our ship cast anchor off Grosse Île on the 30th August 1832, and we were boarded a few minutes later by health officers ...

At Quebec ... the almost ceaseless tolling of bells proclaimed a mournful tale of woe and death. Scarcely a person visited the vessel who was not in black, or who spoke not in tones of subdued grief. They advised us not to go on shore if we valued our lives, as strangers most commonly fell the first victims to this malady.

– Susanna Moodie, *Roughing It in the Bush* (1852; reprint, Toronto: McClelland and Stewart, 1984), 19, 30

To keep typhus from the established communities, the authorities used the quarantine station on Grosse Île, in the St Lawrence River near Quebec City. Immigrants were housed in the island's inadequate buildings, without water or fresh clothing, where the conditions guaranteed that those who did not already have typhus would soon contract it. Six thousand died on the island, and at least an equal number in hospitals or sheds at Saint John, Quebec, Montreal, Kingston, and Toronto. Some would have died in any case, but others were killed by the laws that confined them to the crowded sheds. Furthermore, the barriers did not work: typhus – like cholera – spread well beyond the immigrant group. With the advent of AIDS, Canadians have looked back on these tragic episodes with a sense of shame: a commemorative plaque was raised at Grosse Île in 1989, and the island became a national historic site.

Literary Vignette: Typhus at Grosse Île Quarantine Station, 1847

And then he was trotting back along the deck and down the hatch into the hold ... The smell was staggering. A single oil lamp hung from the ceiling, and in the dim light Lauchlin saw the stalls and the narrow passages between them. Within the stalls were rows of bare berths stripped of their bedding and hardly more than shelves. In an open area, scores of unshaven men and emaciated women huddled together, some weeping. Children lay motionless. An old man sat on the floor leaning his back against a cask and gasping for breath ...

Lauchlin ... stepped back, now seeing as his eyes adjusted to the light all the other people collapsed on the bare boards. They shook with chills, their muscles twitched, some of them muttered deliriously. Others were sunk in a stupor so deep it resembled death. On the chest of a man who had torn off his shirt, Lauchlin could see the characteristic rash; on another farther along, the dusky coloring of his skin.

– Andrea Barrett, *Ship Fever* (New York: W.W. Norton, 1996), 178–9

Prevention without Cause: Smallpox

The history of smallpox shows that knowledge of the biological cause of a disease is not essential for its control or even for its eradication. Endemic in Europe since antiquity, smallpox killed kings and peasants alike. Early modern records indicate that at least 20 per cent of the population had been scarred or blinded by variola. European explorers and traders brought the disease to North America, where it exploded with disastrous effects among the susceptible aboriginals, who lacked the relative natural immunity of the intruders. Not only an accident of contact between peoples of two continents, smallpox was sometimes transmitted deliberately on soiled blankets in a form of biological warfare.

No cure for smallpox exists, although many remedies have been

Smallpox Vignettes

The Death of Louis XV, 1774

[On May 7] ... the king's illness took a turn for the worse. He was racked by a high fever, his face changed. That evening he lapsed into delirium again ... the scabs and dried pustules became black ... and an inflammation of the throat prevented him from swallowing. Within hours, scabs formed on his eyelids and blinded him ... His face swollen by scabs was the color of bronze ... On May 10 ... he remained conscious until noon ... [but] at three fifteen he expired. Immediately the courtiers ran out of the bedroom where the body had already begun to decompose.

> – Eyewitness account by Emmanuel, duc de Couÿ;
> cited in Olivier Bernier, *Louis the Beloved: The Life of
> Louis XV* (Garden City, NY: Doubleday, 1984), 248–9

Smallpox in North America

Could it not be contrived to send the smallpox among these disaffected tribes of Indians? We must use every stratagem in our power to reduce them.

> – British officer Jeffery Amherst to Col. Henry Bouquet, 1763

I will try to inoculate the ———— with some blankets that may fall into their hands and take care not to get the disease myself.

> – Bouquet's reply; both cited in J.J. Heagerty, *Four Centuries of
> Medical History in Canada*, 2 vols. (Toronto: Macmillan, 1928), 1: 43

None of us had the least idea of the desolation this dreadful disease had done, until we went up the bank to the camp and looked into the tents, in many of which they were all dead and the stench was horrid; those that remained ... were in such a state of despair and despondence that they could hardly converse with us ... From what we could learn three-fifths had died of the disease.

> – Journal of David Thompson (1780s), cited in Heagerty (1928), 1: 45–6

tried. Effective prevention, however, long antedated our concept of its transmission. Folk methods relied on two generally accepted principles: first, smallpox was inevitable; second, survivors were immune. If a mild case occurred in a community, families would feed the scabs of the lesions to their children, hoping to provoke immunity with only minor suffering. Others introduced the pus from smallpox vesicles directly under the skin, a technique known as variolization. But deliberately acquired smallpox could be just as relentless, disfiguring, and dangerous as the natural variety.

Of unknown origin, variolization was brought to Western Europe in the early eighteenth century by two Greek doctors, Iacob Pylarino and Emmanuel Timoni. Timoni published in Constantinople, where the technique was observed in 1717 by Lady Mary Wortley Montagu, wife of the British ambassador. Having herself been disfigured by the disease, she determined to inoculate her own child. Montagu's role in the dissemination of the practice is debated, but by 1722 the children of the English royal family had been inoculated, and by the 1740s variolization was common in Britain.

Folk wisdom about cowpox (vaccinia) inspired the discovery of the physician and naturalist Edward Jenner. As a student he had learned that milkmaids who had contracted the mild pustular eruption from infected cows considered themselves immune to smallpox. Common knowledge for milkmaids was news to the young doctor, who pondered its significance for several years. Historians link Jenner's subsequent investigations to the famous advice he had been given two decades earlier in a letter from his former teacher, John Hunter. In reply to Jenner's queries about the anatomy of a hedgehog, Hunter had written, 'But why think, why not try the experiment?' (2 August 1775, Royal College of Surgeons). To test the cowpox hypothesis, Jenner conducted an experiment that would probably fall short of current standards of ethics. He inoculated eight-year-old James Phipps with vaccinia, waited six weeks, then inoculated the boy with fluid from active smallpox – the standard practice in variolization. Young Phipps did not react to variola, and Jenner published his results in 1798. If the boy had died, would Jenner have told the tale?

Fortunately for Master Phipps, for Jenner, and for the rest of the world, the empirical observation was correct: infection by vaccinia prevents subsequent infection by variola. Vaccination soon became standard prevention, but the availability of vaccine lymph was unpredictable, and no legal, medical, or social mechanisms enforced its use. Meanwhile, smallpox had become endemic to the New World. Jenner was aware of the lack of supply. Vaccine lymph reached physician Benjamin Waterhouse at Harvard in 1800, and he set about vaccinating his own family and others with the support of President Thomas Jefferson. The National Archives of Canada holds an autographed copy of the book of instructions that Jenner sent with his gift of vaccine lymph to the 'Chief of the Five Nations' in 1807.

Despite sporadic vaccination, smallpox outbreaks often occurred among native and immigrant populations. The 1885 epidemic in Montreal killed more than 3,000 people. Riots broke out over control measures; some feared that vaccination could spread the disease (see figure 7.6). The conflict was fuelled by class and linguistic tensions between anglophones, who held power and promoted vaccination, and francophones, who were less affluent and were largely unvaccinated for reasons of finance, neglect, or fear. From 1895, when Sweden eliminated the disease, several countries applied vaccination to complete prevention. England and the USSR succeeded during the 1930s. The last Canadian outbreak occurred in Windsor, Ontario, in 1924. The last American outbreaks were in New York City in 1947 and Texas in 1949.

But smallpox persisted in Asia, Africa, and Latin America. In the mid-1960s, the WHO launched a plan to eradicate smallpox by tracking all cases, isolating and supporting sufferers, while vaccinating and quarantining every person exposed. The task was said to be impossible, but workers persevered in the face of disease, famine, and war; some were killed. The last natural case was identified in a twenty-three-year-old hospital cook, Ali Maow Maalin of Somalia, in December 1977. In August the following year, Janet Parker, an unvaccinated staff photographer, contracted the disease in the Birmingham University laboratory where she worked. Her death and the subsequent

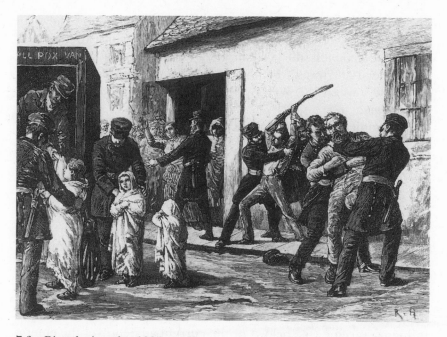

7.6   Riot during the 1885 smallpox epidemic in Montreal. Robert Harris illustration in *Harper's Weekly*, 28 November 1885. Bert Hansen Collection, New York.

suicide of the laboratory director, Henry Bedson, were the last known wages of this great disease.

On 9 December 1979 the WHO formally declared that smallpox had become the first human disease to be eradicated. At the time of writing, scientists are deliberating the ultimate destruction of the remaining samples of variola virus, which are held by laboratories in Russia and at the Centers for Disease Control in Atlanta, Georgia. Some argue for their preservation, questioning the ethics of exterminating a 'living species' and citing the importance of biodiversity. They argue that 'friendly' variola might be needed to combat a possible epidemic caused by an enemy, or by an inadvertent escape from a forgotten freezer somewhere. Untroubled by this possibility, advocates for destruction invoke the huge mortality that could result from any accident in the largely unvaccinated population, and they cite the vast supply of vaccinia as ample protection against oversight or attack. Nevertheless, the 'execution' of variola, originally planned for December 1993, was stayed until June 1995, then repeatedly delayed until 2007, when the WHO postponed taking a decision for four more years.

The eradication of smallpox was a triumph of medical science, but the methods had been in place for two hundred years, long before germ theory or antibiotics. It was facilitated by the fact that humans are the only host. No particular knowledge about the causative organism was required. Similarly, the effective prevention of childbed fever, established by Ignaz Semmelweis in Vienna, did not require germ theory (see chapter 11).

If knowledge of a microbial cause is not essential for prevention of some infectious diseases, what then were the contributions of germ theory, vaccines, or antibiotics on epidemics? Their impact is difficult to demonstrate. Some would argue that these innovations create as many problems as they solve – witness the side effects of the 1976 influenza vaccine (see below) or the current anxiety over the emerging strains of multi-drug-resistant staphylococcus (MRSA). Despite the best of intentions, iatrogenic epidemics are nothing new.

Decline (and Rise) of Tuberculosis: Scientific Triumph or Coincidence?

In the late nineteenth century, tuberculosis was the single most important cause of adult death, a distinction it held for more than a century. Many changes had taken place in the medical conceptualization of this disease. Formerly characterized by its symptoms of wasting, fever, and cough, its anatomical basis was described by R.T.H. Laennec in the early nineteenth century (see chapter 9). Another French doctor, J.A. Villemin, later demonstrated that tuberculosis could be inoculated, and Robert Koch identified its bacterial cause as he established germ theory (see chapter 4). Despite Koch's discovery, notions of heredity persisted, for the disease seemed to run in some families while others were resistant. Tuberculosis pervaded all social classes, and it shaped cultural notions of beauty, art, and genius, as Susan Sontag's *Illness as Metaphor* has shown.

Literary Vignettes: Romantic Tuberculosis in CanLit

What had happened to Ruby? She was even handsomer than ever; but her blue eyes were too bright and lustrous, and the colour of her cheeks was hectically brilliant; besides she was very thin; the hands that held her hymn-book were almost transparent in their delicacy ...

She lay in the hammock, with her untouched work beside her, and a white shawl wrapped about her thin shoulders. Her long yellow braids of hair – how Anne had envied those braids in old schooldays! – lay on either side of her ... The moon rose in the silvery sky, empearling the clouds around her ... [and] the church with the old graveyard beside it. The moonlight shone on the white stones ... 'How ghostly!' she shuddered. 'Anne, it won't be long now before I'll be lying over there.'

– L.M. Montgomery, *Anne of the Island* (1915; reprint, Toronto: Bantam Books, 1980), 79–80, 105–6

Cissy could not get her breath lying down that night. An inglorious gibbous moon was hanging over the wooded hills and in its spectral light Cissy looked frail and lovely and incredibly young. A child. It did not seem possible that she could have lived through all the passion and pain and shame of her story ...

But a spasm of coughing interrupted and exhausted her. She fell asleep when it was over, still holding to Valancy's hand ... At sunrise ... she opened her eyes and looked past Valancy at something – something that made her smile suddenly and happily. And smiling, she died.

– L.M. Montgomery, *The Blue Castle* (1926; reprint, Toronto: Seal Books 1988), 119, 121

Various stringent public health measures, with more or less prejudicial baggage, were enacted to keep the germs of the tubercular
sick, or the potentially sick, away from the more powerful non-sick.
Sufferers were isolated or quarantined in sanatoria. An effective vaccine using the less aggressive Bacillus Calmette-Guérin (BCG) was
developed in Paris in the early 1920s. BCG is still recommended for
certain people in France, England, and other European countries,
but it was never adopted in the United States. Through the work of
R.G. Ferguson and Armand Frappier, BCG became part of Canada's
tuberculosis prevention programs, which were expanded from 1948
until the mid-1960s to include schoolchildren, health-care workers,
native people, and prisoners.

Surgical therapies for tuberculosis were invented to create a poorly
oxygenated environment hostile to the organism. In 1927 the Canadian surgeon Norman Bethune, who had tuberculosis, insisted on
having an experimental operation of artificial pneumothorax (col-
lapsing the lung), against the advice of his physicians at the Trudeau
Sanatorium (the movie version has him administer it to himself).
Antituberculous drugs were greeted with much fanfare; the 1952
Nobel Prize went to the Russian-born American Selman Waksman
for his discovery of streptomycin. Drugs soon eclipsed preventative
measures, but controversies over vaccines and other controls have
not vanished. They are intimately linked to social and political ideals
in individual countries, and they exemplify the wide gap in the relative status of disease treatment over disease prevention in the medical
model.

Tuberculosis mortality declined steadily throughout the twentieth
century, and medical scientists congratulated themselves on what
they seem to have accomplished. In the late 1970s, however, Thomas H. McKeown challenged this medical self-satisfaction when he
demonstrated that tuberculosis mortality had already been waning
long before the advent of drugs; furthermore, the rate of decline had
not altered with the innovations. The germ may have become less
virulent or human resistance may have grown with a rise in wealth,
hygiene, and nutrition (see figure 7.7).

McKeown identified a similar pre-intervention decline in British
mortality from measles, although he acknowledged that diphtheria

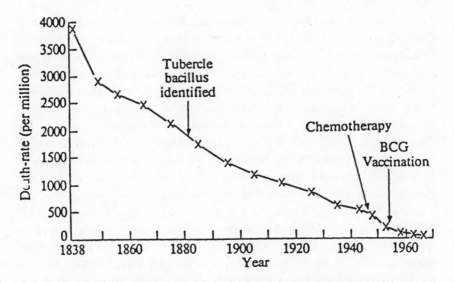

7.7   Rate of decline in tuberculosis mortality does not alter with the advent of specific medical interventions. From Thomas McKeown, *The Role of Medicine: Dream, Mirage, or Nemesis?* 2nd ed. Oxford: Blackwell, 1979, 92

mortality had fallen with medical intervention. But his observations about tuberculosis were sobering. Antibiotics treat individual illnesses effectively, yet they foster resistant organisms, offsetting relief for individuals with their long-term and possibly harmful impact on humankind. The rise in tuberculosis in the early 1990s was correlated with a parallel rise in poverty and homelessness throughout North America.

Historians have made increasingly sceptical judgments about the medical claims of success in treatment and prevention. Allan Brandt and John Parascandola showed that wartime control measures against venereal disease included the demonizing and incarceration of prostitutes, who were equated with infective organisms. Jay Cassel and Peter Neary made similar observations about control measures in Canada. Entrenched medical practices die hard.

Influenza and Polio: Pandemics of the Early Twentieth Century

In mid-1918 as the First World War drew to a close, pandemic influenza swept the globe. The precise mortality is impossible to know: world totals range from 25 to 100 million, with estimates of 7 million deaths in India, 400,000 in France, 250,000 in Britain, 50,000 in Canada, and half a million or more in the United States. In contrast, the four years of war in Europe had killed 20 million civilians and soldiers. Many of the influenza dead were young occupants of military barracks or boarding schools. Also known as the Spanish flu (some things never change), the disease caused fever, pneumonia, and rapid death. It arose on hog farms in the American midwest; Spain was implicated only because it was a non-combatant and the first country to report the disease during the period of wartime secrecy.

Influenza has since returned in pandemic waves, although so far not with such virulence. It has been given adjectival labels indicative of the various viral strains: Asiatic (1890), swine (1931, 2009), Asian (1957), Hong Kong (1968), and avian (1997, 2003–); the latter regularly affects birds with occasional transmission to humans. An influenza vaccine was developed in 1943, but it was only moderately effective because the virus changes often, spreads easily in air, and is refractory to other controls. In 1976 rumours of an emerging strain of virulent swine flu reminded authorities of the great tragedy of 1918 and prompted U.S. President Gerald Ford to recommend a sweeping campaign to vaccinate 50 million citizens. This attempt at prevention produced another iatrogenic epidemic – two hundred cases of Guillain-Barré syndrome of ascending paralysis in those vaccinated against the hypothesized influenza epidemic, which, in the end, never materialized.

Molecular typing of viral strains has been possible since the mid-1980s. The especially virulent H5N1 strains of avian influenza have been threatening a human pandemic since 1997; a few dozen cases have appeared in Asia, moving ever eastward as it is spread by migratory birds, from Hong Kong to Turkey; Vietnam has had ninety deaths. Influenza H5N1 is now the object of a WHO electronic tracking system, and the media are quick to report on affected birds. At the time of writing (late 2009), H1N1 swine flu has reached pandemic proportions with cases in 208 countries.

Poliomyelitis, an enterovirus infection of nervous tissue with fecal-oral transmission, was endemic in early twentieth-century Europe and

North America. Virtually unknown before 1900, its annual outbreaks increased in scope to as high as 100,000 annually in England, 58,000 in the United States, and a maximum in Canada of over 8,800 in 1953. The reasons for its rise are still under debate. Also called infantile paralysis, polio worked its dangerous effects on the very young. About 5 per cent of patients died, but a much higher percentage of survivors were permanently disabled. The epidemic in developed countries was arrested by the vaccines of American virologists Jonas Salk (in 1953) and A.B. Sabin (in 1956).

Polio was the impetus for the iron lung and other technologies designed to compensate for damaged autonomic functions. It also provided a powerful justification for the rise of pediatrics as a specialty and the creation of centres of rehabilitation medicine. Naomi Rogers has shown that it inspired philanthropic action by taking on the identity of its helpless child victims; that President Franklin D. Roosevelt had survived polio was known to many, although his disability was well concealed from the masses.

In 1988, the WHO commited to a global eradication plan: in 1994, the Americas were declared polio free; Europe followed in 2002. While eradication is considered technically feasible, the annual global case rate hovers at just below 2,000 – less than 1 per cent of the rate in 1988, with the highest numbers in Afghanistan, India, Nigeria, and Pakistan.

Controlling polio in developed countries, coupled with the great promise provided by the advent of antibiotics, led to a brief period of optimistic complacency about infectious diseases (see chapter 5). It seemed that modern science had finally solved the problem in the wealthy parts of the world. This naive attitude ignored the fact that humans share most of their infections with other animals and that nature constantly finds new ways to refashion old pathogens. The optimism was short-lived.

AIDS

The arrival of AIDS reawakened many of the old responses to epidemics, including the panic described by Thucydides long ago. Retrospective testing of frozen serum has shown that the virus has been causing disease in humans since at least 1959. In 1981, AIDS emerged, simultaneously in California and New York, as an epidemic among male homosexuals. Initially called a 'plague,' modified by 'gay,' 'Haitian,' 'African,' or 'new' – AIDS was understood to be the creation of (and synonymous with) these people. One of its first medical names was GRID (gay-related immunodeficiency). Affecting people of all ages, in all countries, AIDS has caused more than 25 million deaths worldwide. The burden in Africa is enormous: adding to deaths and illness, it has created more than 11 million orphans and immeasurable social and economic hardship. Intolerance and fear inform irrational proposals for controls, and politics interferes with willingness to seek help.

Compared with legionnaires' disease, a somewhat longer time passed (and more people died) before AIDS was given the credibility of financed investigation. President Ronald Reagan was criticized for not even uttering the word until 1985, well into his presidency and the epidemic. The causative agent was the discovery of the team of Luc Montagnier at the Pasteur Institute – but a priority dispute arose with Robert Gallo of the National Institutes of Health (NIH); later it emerged that Gallo had 'discovered' the virus that had been given to his lab by the French. The stakes were high in many ways: HIV became the basis for lucrative test kits. The scientific community excluded Gallo from the 2008 Nobel Prize – vindicating Europeans and baffling Americans.

As with all other epidemics, control measures for AIDS were laden with expectations from the past. In Cuba, for example, people who were seropositive for HIV were indefinitely and forcibly confined in a closed community called a 'national sanatorium.' Controversial from the outset, it persisted for seven years until 1993 notwithstanding the facts that (1) the 'rest of society' was (or could be) protected with information on how to avoid HIV; (2) seroconversion may take months; and (3) seronegative persons may be equally infective. Observers admitted that the severe response might have had something to do with the relatively low infection rate in that country. The government-sponsored health provisions involved many other helpful modalities, but it took until 2000 for Cuba to focus on male-to-male transmission.

In Britain, Canada, and the United States, despite initial demands to the contrary, those with AIDS or HIV seropositivity were not segregated. Confinement is expensive, and it infringes punitively on the rights of potentially sick people. It could result in the kind of tragedy once seen on Grosse Île, and in the end it would not prevent the spread of a disease which could be avoided. The global infection rate from AIDS peaked in the 1990s, and death rates are starting to fall. In the United States, it remains one of the leading causes of death for adults under age fifty-four. The WHO estimates that in 2007, 2 million died of AIDS worldwide and 33 million are living with the infection – 70 per cent or more of them in Africa. Yet in certain parts of Europe, Africa, and Asia numbers of new cases continue to grow. The levelling off of global statistics shows that the information and interventions work. Clearly, it is important to prevent more infections and to help the sufferers. The millions of dollars spent on AIDS research are well justified.

Medical hubris, blended with entrenched attitudes to the 'sins' of homosexuals and intravenous-drug users, may also explain why more than a decade went by before people focused on thorny questions about the possible role of science in the origins of AIDS. Molecular biologist Peter Duesberg points out that HIV is still unproved as a cause, because current research has failed to satisfy Koch's postulates; no virus can grow in pure culture (see chapter 4). Medical technology itself has been cited as a causative factor. For example, the historian Mirko Grmek suggested that a window of opportunity for the pathogen was created in the natural disease ecosystem (pathocenosis) following the elimination or reduction of other pathogens, such as smallpox, diphtheria, measles, and polio. By 1989 several independent observers began to imagine an even more direct role for science when they asked if AIDS could have arisen in 1957 from the polio vaccines that had been developed by Western scientists in monkey cells and tested on Africans; if the monkey cells harboured simian immunodeficiency virus (SIV), the vaccines would be contaminated. Publicized in America by freelance writer Tom Curtis in the 19 March 1994 *Rolling Stone* magazine and by Edward Hooper in his book *The River* (1999), this hypothesis attracted media interest by implicating the fieldwork of the distinguished scientist Hilary Koprowski. The scientific community quickly dismissed it, using historical and epidemiological arguments. The retrospective serological testing of the old vaccines was not done until September 2000; the results were negative. Koprowski sued writers and the media for defamation and won out-of-court settlements. Nevertheless, the debate continues.

Innocent (and Guilty) Victims

The 1976–7 outbreak of Guillain-Barré syndrome in the United States occurred among 'innocent victims' of a clumsy presidential policy. Legionnaires' disease shared the thoroughgoing respectability of its first victims, and it was given prompt, lavishly funded medical investigation. By contrast, toxic shock syndrome was regarded as punishment for 'guilty,' dirty women; however, as marketing trends soon indicated, it was later perceived to be caused by the menstrual tampons, not their users.

'Innocent victim' is a term that physicians should never use lightly. Yes, it means that some people are sick through no fault of their own, but it can also imply that others are 'guilty' – responsible for and deserving of their illness. Newborns, hemophiliacs, health-care workers, and the heterosexual wives of bisexual men are called the innocent victims of AIDS. But these differences between sick people are defined by moral estimation of their behaviour, not by the biological effects of the germ.

New and Emerging Diseases

New infectious diseases are not usually as new as they first seem. Rarely are they due to the advent or alteration of a causative organism. Sometimes they have been present for decades at a subliminal level. Frequently, they come to medical attention through social circumstances that favour transmission. Nearly always, the identifying characteristics of those in whom the condition is first recognized –

together with our sympathy (or lack of sympathy) for these people – are incorporated into our concept of the disease and what ought to be done about it.

Since 1970, several 'new' epidemic diseases have emerged, although their pathogens have been around for a long time. AIDS is the greatest and most obvious, but it had precursors. In 1976 legionnaires' disease was first identified among the participants of an American Legion conference at a Philadelphia hotel. The Centers for Disease Control traced it to a previously unrecognized bacterium, *Legionella pneumophila*, which now has more than fifty variant species. Toxic shock syndrome, which complicates certain bacterial infections, was originally recognized in young women and – too narrowly (but irreversibly) – linked to the use of menstrual tampons. It turned out to be the effect of known bacteria. When combined with the advent of AIDS, these 'new' diseases tended to destabilize the complacent attitude about infections. But as AIDS became a chronic disease with well-known transmission patterns, the general public slipped back into thinking they were safe. The complacency would not last long.

By 1996, the untreatable neurological condition of variant Creutzfeldt-Jakob disease (vCJD) was detected in a growing cluster of cases in Britain; it was linked to the presence of prions that cause human kuru and bovine spongiform encephalopathy (BSE, or Mad Cow disease), the latter a condition that was reaching alarming proportions in cattle. Unnatural but cost-saving practices had put infected meat into cattle feed, thereby infecting those animals and the humans who ate their flesh; the incubation period could be long. More than 90 per cent of the cases were in the United Kingdom: 180,000 cattle; and approximately 130 people. To control the disease, quell the public outcry, and restore consumer confidence 4.5 million animals were destroyed. International vigilance over zoonoses and food products increased, and prohibitions over who can donate blood were established. Since 2003, pockets of animal infection have appeared in both Canada and the United States, resulting in temporary border closures to beef, actions from frightened consumers and nationalistic lobbies of meat producers and packers, tighter regulations and heightened surveillance. Only two human cases have occurred in North America; both were people who had lived in Britain.

In 1999, West Nile virus appeared for the first time in North America. Spread to humans and animals by mosquitoes, this disease was first recognized in 1937 – but had previously been confined to the eastern hemisphere. Responsible for neurological disabilities in a significant minority of cases, its arrival was met with nervousness and vigorous municipal campaigns against standing water.

In the spring and summer of 2001 a large outbreak of foot-and-mouth disease occurred in the United Kingdom. Although this disease does not affect humans, the staggering size of the outbreak and the heightened sensitivity to those infections that we share with other species guaranteed wide media coverage. Another cull of 7 million animals took place. The images of vast burning pyres of carcasses so soon after the BSE cull further added to the growing unease.

The terrorist attacks of 11 September 2001 in New York and Washington only added to the sense of vulnerability. They were followed by a series of 'anthrax letters,' sent to prominent Americans, that caused at least five deaths. Initially blamed on foreign terrorists, the anthrax investigation settled on an American microbiologist who died of a drug overdose in July 2008, just as charges were to be laid. In the aftermath of 9/11 these events served as a reminder of the horrifying past and frightening future of biological weapons. The threat grew with other devastating terrorist attacks in Bali (2002), Madrid (2004), and London (2005).

Biological weapons have a long history. Some evidence suggests that infected animals may have been set among enemies to spread disease as long ago as the Hittite plague of 1320 B.C. In the Middle Ages, corpses of people who had died of contagious disease were catapulted over enemy walls. Both sides fighting in the Second World War devoted scientific expertise to weaponization of various pathogens, including anthrax, smallpox, and tularemia. Japan is alleged to have released plague-infested fleas in China. Fear that the 'other side' might have the capability first drove this work. A convention against the use of biological weapons was ratified by most major powers in the early 1970s and by Russia in 1992. Terrorists are not bound by such agreements.

Finally, in early 2003, a new disease rapidly spread from Guangdong province in China to provoke illness in more than thirty countries, leaving 774 dead, mostly in China, Hong Kong, Taiwan, Singapore, and Canada. Named for its symptoms, Severe Acute Respiratory Syndrome (SARS) taxed intensive-care facilities and had a predilection for health-care workers. It claimed the life of the Italian doctor Carlo Urbani, who first brought it to the attention of the WHO. Its cause was rapidly identified as a previously unrecognized type of coronavirus. Panic over global supplies of antiviral drugs promoted increased production and reserves. But the novel outbreaks were contained by traditional methods of isolation and quarantine, involving hospitals in all affected jurisdictions and millions of people. The words 'new normal' and 'pandemic planning' entered medical and public vocabulary.

Not All Bad Diseases Are Emergent: Malaria

An ancient disease, malaria still exacts a steady toll of nearly a million deaths, mostly of children, from the 500 million cases each year. With its periodic fever, malaria has been known as 'swamp fever,' 'ague,' and 'paludism' (from the Latin for marsh). The name 'malaria' crept into English from the Italian ('bad air') in the eighteenth century. Malaria was endemic to parts of Europe, where it sometimes killed thousands. During the nineteenth century, it ravaged British colonial troops in India, whence it spread to Canada and south. Shrinking from the northern areas, it remained endemic in southeastern United States until it was eradicated in a 1947–51 campaign.

An Inca remedy called cinchona, or Jesuit bark, was brought from Peru to Europe in the early seventeenth century, and its active ingredient, quinine, was isolated in 1820. In 1880, at the height of British imperialism, the parasite was identified by C.L.A. Laveran. Seventeen years later, Ronald Ross elucidated the role of the anopheles mosquito. Ross and Laveran received the Nobel Prize in 1902 and 1907, respectively.

In 1955, despite fears of overpopulation if malaria were to disappear, the WHO launched an eradication program, based on draining swamps and spraying insecticides, including the 1948 Nobel-Prize-winning poison DDT. Unlike smallpox, however, malaria affects other creatures. Moreover, insecticides and the destruction of wetlands conveyed their own harm. Consequently, these methods were revised in 1969, and by 1980 the WHO was aiming only for control, not eradication. Meanwhile, malarial resistance to the quinine derivative chloroquine arose and spread to most countries, demanding a combination of drugs. This preventable and treatable disease is still endemic to 109 countries or territories containing more than 40 per cent of the world's population. In an effort to obtain better control, some scientists call for a return to DDT.

Northern and western populations concerned have trouble focusing on the great burden of malaria and other problems that seemed to have already been conquered. Measles still kills approximately 0.24 million infants annually; neonatal tetanus kills 0.18 million; and schistosomiasis (bilharzia) is thought to affect 200 million people each year. Inordinate media attention is given to the spectre of frightening diseases: for example Ebola spread from laboratory monkeys to four humans in Virginia in 1989; and in 1998 an airline passenger falsely claimed to have arrived from an Ebola-stricken part of Africa. Ebola is the subject of many books and movies. According to the WHO, that dreadful disease has taken about 1,200 lives in the more than thirty years since its discovery. We focus on what seems to threaten 'us'; malaria, measles, and bilharzia are problems for 'them.'

Twenty-five hundred years after Thucydides' ineffective but eager doctors perished in the plague of Athens, we may have learned less than we think. Indeed, over the past decade, humans rediscovered their intrinsic vulnerability. New plagues emerge. Cures, though highly sought after, may not control epidemics. Interventions can provoke new diseases or worsen existing ones. Reactions to travellers exposed to places with infectious diseases are hauntingly familiar. And the role of social factors has not changed a bit.

Suggestions for Further Reading

At the bibliography website http://histmed.ca.

CHAPTER EIGHT

Why Is Blood Special?
Changing Concepts of a Vital
Humour*

Blut ist ein ganz besonderer Saft. (Blood is a very special juice)

– J.W. von Goethe, *Faust*, I, 1 (1808)

Blood as Magic and Mystery

Blood is important. It has always been important, and it has always *seemed* to be important to everyone. Of the four ancient humours, it alone remains a vital entity, with a status well above that of phlegm or bile of any colour. Most people immediately understand that blood is essential for life. On the other hand, when asked if the spleen, liver, kidneys, or pancreas are essential, they are less certain. People do not think of those organs in the way that they think of blood.

Why has blood always enjoyed a special status? Two reasons. First, it is eminently visible, being the only internal organ that regularly surfaces for perusal; all humans have seen some of their own blood. Every injured person knows that bleeding marks the severity of the wound. Every woman can expect a flow at regular intervals allied to the phases of the moon.

Second, blood is always associated with life. Even children know that when blood is lost in great quantities, death may ensue. In many

*Learning objectives for this chapter are found on p. 453.

languages, it is synonymous with life and health. Some cultures, such as prehistoric peoples of Europe, Africa, and Asia as well as Australian aborigines and the vanished Beothuk of Newfoundland, prepared for burials by colouring bodies or graves with red ochre (containing hematite) to restore the blushlike colour of life. Scholars have analysed how menstruation influenced perceptions of women at various times and places, noting that myths and traditions cast suspicion on those who could bleed regularly without ill effect. For example, Islam and orthodox Judaism forbid sexual relations with a menstruating woman. In Judaic tradition, a woman is unclean following her menses or delivery of a child, until she has taken the ritual *mikveh* bath. K. Codell Carter speculates that in the nineteenth century, menstruation may have served as a model for regular bloodletting in men to provide healthful 'monthly evacuations.'

In ancient Greek mythology, blood was one of the first miracle drugs. Perseus severed the snake-tressed head of the Gorgon monster Medusa and presented the gruesome trophy to the goddess Athena, who placed it on her shield. Athena gave blood from the Gorgon's head to the healer Asklepios (in Latin, Aesculapius), who used it for amazing cures and to raise the dead. The potent treatment led to his deification as the god of medicine. Asklepios's staff, around which a snake is entwined, is the medical caduceus, the symbol of medicine for more than 2,000 years.

Christianity has done nothing to diminish the importance of blood in our culture. Blood is central to the mysteries of the sanctuary: not only is it life and health, it also indicates redemption of sin and eternal salvation. The blood of martyrs symbolizes pain and faith; that of children, the worst of the world's many unjust tragedies. The word 'blood' and its derivatives are mentioned no less than 460 times in the Bible; 'life' is mentioned only slightly more often (487 times). How often does the word 'kidney' appear? Seventeen times. 'Liver'? Thirteen times. 'Bile'? Once. And 'brain,' 'pancreas,' 'lungs,' and 'phlegm'? Never. True, 'heart' is mentioned more often than 'blood' (817 times). The reason relates to the importance of the religious signifiers: if blood was life, heart was love or soul.

Given its ancient connection with life, blood as therapy is also very old. However, blood-medicine was not always convenient. Wine often served as a proxy, taken as a panacea, a stimulant, a depressant, a restorative, a digestive, a hypnotic, or an escape. Rooted perhaps in their visual similarities, the substitution of red wine for blood was further endorsed by the Christian doctrine of transubstantiation: in the mass, wine becomes the redeeming blood of Christ. Renaissance images showed the body of Christ crushed in the 'miraculous press' from which blood trickled into waiting barrels.

The English word 'blood' is neither Latin nor Greek in origin, as are so many of the words used in medical terminology. Medicine makes use of the terms 'hematology' (derived from Greek) and 'sanguinous' (derived from Latin), but words such as these with classical roots are rarely used in regular practice to identify the humour itself. Even the leading journal of the field, published by the American Society of Hematology, is called *Blood*. The word comes from Old English through Nordic and Saxon roots. Language theory holds that as the French-speaking Norman invaders married the Anglo-Saxon women, Latin-derived French words took over the vocabulary of the external environment of masculine authority; however, words pertaining to the interior, domestic, female environment, and to emotions and feelings, were retained – with these words we have 'blood.' The derivation may illustrate blood's special importance to women's work rather than its power. For example, the words 'liver,' 'kidney,' and

---

More along Linguistic Lines

Anglophones appear to have a special subliminal respect for the word 'blood.' Think about the psychic power in its many derivatives: cold blood, blue blood, bad blood, fresh blood, hot-blooded, red-blooded, bloodline, blood red, bloodless, bloodthirsty, blood-curdling, bloody, bloody-minded, bloodshed, bloodshot, bloodstone, blood money, blood poisoning, bloodstain, blood feud, flesh and blood, and lifeblood.

How many similar words can be found for the liver? Liverish, liver spots, and lily-livered – not very impressive words. And for the kidney?

'heart' also come from Old English, possibly because these organs, like blood, are edible parts of animal bodies. Body parts with Latinized names – such as aorta, colon, duodenum, rectum, vagina, tendon, and cartilage – have little or no culinary interest.

If the linguistic argument for the special power of blood is unconvincing, a psychological analysis is difficult to refute. Most patients who are referred to a hematology clinic have no symptoms at all; they are sent for abnormalities picked up during routine testing. Even patients with newly diagnosed leukemia may be symptom-free. Nevertheless, people sent to hematologists are apprehensive: a problem with blood is a problem with life.

Blood as Medical Science

Medical professionals discount magic and myth, finding them quaint but incredible. As blood has been medicalized and objectified by technology, its mystique with scientists may have waned. But blood and its multiple functions still occupy an exalted state – a position that seeks to reconcile the ancient notions of blood's great power with our understanding of modern science.

Blood Therapy: Transfusion

If blood is life, it is only logical to assume that faltering life might revive with a little extra blood. The first 'transfusion' is often said to have been given in 1492 to the dying Giovanni Battista Cibò, who had been elected pope as Innocent VIII in 1484. His Jewish physician, Giacomo di San Genesio, is said to have tried to resuscitate the ailing pontiff by having him drink the blood of three ten-year-old boys whom he had had killed. The evidence for this peculiar treatment is unreliable, and the story is probably an anti-Semitic fabrication, not unlike the rumours of ritualistic child murder that tracked the customs of Passover.

Oral blood had probably been tried many times before, and without the prerequisite of donor death. Moog and Karenberg report on the use of gladiators' blood for epilepsy in late Roman antiquity. Galen held that blood was elaborated from ingested substances; surely consuming blood would facilitate the process of building more. The mouth offered an appropriate, accessible, logical, and comfortable site of administration, and drinking of blood enjoyed faddish popularity both before and after the discovery of circulation.

Interest in vascular transfusion was stimulated by William Harvey's 1628 treatise *On the Motion of the Heart* (see chapter 3). Soon after, experiments were conducted, using quills, bladders, and silver tubes to remove blood from one animal and give it to another. Indirect transfusion entailed the removal of blood into a container and its subsequent administration into the recipient; direct transfusion took place through a connector from the vessel of the donor animal to the vein of the recipient. These experiments captured the interest of many, including the quiet cleric Francis Potter, the illustrious polymath Sir Christopher Wren (architect of London's St Paul's Cathedral), and the physician Richard Lower, who began to transfuse dogs.

Borrowed Blood

At dinner on 14 November 1666, Samuel Pepys learned of a successful direct transfusion between dogs, which had taken place in London that day. The potential of such an achievement did not escape the diners. Pepys recorded their mischievous reaction in his famous diary:

This did give occasion to many pretty wishes, as of the blood of a Quaker to be in an Archbishop, and such like. But, as Dr. Croone says, [it] may, if it takes, be of mighty use to man's health, for the amending of bad blood by borrowing from a better body.

– *Diary of Samuel Pepys*, ed. Robert Latham and William Matthews
(Berkeley: University of California Press, 1970–83), 7: 371

In early 1667 the French physician Jean-Baptiste Denis appears to have attempted the first intravenous transfusion between humans when he gave lamb's blood to a fifteen-year-old boy to calm his nerves.

Not to be outdone by the competition from across the channel, Lower performed his own sheep-to-man transfusion later the same year. Back in France, Denis became a transfusion specialist, but the next year a man died following a failed attempt to give him a third transfusion of animal blood. Denis was sued – but the court decided that the patient had been poisoned by his wife, and the doctor was exonerated. However, the sobering publicity dampened enthusiasm, and transfusion activities were curtailed for nearly a century and a half.

Indeed, blood transfusion was (and still is) a potentially life-threatening intervention, never to be undertaken lightly. Three problems posed serious hurdles: the reactions that were later known as blood-group incompatibility, clotting, and infection.

Transfusion was cautiously revived in the early nineteenth century. The perennial problem of obstetrical bleeding became more obvious to practitioners as childbirth was medicalized (see chapter 11). In the 1820s, James Blundell of Guy's Hospital in London, England, attempted transfusion for uncontrollable postpartum hemorrhage. Using a syringe, he injected the bleeding mothers with blood taken from the resident housestaff; a few lives appeared to be saved. Patients given this heroic therapy were not expected to live; if death resulted from transfusion, it would have been ascribed to the original hemorrhage.

Another stimulus to transfusion came from the urgent need to save bleeding soldiers. During the Franco-Prussian War of 1870–1, direct transfusions were given on the battlefield, soldier to soldier, by medics in the armies of Austria, Belgium, and Russia. Sterile technique was used, but incompatibility and clotting had yet to be resolved, while storage of blood seemed to be virtually unattainable. These problems found solutions in the twentieth century.

Compatibility

The problem of compatibility began to unravel with the work of the Vienna-born Karl Landsteiner, who in 1901 published a short study based on the twenty-two workers in his laboratory: their blood could be divided into three major groups, A, B, and C (now called O). The following year, two of his pupils discovered the fourth major blood

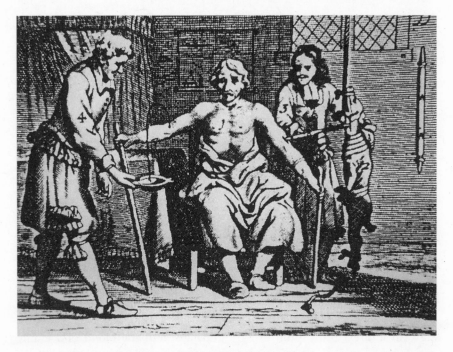

8.1   A direct transfusion from animal donor to recipient (probably hypothetical). From J.B. Lamzweerde, *Appendix ad Armamentarium chirurgicum Johannis Sculteti*, Amsterdam, 1671, 28

group, AB. Landsteiner's work was ignored until just before the First World War. He moved to New York to the Rockefeller Institute in 1922 and became an American citizen. His Nobel Prize was awarded in 1930 when the practical application of his discovery had been realized.

In 1937, Landsteiner and his colleague Alexander Wiener also noticed another blood-type system that they called 'Rhesus' (Rh), because it appeared in experiments between rhesus monkeys and rabbits and was subsequently found to react to human blood too. Although not exactly identical to the factor that now bears the name, this system helped to explain a strange condition of newborn babies called erythroblastosis fetalis: an Rh-negative mother, sensitized by mixing of blood at the birth of a previous Rh-positive child, develops antibodies that travel across the placenta to attack the blood of the

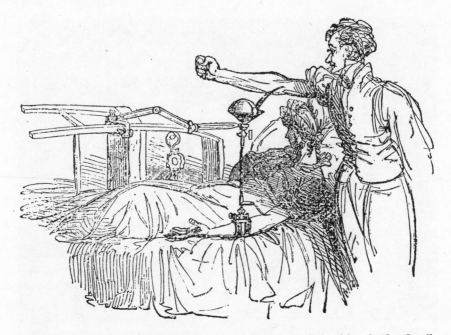

8.2 An indirect transfusion using a gravitator and the blood of a family member who is a house officer. James Blundell, *Lancet*, 13 June 1829, 321

next Rh-postitive fetus. Recognized clinically since at least the early modern period, the disease had been described as a problem of blood in 1932. In the mid-1940s exchange transfusions were attempted to try to save the lives of affected newborns by giving them blood that is Rh-negative; if necessary, transfusions can now be given to fetuses in utero. By the early 1960s researchers were trying to prevent the disease by injecting every Rh-negative mother of an Rh-positive baby with the antibody to 'fool' her immune system into not reacting to her newborn's blood. At first, they used antibody-rich 'raw' plasma from women who had given birth to affected infants; as one of the doctors remembered it: 'these women exemplified the finest in "essential feminine altruism" ... to save their sisters from their own tragedy' (E.G. Hamilton, *Obs & Gyn* 77 [1991]: 957). In 1968, Bruce Chown of Winnipeg working with Connaught Laboratories developed a more practical method of manufacturing Rh serum. The method has prevented the disease in thousands of infants around the world.

Now hundreds of blood groups are recognized, the most important still being the ABO and Rhesus systems. The ability to wash, freeze, and thaw blood safely has made it possible to provide a relatively compatible supply for even the rarest types.

Anticoagulation

As the researchers quickly discovered, untreated blood will clot within a few minutes. Storage depended on finding a method to inhibit this natural property without harming either the product or the recipient. Testing began on techniques for removing fibrin (the clotting protein) and on anticoagulant drugs. Just prior to the Second World War the Russians took advantage of natural anticoagulation – cadaver blood will not clot because it has already clotted and lysed. Cadaver blood and, for similar reasons, placental blood, were also used for transfusion in India and elsewhere.

Now the preferred anticoagulant is sodium citrate, discovered in 1914. It was systematically applied to battlefield needs of the First World War by an American army doctor, O.H. Robertson, working with a British unit. Using only O-positive donors, Robertson demonstrated that citrate combined with dextrose (to nourish the blood cells) allowed safe storage of blood for up to three weeks – the first blood bank. Work on heparin as an anticoagulant for medicine and surgery was the product of Canadian research by Charles Best, Louis B. Jaques, and D.W. Gordon Murray in the early 1930s.

Blood Components

With the problems of compatibility and coagulation under control, hospital blood banking began. By 1927, plasma was usefully extracted from outdated blood by centrifugation. The Mayo Clinic of Rochester, Minnesota (1935), and Cook County Hospital in Chicago (1936) vie for the honour of being the first American hospitals to run blood banks. The controversy arises because individuals had been transfused there and elsewhere for several years, and sometimes the blood had been stored. The Canadian surgeon Norman Bethune helped to establish a mobile unit for plasma transfusion in December 1936 during the Spanish Civil War. Plasma for shock and clotting factors became the mainstay of emergency treatment in the Second World War. Component therapy, the use of specific parts of blood – red cells, platelets, white cells, factors, and plasma – is now standard practice.

After 1945, blood banking became a regular practice in countries all over the world and could be cited as the beginning of hematology as a distinct professional entity. In the United States, city-, state-, and nationwide services were created with the help of non-physician volunteers. For example, after serving at Pearl Harbor, Bernice Hemphill returned to work in a San Francisco blood bank; from 1948 until 1953 she was instrumental in extending the blood-bank cooperation across California, and eventually to the entire country. The National Blood Service of England began in 1946, with separate agencies for Scotland, Wales, and Northern Ireland. In Canada, as in several other countries, the blood transfusion service was run by the national Red Cross from 1947 until 1998. Blood collection, storage, and transfusion was only one of many peacetime services offered by that organization, but its role in Canadian blood banking came to an abrupt end with new controversies over infection (see Krever commission below; on the Red Cross, see chapter 10). Since 1998, the non-profit organization Canadian Blood Services fills this function and oversees a stem cell and marrow registry; HémaQuébec handles the equivalent tasks in Quebec. The Red Cross is still involved in collection as the sole organization or with others in several other countries of Europe, Australia, and the United States.

Infection

Sterile technique for handling blood has been in place for more than a century; however, infection has been a serious problem and is currently the object of public anxiety. Syphilis, several forms of hepatitis, West Nile virus, and AIDS are among the many infections that can be transmitted by blood. Serological testing has reduced the risk. Hepatitis remained the most frequent of the transfusion infections until the early 1990s, when testing finally became available for what is now known as hepatitis C. Vaccination against hepatitis B, which received U.S. Food and Drug approval in late 1981, is an important consideration for medical personnel who can accidentally be exposed to the blood of others. In countries where equipment may not be sterilized properly, donors can transmit infections to each other. And when donors fear infection, supplies falter.

Members of the Christian religious group Jehovah's Witnesses base their stand against transfusion on an interpretation of biblical passages forbidding consumption of blood. The same passages are cited as an origin of kosher butchery methods in the Judaic tradition. They also illustrate how the story of the Last Supper and the tenets of the Catholic mass, especially transubstantiation, could be seen as a surprising rupture. Concern over infection, added to steady pressure from those who have philosophical objections to transfusion, has stimulated research into blood surrogates such as plasma expanders, hemoglobin, and clotting-factor substitutes.

Blood Is Life, but You Should Not Eat It

Only you shall not eat flesh with its life, that is, its blood.

– Genesis 9:4

If any man of the house of Israel ... eats any blood, I will set my face against that person who eats blood, and will cut him off from among his people. For the life of the flesh is in the blood.

– Leviticus 17:10–11

Only be sure that you do not eat the blood for the blood is the life, and you shall not eat the life with the flesh.

– Deuteronomy 12:23

The shape and image of blood banking and transfusion have been altered. No longer 'the gift of life,' blood therapy is mistrusted, especially in the United States, where until the late 1970s donors could be paid. In France, a lengthy inquiry into policies surrounding blood products resulted in the 1992 conviction with a four-year prison sentence for the physicians who had directed the national blood service,

Michel Garetta and Jean-Pierre Allain. France was said to have kept using blood known to be contaminated and delayed AIDS testing with an American product until October 1985 in order to allow the French version to catch up; the investigation continued to the end of the decade. In Canada, a royal commission into the issue of transfusion-related infection, chaired by Justice Horace Krever, began hearings in 1993. It resulted in many changes to the blood system and allegations of wrongdoing by politicians and Red Cross officials. The former national director, Roger Perrault, endured years of RCMP investigation, criminal charges, and a long trial, which he won; his complete exoneration did not occur until 2008, when outstanding charges were dropped.

Entrepreneurial persons have taken advantage of the situation to open private blood banks, where the anxious can stock their own blood for future surgery or a disaster that occurs within convenient reach of the freezer. A similar situation prevails with respect to umbilical cord blood, which since 2000 is banked both publicly and privately in many countries throughout the world, prompted by expectations for stem cell research. Private procedures are a grey area legally and they are inaccessible to many citizens. If tolerated, they will replace the previously imperfect but equitable system with a two-tier system. Donation experts worry that reporting of high-risk behaviours could decline with added pressure for family contributions.

Marrow transplantation can be seen as the ultimate form of component transfusion. It was developed during the 1970s in Seattle, Washington, under the direction of E. Donnall Thomas, who used the principles of anticoagulation and intravenous infusion, and the cell-cloning techniques of Canadian researchers J. Till and E.A. McCulloch. Marrow transplant offers hope for chronic anemias and malignancies. As a side effect, the new iatrogenic problem of graft-versus-host disease arose. To help those who did not have suitable donors, autologous (self-) transplantation was developed; however, because the graft-versus-host side effects do not occur with the patient's own cells, this method is widely used in other situations – for example, to 'rescue' a person's blood-making ability following the ravages of strong treatments for cancers and autoimmune disease. The ultracentrifuge technologies of cell separators allow for the selective collection of stem cells, so that a 'transplant' may now involve more specificity and a smaller volume of cells. E.D. Thomas shared the Nobel Prize in 1990. For their 1960 discovery of hematopoietic stem cells, Till and McCullough received the Lasker Award in 2005.

Blood in Diagnosis: What Is Normal Blood?

Today's physicians have few opportunities to look at their patients' blood. Blood is visible in surgery and emergencies, but these settings do not allow for contemplation. Nurses, IV teams, laboratory technologists, blood banks, computerized analysis, and printed reports have distanced the doctor from the physical realities of blood. Not so in the past. From antiquity until the mid-twentieth century, bloodletting was standard treatment, and all doctors regularly examined their patients' blood for the changes that took place in it upon standing.

Bloodletting seemed to be beneficial in fevers: it lowered the pulse, lessened plethora, and calmed agitation. The let blood soon coagulated and separated into several easily distinguished components, in which could be visualized the four ancient humours: yellow serum above, dark (deoxygenated) blood below, a rim of bright red (oxygenated) blood in the middle, and above it a pinkish-beige layer called the 'buffy coat' or 'web,' containing white cells and clotting protein. After performing a bloodletting, doctors noted the colour and quantity of each component and were able to link the appearance with diagnosis and prognosis. Dark blood was a poor prognostic sign in pneumonia. A thick buffy layer with a concave configuration (called 'buffed and cupped') was a sign of acute inflammation.

Red Cells: Linking Blood to Air

Hemoglobin and oxygen. With his early microscope, Antonie van Leeuwenhoek observed the tiny 'particles' now known as red cells. Their existence, however, was controversial; those who saw them could not explain their function. Around the same time, both the French chemist Nicolas Lemery and Richard Lower of transfusion fame noticed that iron was a constituent of blood. Lower also described the change in colour of venous blood, from dark to bright red, on exposure to air. Some years later, iron became a treatment for anemia after the 1725 observations of the Russian military doctor Alexei Bestouyev-

Rioumine. But neither iron nor the colour change were connected to the little globules, and oxygen had yet to be described.

In 1668 John Mayow demonstrated the life-sustaining properties of some air (see chapter 3), but one hundred years passed before the vital air could be identified. In the 1770s oxygen and 'laughing gas' were isolated by Joseph Priestley, an English theologian and chemist, and a sympathizer with the revolutionaries in France. Uncertain of his findings, he explained his discovery to his friend, the French aristocrat Antoine-Laurent Lavoisier, who quickly recognized its importance. With his personal fortune and the help of his wife, Marie-Anne-Pierette Paulze, Lavoisier experimented on respiration, combustion, and oxygen. By 1777 he had formulated a chemical theory of life as a process of oxidation. But the French Revolution put an end to their work: Priestley's church was sacked, and he fled to the United States; Lavoisier was guillotined.

If life had now become the chemical consumption of oxygen, then oxygen had to be linked to blood, because it too had been equated with life since prehistoric times. This vast scientific project began in the late eighteenth century and extends into our own time. Hemoglobin was identified as the 'red pigment' in the globules in 1851 by the German physiologist Otto Funke. His compatriot, Felix Hoppe-Seyler, proved that the pigment could take up and discharge oxygen. Two independent ideas – one ancient, the other relatively new – had been brought together in the red blood cell: blood was life; life was the combustion of oxygen.

A Tragedy Links Blood, Oxygen, and Life

In 1875 the French physiologist Paul Bert sent a hot-air balloon, the Zenith, to 7,900 metres, the highest altitude yet reached by humans. When the balloon descended, two of the three-man crew were dead. Bert concluded that for survival at low pressures, *supplemental* oxygen was needed to ensure adequate uptake by the blood. His insight laid the ground for the theories of partial pressures in the lung and helped resolve the mystery of the well-known but poorly understood condition called mountain sickness.

An elegant contribution to the characterization of hemoglobin function was the oxygen-transport work of the Danish scientist Christian Bohr, whose son Niels and grandson Aage are both Nobel laureates in physics (1922 and 1975, respectively). Bohr used mathematics to express the relationship of oxygen to hemoglobin. His oxygen dissociation curve describes a remarkable property of blood – its variable affinity for oxygen. The curve is sigmoid; the dips above and below a straight line show how hemoglobin picks up oxygen more readily when it is plentiful (for example, in the healthy lung) and releases it more readily when it is scant (for example, in the healthy tissues). These affinities are ingenious, especially compared with those of a mundane transport protein sporting a banal linear relationship to its object. Moreover, Bohr's curve shifts right or left, according to the environment in acidosis or alkalosis, to favour the transfer of oxygen to the host. The curve also illustrates the dangerous 'point of no return' situation that can occur in severe lung damage, where low concentrations of oxygen 'on the shoulder of the curve' can cause hemoglobin to release rather than take up oxygen.

Hemoglobin was the first protein to be chemically identified. Using X-ray crystallography, Max Perutz, John Kendrew, and colleagues elucidated the primary, secondary, and tertiary structure of the hemoglobin molecule in 1960. Its genetic basis was so well understood that researchers could define the molecular substitutions, in both protein and DNA, that are responsible for many abnormal hemoglobins. For example, in 1957 Vernon M. Ingram demonstrated that hemoglobin in sickle-cell disease involved the substitution of a single molecule. Variations in hemoglobin structure were related to changes in function. Altered control over the genetic production of hemoglobin explains the common and devastating thalassemias.

This vast restructuring of knowledge into biochemical terminology promises new therapies for abnormal hemoglobins, through reduced-intensity marrow transplants and genetic engineering; but at the time of writing, little change has taken place in the therapy of most afflicted persons. The field is still very messy. Only 10 percent of people with sickle-cell disease are likely to have an unaffected sibling donor. And as several historians have shown, the elegance of molecular discoveries do not soften the hard realities of social construction on the basis of race. For people suffering in sickle-cell crisis, we still provide the old remedies of analgesics, hydration, oxygen, and trans-fusion; for thalassemia, transfusion. These treatments generate new iatrogenic problems, which require secondary therapies, including chelation of excess iron following multiple transfusion, social sup-port for addiction to analgesic drugs, and management of infections. It was an industry-sponsored clinical trial to assess a chelating agent in thalassemia that resulted in a famous case of scientific harassment in 1996, when Toronto hematologist Nancy Olivieri dared to warn her patients of side effects (see chapter 5).

Morphology and a bevy of fathers. Extending the microscopic observa-tions of van Leeuwenhoek, William Hewson measured the size and shape of blood cells in different animals. He found that the red glob-ule is usually flat, not spherical, and he recognized that coagulation is a process of change in plasma, not red cells. Hewson died in 1777 of an accidental scalpel wound which he sustained while performing an autopsy. For his precise observations and his romantic end, he has been called the father of hematology, especially by the British.

Despite Hewson's elegant studies, cell theory was not established until late in the nineteenth century. The vista presented by early microscopes was unreliable. Only after the achromatic lens and com-pound microscope became available in the 1830s did observers begin to trust their eyes and turn their attention to the cellular components of blood. Gabriel Andral and Alfred Donné, both of France, pio-neered quantitation in hematology by linking various illnesses with the number, concentration, size, and shape of red cells. These men too have been called fathers of hematology, mostly by the French.

Andral was the first to suggest that anemia could occur if red cells were destroyed (hemolysis), and he described anemia as a decrease in the number of red cells. He associated anemia with pregnancy and with chlorosis. Once called the 'green sickness of virgins' for the peculiar cast it gave to the complexion, chlorosis had been described in the sixteenth century by Johannes Lange, who recommended mar-riage as therapy. It has come to be synonymous with what we would now call iron-deficiency anemia, although it also resembles anorexia nervosa. Andral was the first to observe the small size of red cells in chlorosis. Here was a capital discovery: a diagnosis formerly bound to a patient's subjective account of vague symptoms and a doctor's opinion of her complexion could now be reduced to an accessible, objective test: red cell number and size.

Insight concerning red cells sometimes emerged from intensely practical observations. The American George Minot, for example, noticed that fewer than expected red cells were found in patients with the aggressive and uniformly fatal disease pernicious anemia (also known as Biermer's anemia, for the German physician who described it in 1868). In 1926, Minot reported that red-cell production increased with a diet containing up to half a pound of raw liver daily. Pernicious anemia is now linked to an inability to absorb vitamin B12. At the time of Minot's celebrated cure, however, the existence of vitamins was still under dispute (see chapter 13). Minot's diet was yet another example of empirical success, advocated before the definition of the chemical errors in the disease: intrinsic factor was described in 1929 by W.B. Castle; vitamin B_{12} was isolated in 1948 by E.L. Rickes and K.A. Folkers.

Red-cell chemistry. Red cells are unusual. They have no nuclei and no mitochondria. They are tiny, 'brainless' packages whose 120-day lifespan is dedicated to the transport of oxygen and carbon dioxide between the lungs and the tissues. Their other functions include buffering, but their physiology is largely devoted to maintaining the integrity of their hemoglobin and cell walls to provide safe, efficient passage of their precious cargo, oxygen or carbon dioxide. Enzymes are the key.

Red cells were known to be consumers of glucose, but how they could use sugar without indulging in oxygen was not understood until the work of three German scientists: Otto Warburg, his student Otto Meyerhof, and Gustav Embden. The three researchers uncovered two enzyme pathways: the hexose-monophosphate shunt, which provides energy to repair damaged hemoglobin; and the glycolytic pathway, which generates energy for the cell itself. Warburg and Meyerhof are both Nobel laureates.

In 1911, during this wave of 'chemicalizing' the red cell, H. Günther characterized the porphyrias, hemolytic diseases that result from an absence of enzymes that govern the production of hemoglobin. Soon after, physicians who are fond of using the 'retrospec-toscope' invoked porphyria to account for strange behaviours of the past, ranging from the intermittent madness of King George III of Britain to the werewolf legends of Transylvania.

Later in the century, Canadian Maxwell Wintrobe invented useful instruments, such as the hematocrit, and made practical observations about erythrocyte morphology and behaviour in health and disease. Raised by an Austrian-Jewish family in Halifax, he completed his MD at Winnipeg and went on to New Orleans, finally settling in Salt Lake City, Utah. He was the sole author of the first six editions of the authoritative textbook *Clinical Hematology* (1942–68). Its bibliography could serve as a model of thoroughness and historical sensitivity. Canadians and Americans alike may be understood (if not forgiven) when they cite him as the father of twentieth-century hematology.

The idea that human illness could derive from modifications in the biochemistry and survival of red cells came during the Second World War. Sources of quinine for malaria prevention in the Allied troops of the Pacific theatre had been stopped and alternative drugs had to be found. The new antimalarial agents provoked hemolytic anemia in some soldiers, mostly black males. A similar phenomenon took place in the Korean War when primaquine was used for malaria prevention. In the mid-1950s, using volunteers from the Stateville Penitentiary near Chicago, the American army scientists Alf S. Alving, Paul Carson, R.J. Dern, and Ernest Beutler demonstrated that the red cells of hemolysis patients were inordinately sensitive to the drug because they lacked the X-linked, reducing enzyme glucose-6-phos-phate dehydrogenase (G-6-PD). Not only did the discovery explain a new drug problem, but it also provided a scientific basis for favism, an ancient disease triggered by eating fava beans. Each of the many red-cell enzymes was discovered when a fortuitous accident of nature provided a mutant in whom the enzyme was missing.

White Cells

First described in the eighteenth century, white blood cells were neglected until the nineteenth-century work of the British physician Thomas Addison and the German pathologist and statesman Rudolf

Virchow. Addison noticed that 'colourless corpuscules' passed through the walls of blood vessels to form pus in inflammation. In 1845 Virchow described leukemia – literally, 'white blood.' The thick buffy layer in these patients was like pus, but without the usual inflammation; he suggested that it was due to an inappropriate production of abnormal cells at the expense of normal ones (see also chapter 4).

In the late nineteenth century, new staining techniques facilitated white-cell morphology. This technological change was a by-product of a search for new treatments. Paul Ehrlich had been seeking dyes that could act as chemotherapy for infections by bonding with, and specifically killing, bacteria (see chapter 5). In 1880 he described white-cell types, inventing names based on their staining properties, for example, neutrophil, eosinophil, basophil. Ehrlich believed that white cells played a role in protecting the body from invasion by the newly discovered bacteria.

Elie Metchnikoff shared Ehrlich's opinions about the immune functions of white cells. A Russian working at the Pasteur Institute in Paris, Metchnikoff discovered the capacity of phagocytosis. To some, the notion of one kind of cell gobbling up another seemed ridiculous – and befitting the Russian's strange character. The molecular biologist André Lwoff recalled Metchnikoff on visits to his childhood home – lively, but disorderly, with test tubes of blood and other unusual substances poking out of his pockets. But Metchnikoff's insights were in concert with the new immunology, and he was awarded the Nobel Prize in 1908. The ancient idea that 'bad blood' brought disease had been rephrased in a three-dimensional chemical and physical package that was consonant with contemporary science.

From 1890 to 1910, serotherapy (or serum therapy) – the use of blood or blood components containing what we would now call specific antibody – was advocated as treatment for diphtheria, cholera, tetanus, meningitis, and other infections caused by bacterial agents. Emil von Behring and his Japanese colleague Shibasaburo Kitasato, working in Germany, explored the production of antitoxins by exposing animals to specific infections, such as diphtheria, and extracting the sera they elaborated. Once again, the constitution of these sera was unknown, but they were effective.

A study of lymphocytes and their manufacture of antibodies led to a biochemical explanation of immunity and clone theory. Niels Jerne observed a background production of many different antibodies, but when the test animal was exposed to a specific antigen, large amounts of specific antibody would result. Clone theory arose from an extrapolation of the ideas of Virchow and Jerne. The Australian Frank Macfarlane Burnet made two postulates: first, each cell could react to only one antigen; second, in the course of development, millions of potentially reactive cells arose. Clone theory explains normal immune function and provides a model for some hematologic malignancies – multiple myeloma, chronic myelogenous leukemia, polycythemia rubra vera, and essential thrombocytosis. With the advent of the ability to detect gene rearrangement, many more malignancies are shown to have clonal components.

Platelets

After the technical problems of light microscopy had been resolved, the existence of the tiny cells that came to be called platelets was under dispute. In 1868 the Italian anatomist Giulio Bizzozero reported that these tiny blood cells originated in bone marrow and represented a separate cell line. Bizzozero distinguished between thrombus formation and precipitation of clotting factors, and he thought that platelets could trigger the clotting cascade. Knowing of Bizzozero's work, the twenty-four-year-old Canadian William Osler soon joined the debate. He reported that these bodies were 'sometimes' found in normal persons, and he speculated on their relationship with bacteria.

The Frenchman Georges Hayem devoted much of his career to a series of elegant experiments that linked platelets to hemostasis. Against his own evidence to the contrary, however, he viewed platelets as a by-product of red cells. One historian has speculated that Hayem's error was the result of 'the unimaginative burden thrust on those, who like him, come early to positions of authority' (T.H. Spaet, in M. Wintrobe, *Blood Pure and Eloquent.* New York: McGraw-Hill, 1980, 553). More likely, Hayem's ideas stemmed from preconception – the 'epistemological obstacle' that has allowed many fine researchers to find precisely what they seek. The French look on Hayem, together with Donné and Andral, as yet another father of hematology.

Platelets occupy a huge literature with a high profile in our society, where cerebrovascular and cardiovascular thromboses are the leading causes of death. The genetics and biochemistry of platelet function are used to predict the antiplatelet effects of drugs. Many longitudinal studies of antiplatelet drugs have been conducted over fifty years; by 2000, the old off-patent drug aspirin was finally shown to be effective in primary prevention of cerebrovascular disease. However, because aspirin has many side effects (and costs very little), new (more expensive) antiplatelet drugs have been introduced to become bestsellers (see chapter 5). In the interests of the rising burden of lifestyle disease in developing countries, yet another protocol to review whether or not the benefits of affordable aspirin outweigh its side effects is underway at the Cochrane Collaboration.

Plasma and Coagulation

The tendency to bleed has been recognized since antiquity. Writers of the Talmud seemed to know that male bleeders inherited the problem from their mothers, and they exempted from circumcision the next son of a mother who had already lost two or three boys to hemorrhage (Yebamot, 64b). Well before classical hemophilia had been characterized in chemical terms, it was used as a model by the American geneticist Thomas Hunt Morgan for his Nobel Prize–winning work on sex linkage.

In his immensely popular book of 1968, *Nicolas and Alexandra*, historian Robert K. Massie suggested that hemophilia helped to fuel the Russian Revolution with the stresses it produced in the family of Tsar Nicholas II. The tsarevitch Alexei suffered from hemophilia, which he had likely inherited from his great-grandmother, Queen Victoria, via his mother, Alexandra. The relationship between a hemophiliac and his mother is poignant: she is doubly tormented, by her child's pain and by the ancient idea that the problem was passed through her blood. Desperate to help her son, Alexandra turned to Rasputin, a self-styled spiritualist healer (in)famous for his excessive appetites in all things sensual, from cuisine to sex. Rasputin could calm and comfort the boy, and he also appeared to control the bleeding. Against advice, the 'foreign' tsarina continued the consultations; detrimental rumours about her relationship with Rasputin further eroded public respect for the throne.

Bleeding problems were defined by measuring the length of time for a clot to form in whole blood or plasma. Hemophilic blood took a long time to clot, if it did so at all. In the late 1930s, when component transfusion was first implemented, it was discovered that the clotting defect in hemophilic plasma could be corrected by mixing it half-and-half with normal plasma. Researchers postulated the existence of a vague but essential 'anti-hemophilic factor' (AHF) in normal blood. By more mixing experiments, they learned that not all bleeders were the same.

In 1947 an Argentinian team noted the 'paradoxical fact' that mixing plasma from two different bleeders sometimes resulted in mutual correction. In her classic paper published at Christmas 1952, Rosemary Biggs presented seven bleeders whose plasma could correct the defect in other hemophiliacs. She reasoned that these patients must have a different disease, which she named Christmas disease, both for the season and for the 'patronymic' of her five-year-old Canadian 'patient no. 1,' Stephen Christmas, son of the actor Eric Christmas.

Mixing studies continue to be the basis of coagulation screening and the means of identifying new clotting factors. In 1953 the railwayman John Hageman was admitted to a Chicago hospital for elective ulcer surgery. He had no history of bleeding, but his blood clotted poorly on a routine test, and his surgery was cancelled. Hageman's defect could be corrected in the laboratory by mixing his plasma with either normal or hemophilic plasma. His doctors concluded that the plasma of both normals and hemophiliacs contained something that Hageman did not; it was Factor XII.

Each factor in the seemingly complicated 'coagulation cascade' has been found in the same way: someone comes along with a defect that can be corrected by normal plasma *and* by all other known factor-deficient plasmas. At first, clotting factors were named after the patients who lacked them (e.g., Christmas factor, Hageman factor, Fletcher factor, and Stuart factor). Later, they were numbered to reflect our understanding of their place in the reaction cascade. Mixing studies are basic to coagulation research and service. In the future, new factors will be identified in the same way.

A boon to hemophiliacs, the special clotting properties of cryo-precipitate – a blood component collected by freezing plasma – were recognized and made available in 1964. At that time, researchers still did not know whether the tendency to bleed (the so-called absence of AHF) was caused by a defective molecule, an absent molecule, or the presence of an inhibitor. In 1970–1 classical hemophilia was attributed to a defective Factor VIII molecule. As for the hemoglobin-opathies, associated molecular substitutions in DNA have now been defined. In terms of treatment, lyophilized (freeze dried) products were easier to store, use, and carry about, but they were made with pooled plasma, greatly increasing the risk of transmitted infection. The success of blood products in the management of bleeding disorders led to a temporary revolution in pain management and life-style, but it soon brought a tragic reminder of the dangers of blood therapy.

Forty years after his diagnosis, a Canadian team published the precise molecular substitution to account for the coagulation problem in Stephen Christmas, but their work could do nothing to prevent his death from AIDS on 20 December 1993. About half of hemophiliacs in developed countries converted to HIV seropositivity before 1985; many have died. In Britain and the United States, the number of seropositive hemophiliacs is estimated at 5,000 and 10,000 respectively. In Canada by 1997, 400 hemophiliacs had died of iatrogenic AIDS, and another 1,000 were infected with HIV and/or hepatitis.

With transfusion-related HIV or hepatitis we hear again the term 'innocent victim' (see chapter 7). Many drugs, diagnostic procedures, and surgical interventions cause sickness, even death; yet the value-added outrage expressed on behalf of those harmed by 'tainted' blood seems to proclaim the primal significance of this fluid in our world.

Blood and Drugs

The hematologic malignancies of lymphoma and leukemia – though far from being the most prevalent – distinguished themselves early from all other cancers as being responsive to treatment: first by radiation, then by drugs. Almost all these therapies have fascinating histories intimately connected to the scientific discoveries of the late twentieth century. Cures once thought impossible for conditions like Hodgkin's disease and childhood leukemia are now within the realm of the ordinary, usually with a combination of drugs and radiation. Radiation was accomplished by X-rays and radioactive elements such as radium and cobalt. After 1945, nuclear reactors were built in many places, making it possible to produce radioisotopes for medical uses, such as radiophosphorus (^{32}P) and radioiodine (^{131}I).

One of the earliest cancer drugs was nitrogen mustard; its cell-killing (cytotoxic) effect on blood had first been observed in soldiers gassed with mustard in the First World War. In 1950, researchers in England released versions that were relatively safe for medical use, called alkylating agents. These products famously cause hair loss, stomach upset, and bone marrow depression. Around the same time, the hormone of the adrenal cortex (cortisone) was discovered; it produced rapid but short-lived disappearance of lymph masses. When cortisone was combined with the cytotoxic drugs, it produced complete remissions, and even cures. Killing cells in a variety of ways seemed to wipe out tumours so that a small nest of resistant cells could not reactivate the disease; thus the spindle poisons were developed, beginning with the extraction of vinblastine from Madagascar periwinkle in London, Ontario, in 1958. Their application to childhood leukemia resulted in the first cures. Other 'spindle poisons' include paclitaxel (Taxol®) derived from the Pacific yew tree. Combination chemotherapy became even more effective with application of the first rational derivatives or designer drugs, which garnered the Nobel Prize in 1988 (see chapter 5). Virtually all these remedies, once proven effective on blood conditions, were applied to other diseases.

A growth factor (or hormone), called erythropoietin is made in the kidney and promotes red cell production in the bone marrow and in the lab. It was purified in 1977, having been hypothesized many years earlier. By the 1980s it was used to treat people with the anemia of kidney failure. In 1989, a synthetic version made by recombinant DNA was patented in the United States, making it possible to manufacture the drug for wider use and to reduce the need for transfusion. For two decades now it has been applied to a host of red blood cell deficiencies that occur naturally or because of chemotherapy; sadly, it has also become one of the drugs abused in high-performance athletics.

Similarly, white blood cell growth is governed in humans by a stimulating factor (or hormone) that has also been synthesized in bacteria using the techniques of recombinant DNA. The drug, called filgrastrim (Neupogen®), is widely used to help patients recover from chemotherapy. It costs several thousand dollars for each monthly cycle and is governed by a patent due to expire in 2013; 'follow-on' successors are already in trials (see chapter 5).

Most recently, scientists have designed specific drugs in the form of antibodies that attack the molecular markers and pathways produced by defective genes in malignant cells. They result in stunning success rates with relatively few side effects in leukemias, lymphomas, breast cancer, and autoimmune diseases: examples include Rituximab (Rituxan®, launched 1997), trastuzumab (Herceptin®, launched 2000), imatinib (Gleevec® or Glivec®, launched 2001), and the 'follow-on' for imatinib, called nilotinib (Tasigna®, launched in 2008). Each singular discovery is greeted with tremendous public fanfare, and patients clamour to be treated. The drugs promise to make chemotherapy ever more effective and better tolerated, but the cost of their development and use is exorbitant. Finding affordable access to these lucrative remedies is already resulting in appeals from developing countries.

Blood Is Still Special

The exciting achievements of the last fifty years transformed diseases with gloomy prognoses into curable problems and put blood on the cutting edge. Long considered to be a subdivision of internal medicine or pathology, hematology has grown to become its own specialty with sub-specialties. Specialist examinations in England, Canada, and the United States were implemented in the late 1960s and early 1970s. Soon, oncology arose out of those branches of hematology dealing with malignancy to carry the tools into other organ systems,

and creating moments of rivalry. National and international societies exist, the largest of which is the American Society of Hematology
founded in 1958 with 300 delegates; now it boasts 15,000 members
and its annual meetings feature more than 500 papers and 2,500
posters and are attended by more than 20,000 delegates.

Despite its lofty stature as a subject of professional and scientific
activity, blood is still venerated for its magic and mystery. We may
no longer deify great healers like Asklepios, but we do 'canonize'
them with the Nobel Prize. Blood research is disproportionately represented among the Nobel laureates even if it is labelled immunology
or genetics.

In demystifying blood, new mechanisms are proposed in different,
perhaps less magical-sounding words, but the ancient concepts have
simply been rephrased; their essential features are unchanged. Galen
said that blood exposed to air was charged with the life force. Now,
blood is still seen as the equivalent of life, through its links to oxygen
and respiration, while its balance, like that of its ancient Greek precursor, is essential for the preservation of health.

Suggestions for Further Reading

At the bibliography website http://histmed.ca.

CHAPTER NINE

Technology and Disease: Stethoscopes, Hospitals, and Other Gadgets*

Concern for man himself and his fate must always form the chief interest of all technical endeavours.

– Albert Einstein, speech at California Institute of Technology, 1931

Technology (derived from the Greek word for 'craft') refers to the tools in the service of an intellectual enterprise. Tools can be objects, practices, or even ideas; social and conceptual factors both influence their invention. Once established, technologies not only alter practice, they also change perceptions of illness, patients, doctors, and disease. The last two hundred years have witnessed an unprecedented burgeoning of technology, partly because of the demands of keeping medicine 'scientific,' defining professional identity, and satisfying an innate human love of gadgetry.

A wide variety of devices have ancient roots as therapeutic technology: for example, sticks for walking, horns for hearing, and surgical instruments (see chapter 10). The oldest diagnostic instrument is probably the vaginal speculum, which can be traced to Roman antiquity. Printing was rapidly applied to the dissemination of medical knowledge from its invention in the fifteenth century. Some scholars have studied the uses of various images as technologies for teaching and communication. The numerous scientific inventions of the sev-

*Learning objectives for this chapter are found on pp. 453–4.

enteenth century, such as the microscope and thermometer, initially had little to do with the day-to-day practice of medicine. After 1800, however, the new emphasis on anatomy caused a reordering of medical knowledge, which fostered technological creation around visualization. Some historians argue that the molecular revolution of the late twentieth century is creating a different structure for technological organization. In this chapter, the discovery and impact of some technologies will be explored, using the example of the stethoscope as a starting point.

Antecedents to Discovery

Discoveries often seem to have taken place in a flash, a moment of lucky inspiration. Usually, however, they have a long prehistory, during which the inadequacy of old ways – the 'need' – is defined. Conditions that favour scientific discoveries are related to changes in ideas about the body, but they also incorporate factors from society, politics, economics, culture, and philosophy. In this sense, a discovery does not explode on a scene so much as it emerges from a milieu. Consequently, attributing priority is often a delicate matter. The discovery of auscultation and the invention of the stethoscope by René T.H. Laennec illustrate these principles well.

Sociopolitical Antecedents to Auscultation

This story involves the French Revolution, the First Empire of Napoleon Bonaparte, and the Restoration of the Bourbon monarchy. These events profoundly altered the personal lives of French citizens and brought changes in the way society organized the professions and education.

For centuries, European medicine and surgery had been separate. Physicians learned in the universities, through lectures and books. Surgeons, on the other hand, were allied into special guilds with the barbers, and they received practical training through apprenticeship (see chapter 10). Since the Middle Ages, hospitals had been places where patients could seek refuge, comfort, food, and care. They were not sites of learning or research. Only rarely were medical or surgical students taught on the wards.

The French Revolution has been described as an uprising of the lower classes, but the revolutionaries included elite intellectuals with radical opinions about politics and professional education. They thought that medicine and surgery could profitably combine; hospitals should be used in teaching; anatomy was important in the clinical setting; and doctors should maintain the health of the populace as well as treating the sick.

In 1789 the French medical faculties were abolished. The Paris school did not reopen until 1794, when it was revived under the enlightened (and short-lived) name École de Santé (School of Health). But there were no graduates for another five years. Among the new professors were a few of the previously excluded radical sympathizers, who immediately put their ideas to work. The old college of surgery was amalgamated with the remnants of the medical faculty; students were taught in the hospitals; and opportunities for the dissection of cadavers were increased to such an extent that supply could scarcely meet the demand.

Intellectual and Philosophical Antecedents

When the revolution began, diseases were elaborate constellations of symptoms, and their detection had little to do with anatomy (see chapters 2 and 4). Because diseases were fabricated from the pattern, sequence, and qualities of the subjective illness as told to the physician, a patient could not have a disease without feeling sick. Meticulous history taking and careful observation of the symptoms were the essential tools of diagnosis. Physical examination was cursory: the facies, the pulse, perhaps palpation of the abdomen and inspection of urine, stools, sputum or vomitus. This emphasis of unassisted observation over reasoning – empirical wisdom over theorizing – characterized the philosophy of knowledge called sensualism.

Normal anatomy and pathological (abnormal) anatomy had been cultivated for centuries, but the relevance of organic changes to bedside medicine was not obvious. In challenging the accepted wisdom that anatomy could not be made to fit in clinical medicine, the newly revived Paris school owed as much to contemporary philosophy as it did to the social and political climate. Hippocrates was resurrected as a founding champion of medical observation, and his wisdom was contrasted with the discredited and 'overly theoretical' views of Galen.

Anatomy conformed to the ideals of careful observation through the senses. French physicians began to imagine that the barrier between symptoms and structure could be broken by painstaking study and description of bodies both before and after death. Daily ward rounds followed by autopsies became the teaching format of the Paris hospital clinics. New journals were founded to broadcast the 'anatomo-clinical' discoveries.

Jean-Nicolas Corvisart des Marets was one of the new professors in the Paris school. He was a supporter of the revolution, a religious sceptic, and hostile to classical languages and the church. He taught internal medicine in the Charité hospital. In the 1780s he learned of 'percussion' – tapping with the fingers to examine the chest. Resonance indicated healthy, aerated lungs; dullness indicated fluid or pus. The source was a little-known work, *Inventum novum* (A New Invention), published in 1761 by the Austrian physician Leopold Auenbrugger. The musical son of an innkeeper, Auenbrugger had been inspired by his father, who tapped on casks in the family cellar to determine their content of wine. Auenbrugger applied the technique to the rigid barrel of the human thorax.

After twenty years of experimenting with percussion in his own practice, Corvisart published his translation and revision of Auenbrugger's treatise. Students flocked to his rounds and crowded into the autopsy theatre to watch him examine patients and cadavers as he gathered evidence for his book. He could predict anatomical findings with surprising success, and students believed that they were witnessing an exciting transformation of bedside medicine. In April 1801 Laennec joined Corvisart's clinic.

Personal Antecedents

René-Théophile-Hyacinthe Laennec came from Quimper, Brittany, in western France. His mother had died in 1786 when he was five years old, and his lawyer-poet father abandoned him to the care of his brother, a physician. Laennec's youth was played out on a background of revolution, terror, and war. Often working alone, he studied music, Greek, and Breton, and at the age of fourteen he enlisted as a surgical aide in the army, planning to follow in his uncle's footsteps. Because the revolution had closed the medical faculty in Nantes, he willingly set out for the capital.

Having already spent seven years in the study of medicine, Laennec excelled in Paris. He supplemented his meagre stipend by working as a student editor on Corvisart's new *Journal of Medicine*, where he published his own discoveries in pathological anatomy. His lengthy article on peritonitis appeared in 1802, during his second year of Paris training; it has since been recognized as the first description of that disease. He also taught private courses in dissection and began a never-to-be-finished treatise on pathology. In 1803 Laennec took first prize in both medicine and surgery, and in 1804 he became a doctor after defending his thesis on Hippocrates.

Despite the academic success, Laennec and his teachers regarded one another with only qualified esteem. Swayed by the political and religious conservatism of his friends, Laennec cultivated the classics, followed religion, and openly supported a return to the monarchy. To find a job in the liberal, atheist climate of postrevolutionary medicine, he needed more than his prizes and his precocious publications. For twelve years he struggled with his research, living from the proceeds of a private clientele. His fortunes did not improve until Napoleon was defeated at Waterloo in 1815 and the throne was restored to Louis XVIII, brother of Louis XVI, who had been decapitated in January 1793.

Discovery: Myth and 'Reality'

> I have tried to place the internal organic lesions on the same plane as the surgical diseases with respect to diagnosis.
>
> – R. Laennec, *Traité de l'auscultation médiate* (1826), 1: xxv

In September 1816, just one year after the restoration, Laennec was finally awarded (or rewarded with) an official position in the Necker hospital. During that fall or in the early winter, he made the observation that established his reputation. According to his own account, he was examining a young female in whom he suspected a heart problem, but because of her stoutness, percussion was unhelpful. He thought of placing his ear directly on her chest to learn more about her heart, but decorum dictated restraint. Rolling a notebook into a cylinder, he placed one end on her chest, the other to his ear, and was astonished to hear the beating of her heart.

Years later this tale was embellished by J.A. de Kergaradec, a former student of Laennec, who wrote that just before the consultation, Laennec had been crossing the courtyard of the Louvre, where he saw children playing an acoustic game with a log. When the ear was applied to one end of the log, a pin tapping at the other end could easily be heard.

The 'discovery' at the bedside of the well-endowed young patient was simply the rediscovery of a phenomenon: sound can be transmitted through a mediator. Interpretation of these transmitted sounds consumed Laennec's attention for the next two and a half years; the hospital patients were his focus. His new instrument allowed him to listen at a discreet distance that satisfied both modesty and hygiene.

Laennec's method was clinicopathological correlation. Initially, he busied his students with rolling notebooks into tight 'cylinders,' as he called the first stethoscopes, sealed with gummed paper and string. Then he examined patients by percussion and 'mediate auscultation' (active listening through a mediator) (see figure 9.1). The history and physical findings were carefully recorded. Laennec had to invent words to describe the sounds he heard: rales, crepitations, murmurs, pectoriloquy, bronchophony, egophony. When a patient died, the autopsy was correlated with the clinical findings.

Laennec later named his cylinder 'stethoscope' (from the Greek words for 'chest' and 'to explore'). In less than three years, he had established the anatomical significance of most of the normal and abnormal breath sounds still in use today. His book *De l'auscultation médiate* (On mediate auscultation) was written by February 1819, published in July, translated into English by 1821, and republished in the United States by 1823. A few doctors preferred the pathology in his treatise to the 'gimmick' of the stethoscope, but their opposition soon melted away.

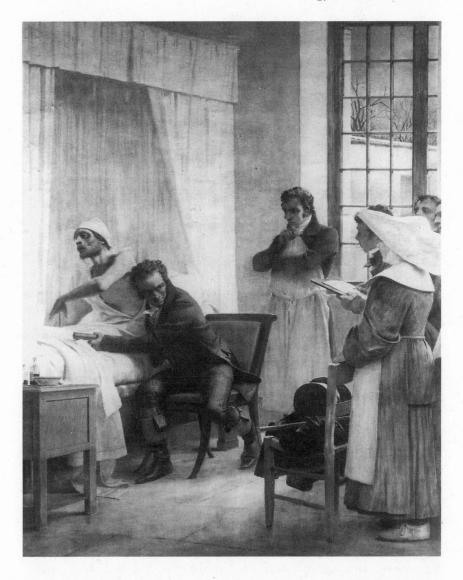

9.1   Laennec practising direct auscultation on a patient in the Necker hospital. Laennec preferred to use his stethoscope (which he is holding in his hand) because he was more comfortable at a distance from patients of differing sex and class. Mural by Théobald Chartran, late nineteenth century. Sorbonne, Paris

---

Laennec's Reaction to a Critic

I especially like the disadvantages that [Mérat] finds in a purely
mechanical technique, which will tend to turn physicians
away from skillful conjectures over the pulse, the facies, and
excrement. It is the same as refusing to dash around Paris in a
cabriolet for fear of losing the ability to tiptoe over droppings
in the street.

– Laennec, letter to his cousin, 24 April 1820; cited in J. Duffin,
To See with a Better Eye, Princeton U Press (1998), 218

Laennec also described the heart sounds and murmurs, but his
interpretation differed from ours. He thought that the first heart
sound represented ventricular contraction because of its synchrony with the carotid pulse; he assumed that the second sound must
be due to atrial contraction. Some historians wonder how Laennec
could have been 'right' on the lung and so 'wrong' on the heart;
however, three more decades of research, including the advent of
cardiac catheterization, were to pass before the valvular synchrony of
the sounds could be established with confidence.

Laennec enjoyed many favours from his royalist connections: a
professorship in the medical faculty, a chair at the Collège de France,
and an appointment as court physician. With the growing fame of
auscultation, he soon attracted a following of foreign students. In
response to criticisms, a considerably rearranged second edition
of his book was released in May 1826. But three months later, the
author was dead of tuberculosis at age forty-five. During his last illness, friends had examined the inventor with his stethoscope, but
they concealed their findings to keep up his spirits. His Parisian colleagues did not eulogize him until more than a decade had passed.
Most historians ascribe the hostility to religious and political differences, but medical philosophy also played a role.

The Inventor's Doubts

Nicknamed 'cylindromaniac,' Laennec was thought to be overreliant on his new invention; however, close study of his writings does not support the contention. His doubts about anatomical medicine and his ideas about the connection between *psyche* and *soma* brought him more disrepute than did his religion or politics. He believed that a person's mental state influenced health and that the causes of diseases such as asthma, angina, tuberculosis, and cancer did not lie in anatomy alone. Something else must precede the physical change. To explain these illnesses, he cited the psychic trauma of the Reign of Terror and the Napoleonic Wars. Auscultation and anatomy were limited, he reasoned, because they could detect only some of the myriad causes of disease.

Laennec warned his colleagues against relying too heavily on organic explanations. To his contemporaries, this 'vitalistic' philosophy from an innovator was paradoxical and reactionary (see chapter 3). By advocating that doctors listen not only to their patients' chests but to their stories as well, Laennec appeared to reject the very revolution that his stethoscope had endorsed. But his personal doubts were swept away and forgotten in the new-found enthusiasm for his method.

Impact of the Discovery

The stethoscope was the first diagnostic instrument to achieve rapid international popularity. Even Laennec's enemies adopted the stethoscope, impressed by how easily and accurately it detected signs of internal change. Within a short time, it was transported across Europe and to North America by the numerous foreign students. Robert Carswell, John Thomson, and James Clark of Britain and James Kitchen of the United States visited Laennec's clinics, lectures, and autopsies to become early advocates. Pierre de Beaubien, a Montrealer who studied in Paris, referred to the instrument in his 1827 thesis, and he likely was the first to bring it to Canada.

Anatomy had suddenly been made to fit into clinical medicine. The state of internal organs could now be 'explored' long before the patient became a cadaver. Laennec began to define lung diseases by their anatomical lesions rather than by the symptoms. Using Greek and Latin derivatives, he coined the terms 'bronchiectasis' and 'pulmonary edema,' while 'consumption' soon became 'tuberculosis' (a name change attributed to J.L. Schönlein in the mid-1830s). Together with the older terms 'emphysema' (puffed up) and 'empyema,' these new words signified diseases in the living rather than pathological change in the dead.

Medical professionals quickly learned to identify disease by the signs of anatomical lesions, many of which were dragged from the realm of curiosity to diagnostic sine qua non. The process extended beyond the chest. Appendicitis, gastroenteritis, cholecystitis, and chlorosis were soon described as separate clinical entities with specific anatomical, microscopic, or chemical definitions. Proponents of neurology and phrenology began correlating behaviour, function, personality, and deviance with lesions in the brain or spinal cord, and with bumps on the head.

Some doctors enthusiastically predicted that all diseases would soon be linked to internal organic changes. This medical philosophy, called organicism, dominated research in the early nineteenth century: diseases were equated with and reduced to their anatomical change, and that change also became the cause. New technologies were devised to serve this new agenda, and the patient's account of symptoms paled in comparison with the objective search for inner change. Laennec had used his ear to 'see' inside the body – visualization of the small inner workings was the agenda. This process continued into the twentieth century.

The stages in the history of this single technology are relevant to all other technological innovations. No discovery is made in isolation without a rich context of antecedents and milieu; no invention will succeed without a perceived need; and no device can be widely employed without also changing its setting, sometimes in unexpected ways.

Technologies and Technopolies – More Gadgets

If a mediator helped in listening to the chest, other instruments might help with percussion, visualization, and measurements of all kinds. Old instruments were redesigned and new ones invented. The durability of each invention relied on its power to demonstrate previously invisible material change to the senses of hearing, touch, and especially sight. Some of these technologies have direct descendants; others disappeared quickly. For example, in 1826 Pierre-Adolphe Piorry invented the pleximeter to improve percussion; a small plate and a hammer, it was more cumbersome than useful, and its popularity was short-lived.

Stethoscopes were modified to adapt to differing circumstances, always with an eye to aesthetic form. The rigid cylinder gave way to slender curved models, then to a flexible monaural (one earpiece) stethoscope by 1843, and in 1852 G.P. Camman of New York proposed a binaural (two earpieces) model. After the 1895 discovery of X-rays, the fluoroscopic stethoscope, called 'see-hear,' or 'stethophone,' allowed examiners not only to hear but also to see inside their patients' chests.

Auscultation relied on the examiner's hearing, but the sounds evoked visual images of internal anatomy: for example, pectoriloquy indicated a cavity in the lung. In this manner, the stethoscope is akin to a speculum. Newer diagnostic instruments also appeal to vision (see table 9.1). Some catered to the sense of sight either directly or indirectly by the use of mirrors. Among these were the first illuminated endoscope (1807), the laryngoscope (1829), the ophthalmoscope (1851), and the bronchoscope (1897). Canulas, fibre optics, and lasers have extended this technology beyond the realm of diagnosis into surgical therapeutics.

Microscopes, X-rays, and Imaging

Priority is difficult to assign. The microscope is usually described as the invention of the Dutch naturalist and optician Antonie van Leeuwenhoek in 1670, but magnifiers of small objects date back to the family of Zacharias Jansen of Holland in the sixteenth century and to Galileo Galilei of Italy and Robert Hooke of London. Until Laennec's time, however, doctors may have been ready to ponder anatomy at the level of tissues, but they mistrusted the microscope. They preferred the naked eye, assuming that less visible changes were inconsequential.

With the new anatomical focus of the 1820s and 1830s, efforts were made to improve the microscope. Compound lenses, correc-

Table 9.1
Advent of some diagnostic technologies*

Year	Technology	Inventor	Nationality
1590	microscope	Jansen	Dutch
1614	thermometer	Santorio	Italian
1670	microscope	van Leeuwenhoek	Dutch
1807	light endoscopy	Bozzini	Italian in Germany
1819	stethoscope	Laennec	French
1826	pleximeter	Piorry	French
1829	laryngoscope	Babington	English
1830s	compound microscope	Donné, Addison	French, English
1851	ophthalmoscope	von Helmholtz	German
1865	microtome	His	Swiss German
1867	clinical thermometry	Wunderlich	German
1881	syphgmomanometer	von Basch	Austrian
1895	X-rays	Röntgen	German
1897	bronchoscope	Killian	German
1903	ECG	Einthoven	Dutch
1925	EEG	Pravditchi-Neminsky	Russian
1938	^{131}I in thyroid	Hamilton and Soley	American
1940	cardiac catheterization	Cournand	French
1952	radio-isotope scanning	Heilmeyer	German
1954	echocardiography	Edler and Hertz	Swedish
1957	gamma-camera	Anger	American
1962	^{99}Tc	Harper	American
1971	computerized imaging (CT)	Cormack/Hounsfield	American, British
1974	recombinant DNA	S. Cohen/H. Boyer	American
1983	MRI	Lauterbur/Mansfield	American, British
1983	polymerase chain reaction (PCR)	Mullis	American
1991	functional MRI – brain	Belliveau	American
2000	PET scan	R. Nutt/D. Townsend	Swiss

*Dates are approximate and apply to invention, patent, use, or publication.

tions in spherical aberration, the advent of histological stains (1840), and immersion microscopy (1844) enhanced magnification and improved visualization. The result was a new pathology of microanatomy – tissues, cells, and organelles. The electron microscope, first constructed in 1931 by German physicists Max Knoll and Ernst A.F. Ruska, extended the visualization to the level of molecules. Fifty-five years later, Ruska shared the Nobel Prize in physics for this work.

In December 1895, Wilhelm Conrad Röntgen gave his first formal lecture on the properties of X-rays. Scholars contend that this powerful discovery has influenced medicine more profoundly than any other technology. The very size of the machines determined a physician-centred locus of practice. The news spread rapidly around the world – for example, just a few weeks later, in February 1896, X-rays were taken in Kingston, Ontario. Soon the anatomical exploration of the chest could be accomplished by images as well as sound. Thomas Edison devised fluoroscopy, making it possible to view the images in real time. Ingenious applications of contrast media, including air, barium, and dyes, resulted in miraculously clear definition of tumors, spinal disorders, and vascular lesions. The interior of the brain could be investigated with carotid angiography, developed in 1941 by A.F. Cournand. Some radiographic tests, such as the pneumoencephalogram (1919), were painful and risky for the patient.

Technologies that are the direct descendants of radiography enhanced the visualization of soft tissue and reduced the need for invasive procedures; they contributed greatly to patient comfort even as they extended diagnosis. Echocardiography (1954) was derived from the ultrasound principles used to track submarines in the Second World War; it has proved particularly useful in assessing heart valves and muscle. Computerized axial tomography, which provided astonishing detail of lesions as small as one centimetre, was the invention of Allan M. Cormack and Godfrey N. Hounsfield; the first scanner was used at Wimbledon, UK, in 1971. Extending this success theoretically and technically, nuclear magnetic resonance was proposed and demonstrated as an imaging technique (nMRI) in the early 1970s, but it was not practicable until the late 1980s, and brain applications came in 1993.

Many of these achievements won their inventors the Nobel Prize: Röntgen in 1901 (physics); Cournand in 1956; and Cormack and Hounsfield in 1979. Three Nobels were awarded for MRI: R. Ernst in 1991 (physics) and Paul C. Lauterbur and Peter Mansfield in 2003. (The 2003 prize was hotly contested, confirming the observations above about antecedents and priority.) The short interval between these discoveries and the Nobel honours indicates the rapid acceptance of these contributions. Some inventions were adopted even before their value had been clearly established – perhaps because they seemed to fill long-recognized needs and because they upheld the image of medicine as 'science' and doctor as 'scientist.'

Thermometers, Kymographs, and Other Devices for Seeing the Invisible

Still others instruments, such as thermometers and kymographs, translated information of a non-visual nature into a visual display with graphs, charts, and numbers (see chapter 3). The early thermometers, as invented by Santorio Santorio in the seventeenth century, were too unwieldy for clinical use. But by the 1870s, Karl Wunderlich and Edouard Séguin had used statistical data to write their influential treatises on the visual assessment of body heat; now perceived to be of clinical value, the instrument was reduced to a tiny rod that could be slipped into a pocket.

In 1861 Jean-Baptiste A. Chauveau and E. Jules Marey took Karl Ludwig's 1846 invention of the kymograph and applied it to recording pressure changes in vessels and in the catheterized hearts of living animals. Twenty years later, S.S. von Basch devised a sphygmomanometer, and in 1905 Nicolai S. Korotkov demonstrated how it could be used with the stethoscope to measure blood pressure. The result was the creation of the new and previously inconceivable disease that now reaches epidemic proportions in an aging population – hypertension.

By 1903, Willem Einthoven had invented an electrocardiograph to translate the electrical function of the beating heart into a visual tracing for easy analysis. This electrical pattern refined the clinical diagnosis of angina and myocardial infarction. Previously detected only at autopsy and debated even then, myocardial infarction emerged from a vague set of earlier diagnoses, including acute indigestion and apoplexy. Einthoven was awarded the Nobel Prize in 1924. His work is often cited as the beginning of modern cardiology.

Like the stethoscope, all these diagnostic technologies were invented to 'see' beyond the patient's story into the patient's body to identify a material basis for the symptoms. Insurance companies quickly embraced the technology revolution, welcoming the predictive value of objective signs of disease in subjective states of health. If visual norms could be found, then a range of deviations could be established; physical examination of the healthy became routine. The word 'natural' to denote health was slowly replaced by the more numerical word 'normal' (see chapter 4). Instrumentation satisfied the objectives of a knowledge system that increasingly valued numbers. Changing disease concepts drove the search for new technologies; in turn, the new technologies drove disease concepts by finding new disorders and discrediting others.

Hospital as Machine

As places of care for sick or poor people who could not look after themselves, hospitals are ancient. In antiquity the hospital may have been more like a 'hotel' for ailing travellers located near a healing temple: a 'xenodochion.' The Romans created special 'valetudinaria' for sick soldiers and wounded gladiators, but these buildings did not serve ordinary citizens, women, or slaves, nor were they widespread. Scholars debate whether or not ancient south Asia had early precursors for the hospital. As a house of care in Europe, the hospital was inspired by Persia and Arabia. Crusaders returning to Europe from Palestine brought back the concept of 'mauristan' and the idea of grouping the sick for their physical and spiritual well-being. Historian Timothy Miller argues that, en route, the medieval versions may have lost the curative goals of their Byzantine precursors.

From the eleventh century, monasteries and convents all across Europe developed hospitals within their precincts; one of the main functions of the religious became care of the sick and shelter for those awaiting death. Often the vast ward would feature an altar for religious services and a nearby garden for medicinal herbs as well as food. Certain orders specialized in hospital work, which they conducted on the basis of charity with church approval. Some hospitals focused on diseases that others would not admit – leprosaria and pest-houses. Municipalities also designated dwellings for the care of the sick in times of outbreaks, and the functions sometimes continued when the danger was past. To sustain these activities, civilians would form confraternities, like the service clubs of today – almost always with a saint as patron, if not the deity himself – l'Hôtel Dieu. With few exceptions, these hospitals were small: at least 1,200 were founded in England and Wales, and thousands more in France. According to historian Daniel Hickey, every region, most towns, and even some villages had a hospital. Gradually some specialized in housing certain people: soldiers, women, or children. Rules governed eligibility for admission; food was simple; beds were shared. Wealthy people avoided hospitals at all cost.

In the new world, hospitals appeared with the first European settlements – although not all have survived; they were modelled on their religious predecessors in the colonizing countries. In Mexico City, Hospital de Jesus Nazareno claims to be the oldest hospital in the western hemisphere, founded in the early sixteenth century by the conquistador Hernán Cortés; portions of its present architecture dating from the seventeenth century are tourist attractions. The Hôtel-Dieu hospital of Quebec City began in 1639; three years later another Hôtel-Dieu opened in Montréal founded by the French-born Jeanne Mance, now a candidate for beatification (see figure 9.2). Both hospitals maintain fascinating museums. Pennsylvania Hospital of Philadelphia, founded by Benjamin Franklin in 1751, is the oldest in the United States; it carefully maintains the original building with a library and operating theatre.

By 1800 in many European countries these sites of charitable care had become the locus of medical education, especially in large cities. Political revolutions, as described above, wrested the ownership of great hospitals from religious caregivers, although in many cases the nuns and monks were retained because no one else would provide care. Wealthy benefactors established charitable institutions as a public testament to compassion and civic pride. (On the special case of asylums and mental hospitals, see chapter 12.)

Friction arose when doctors came into the wards to teach, especially with their interest in dissection. The rise of anatomy provided yet another reason for people of means to avoid hospitals. New attention to hospital architecture, light, and space, was turning the religious sanctuary into a purpose-built place of research and education, if not healing. In the vision of the French health reformer J.R. Tenon, the hospital itself was a medical machine – 'un instrument qui facilite la curation' (cited in D.B. Weiner, *The Citizen-Patient in Revolutionary and Imperial Paris*, Johns Hopkins U Press, 1993, 373). As a result, Michel Foucault and others referred to hospitals as 'les machines à guérir' (machines for curing).

Several important events in the late nineteenth century consoli-

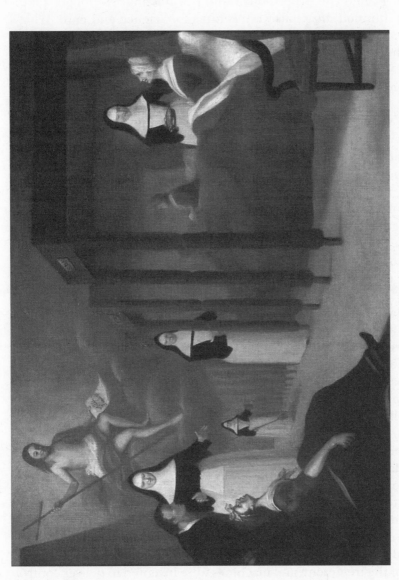

9.2 Hospital as a site of healing. Patients in the Hôtel-Dieu in Montreal being cared for by the nuns under the watchful eye of their saviour. Anon., ca 1710. Musée des Hospitalières de l'Hôtel-Dieu, Montreal

dated this transformation: anesthesia, antisepsis, germ theory, bacteriology, and the professionalization of nursing. No longer places to be shunned, hospitals were centres for science and cure. What's more, some of the new achievements, such as laboratories, operating theatres, and X-ray machines, were far too big and specialized to be found anywhere but the hospital. Now wealthy people needed – even wanted – the hospital. Special new provisions had to meet their expectations – private rooms above all; philanthropic initiatives, many sponsored by middle-class ladies, often doctors' wives, sought to elevate standards of food, linen, privacy, comfort, and hygiene. Hospitals were under pressure to keep up with technology, and the aid societies committed to fundraising. With no government sources of fundings, hospitals were torn between two obligations: the demand for up-to-date medical services and the need to serve the indigent population. Following the Second World War a construction boom and the possibility of health insurance led to more and bigger hospitals.

By the mid-twentieth century, new definitions of neurological, respiratory, and cardiac failure prompted investigation and management by special machines that were available only in hospitals (see table 9.2). The walking well would be admitted – sometimes for several weeks – to undergo diagnostic 'tests.' Instruments to replace the work of breathing were invented to help tide people over temporary incapacity. Although attempts to resuscitate near-dead newborns and drowning victims can be traced to biblical antiquity, the epidemic of poliomyelitis stimulated further development of intubation, iron lungs, and ventilators, now applied to many other situations. The number of patients ventilated for more than twenty-four hours at the Massachusetts General Hospital increased from sixty-six in 1958 to more than two thousand by 1982 (Snider 1989). Soon bypass machines could also temporarily replace the work of heart and lungs rescuing people from devastating pneumonias and permitting ever more elaborate surgeries to repair heart problems.

Radiation technology not only detected tumour masses, it became part of the treatment, and machines were invented to deliver controlled doses. At first, techniques relied on brachytherapy (treatment at short distance), with radium and later cesium applied to tumours

Table 9.2
Advent of some therapeutic technologies*

Year	Technology	Inventor	Nationality
1881	neonatal incubator	E.S. Tarnier	French
1898	radium	Marie Curie	Polish-French
1929	iron lung	P. Drinker	American
1934	heart-lung machine	M.F. DeBakey/J.H. Gibbon	American
1940	^{32}P for polycythemia	J. H. Lawrence	American
1941	^{131}I for hyperthyroidism	S. Hertz/A. Robert	American
1943	renal dialysis	W.J. Kolff	Dutch-American
1950	IPP ventilators	many models	American-British
1951	Cobalt^{60} teletherapy	H.E. Johns	Canadian
1953	linear accelerator P. Howard-Flanders	D. Fry/ C. Miller,	British
1956	membrane oxygenator	G.H. Clowes/W.J. Kolff	American
1958	implanted pacemaker	R. Elmquist/A. Senning	Sweden
1968	total parenteral nutrition	S. Dudrick	American
1975	ambulatory dialysis	R.P. Popovich	American
1980	recombinant DNA	S. Cohen/H. Boyer	American
1982	artificial heart	R.K. Jarvik	American
1982	synthetic human insulin	Genetech & Eli Lilly	American
1983	cochlear implant	Graeme Clark	Australian
1985	laparoscopic cholecystectomy	E. Mühe	German

* Dates are approximate and apply to invention, patent, use, or publication.

inside needles, tubes, and plaques. Later, teletherapy (treatment at long distance) was developed, characterized by high-energy beams from X-ray machines, cobalt units, or linear accelerators.

As the new diagnostic machines further refined the problems, yet more technological invention was needed to solve them. The analysis of cardiac arrhythmias, blood gases, respiratory function resulted in new methods to manage these previously unimagined conditions. For example, the clinical definition of ventricular fibrillation subtended a role for defibrillators. Similarly, an understanding of metabolic imbalance, diffusion properties, and anticoagulation revised the treatment of kidney failure by dialysis. Elegant monitors, catheters, respirators, and pumps occupy the newly vested sanctuaries of healing – units for intensive care, coronary care, respiratory care, neonatal care, kidney dialysis, and cancer clinics. Hospitals had become very expensive.

With the financial crisis of the 1990s, the prevalence of in-hospital care and investigation was questioned. Economists showed that if any bed was available, it would be occupied, costing money. Indeed, in the United States, with its market-based approach to hospital care, beds *should* be occupied to keep income higher than expenses. Elsewhere, to reduce costs small hospitals were closed and numbers of acute-care beds were reduced with a concomitant centralization of investigative and treatment technologies. The biggest reductions took place in countries where the state had most control and the bed-per-capita ratio was high: in the former Soviet Union, Scandinavia, Western Europe, and Canada. In Great Britain, acute-care beds were replaced by more chronic-care beds, but in most other countries promises for more long-term and home-care facilities were not kept. These changes often met with public outcry; people resented the loss of jobs, security, and prestige afforded by the venerable institutions central to their communities. Research on the reductions has mostly come from Canada, where it has yet to be correlated with an anticipated rise in mortality or decline in health indicators.

According to the Organization for Economic Co-operation and Development (OECD) acute-care hospital beds per capita have been declining since the mid-1970s in all wealthy countries at rates directly proportional to the original density. The capacity varies enormously from country to country. Canada, the United Kingdom, and the United States now have between 2 and 3 beds per thousand population, but Germany has more than 6, and Japan 8.2, a drop from 12.3 in 1993 – a density well above any documented for other wealthy countries.

The biggest problem is that, despite a half-century of research on the issue, no one knows the 'right' number of beds for any region. On the one hand, ideal numbers depend on the country and its prevalent diseases; on the other, technologies and diseases are constantly changing. No precise formula can be obtained, and it is likely that at any given moment, need and availability do not match.

By 2000, the hospital had become a place for scientific investigation and cure, furnished with expensive equipment and essential to rich and poor alike. The very sick needed the life support that could be provided only there. Those who were not sick at all occasionally entered the hospital for diagnosis, but the tests could be done on short visits. The chronically ill, the homeless, the poor, and the disabled – the very people who once populated the hospitals – were less welcome. 'Les machines à guérir' are now looking for ways to recover and fulfil their original purpose as charitable houses of care.

Biotechnology

In February 1975, a group of scientists gathered at Asilomar conference centre on the California coast to discuss the future and responsible uses of recombinant DNA. Discovered in the previous year by Stanley Cohen and Herbert Boyer, the process was already awaiting a patent, which would not be awarded until 1980. The technique allowed bits of human genes to be copied and spliced into the DNA of other organisms, such as bacteria, which would then produce human proteins. These scientists were already aware that something completely new was about to happen: the long-promised genetic engineering was about to become a reality with myriad experiments, investigations, and treatments. The scientists also knew that money could be made from the genes of others, raising concerns about possible abuses. Many cite this moment as the beginnings of biotechnology and refer to it as 'Asilomar.'

Cohen stayed in academe; Boyer joined with a venture capitalist to found Genentech, the world's first biotech company; its first drug product was synthetic human insulin, made in 1978 and patented in 1982.

The next exciting step in this new trend was the discovery of polymerase chain reaction (PCR) by Kary Mullis in 1983. This technique made it possible to quickly replicate (or amplify) large amounts from a single strand of DNA, rather than waiting for generations of bacteria to grind out the precious products.

These achievements were applied to diagnosis – of tumours, of cells, of bacteria and viruses – and to treatment, as 'drugs' matched to human proteins are made to react to these new genomic types, vaccines, hormones, and anti-cancer drugs. In the first decade five biotech agents received approval: insulin (1982), human growth hormone (1985), hepatitis B vaccine (1986), tissue plasminogen activator (tPa, 1987), and alpha-interferon (1990). By 2004, thirty-two new agents were approved in a single year. Within the first two decades, revenues of the biotech industry in the United States soared from nothing to $30 billion annually (see chapter 5). The interest in stem cells is fraught with ethical difficulties, especially in the United States, reminding us that bioethics grew as a discipline in conjunction with this rise in biotechnology and clinical trials (see chapter 6).

The new techniques also meant that visualization, so deeply entrenched for two centuries as a leitmotif in medical technology, was gradually being displaced by molecular identity. Some historians believe that biotechnology has created an entirely new paradigm in the conception of disease and in medical practice – a paradigm that eclipses the anatomical, body-based medicine of the last two hundred years. Tumours, bacteria, and viruses are now being classified and subdivided by genetic characteristics, and new drugs are generated to target those signature molecules. 'Patients' are identified by their molecular makeup –rather than by their symptoms or even their physical findings, while the notion of risk has itself become a disease that demands treatment. This chapter is still being written, and perhaps it is too early to tell if those historians are right.

Distance between Doctor and Patient

> Since I do not foresee that atomic energy is to be a great boon for a long time, I have to say that for the present it is a menace.
>
> – Albert Einstein, *Atlantic Monthly*, November 1945

Early detection of disease and diagnostic precision have irrefutable benefits, but they come at a price that critics of modern medicine have called the 'tyranny of the normal.' Prior to the stethoscope, patients could not be sick unless they felt sick. After the stethoscope, it was possible to have a serious disease and feel fine. The patient was no longer the chief authority on his or her own well-being.

In our hypermedicalized world, these principles are deeply ingrained. Most people with hypertension have no symptoms at all, but they readily accept a machine's diagnosis even when it obliges them to take pills for many years. With the advent of biotechnology, the line between normal and abnormal becomes blurred because we now know that many gene variants can exist without causing harm. Which ones should be treated ? Whose genes count as normal?

Only the psychiatric diseases have no objective organic or chemical correlatives (see chapter 12). Patients who feel sick but in whom no material sign of disease can be found have 'merely functional' ailments or are mentally disturbed. And they are considered less seriously ill than those who may feel completely well but have technologically defined diseases.

Just as critics of medical ideas deplore the devaluing of subjective accounts of illness, critics of medical technology lament the distance interposed between the doctor and the patient. They complain that medicine treats the data, not the person. Dissatisfaction with impersonal technology generates interest in alternative medicine and holistic explanations. Technology also separates the patient from his or her disease, elevating it to the status of a living enemy that must be hunted and destroyed. If the disease is chronic or congenital, then attacking it seems unnecessary and even self-destructive; for example, vigorous opposition to cochlear implants arose from the deaf community, which viewed the rigorous application of this technology as a form of cultural genocide.

Some critics, like writer Neil Postman, situate the origin of medicine's loss of empathy in Laennec and his stethoscope, but they do not realize that the inventor harboured doubts about the trend that he is said to have launched. In adjusting to the high-tech world, many physicians meditate on losses and gains. Historian Joel Howell studied the hospital use of blood tests, urinalysis, and X-rays, and noted an irony: technologies may save time, but doctors now spend less time with patients than they did before. Similar ironies have been observed by other historians of science: Edward Tenner wrote how computers had promised to save paper but, instead, have vastly increased its consumption; historians of 'women's work' have shown that the 'labour-saving devices' for homemakers did not live up to their promise. Technologies can backfire, but their tremendous advantages make their side effects seem like the norm.

The history of technology is just beginning. It will demonstrate the ingenious solutions and marvellous potential of medical invention. It will reveal how each new technology created new diseases where none had been conceived. And it will uncover more fascinating discrepancies between the aspirations of inventors and the applications that their instruments subsequently find.

Suggestions for Further Reading

At the bibliography website http://histmed.ca.

CHAPTER TEN

Work of the Hand: History of Surgery*

Any fool can cut off a leg. It takes a surgeon to save one.

– George Ross of Montreal

Recurrent Themes

Surgery and medicine are now mutually dependent; however, in the past they were separate. The so-called surgical personality originates in the perceived difference between surgical and medical work. The word 'surgery' is derived from the Greek for 'work' and 'hand.' Some cultures looked on handwork as menial and ranked it below that done by the mind. Others, more like our own, have prized it above all other skills. Variations in the relative status of surgery and medicine will be a theme of this chapter.

Surgery may be the oldest of all medical activities. Cave paintings of injured hunters show that prehistoric people responded to the accidental trauma of existence. But not all trauma is accidental. Neolithic peoples used arrows and rocks to injure enemies deliberately, and they devised procedures to treat wounds. The dangerous technologies of warfare generate a need for compensatory surgical techniques, which then find peacetime applications. This, too, is a recurring theme in surgery's past.

*Learning objectives for this chapter are found on p. 454.

Two other themes can be traced throughout this history. First, the profession of medicine as a whole shaped its structure and values from surgical models. Second, elective procedures – those done by intention and not of necessity – gradually became more frequent through time and are now the result of complex, cautious choice.

Prehistoric and Ancient Surgery

Prehistoric medicine is said to have involved cooking and mixing foodstuffs, but early traces of this activity are scarce. In contrast, evidence from paleopathology and comparative anthropology testifies to the prevalence of surgery. Bark splints for setting fractures date back to at least 2450 B.C. Similarly, skulls from the Neolithic period (10,000 to 5000 B.C.) indicate the great antiquity of the elective procedure of trephination, in which a flap of bone was removed.

Why were early peoples motivated to drill holes in the skull? Answers can only be conjectured. Attention may have been directed to the cranium, perhaps by headache or seizures, or by loss of consciousness following a blow. Observers, who possibly had noticed survival in victims with open fractures, might have decided to open the skull deliberately by boring holes with stone implements. The practice may have been justified by ideas such as releasing of pressure or dispelling of evil humours and malevolent spirits. Fossil remains with bony healing show that the treatment, if not curative, was at least survivable. Between 3000 and 2000 B.C., trephination was relatively common in South America, Western Europe, and Asia. Today, bore holes are indicated when an epidural or subdural hematoma is suspected, but no evidence tells us if prehistoric surgeons conceived of those conditions.

Other sources of information about prehistoric surgery derive from present-day cultures that are isolated from modern technology. For example, biting insects continue to be used as sutures in parts of Africa and South America. The edges of the wound are brought together and an ant is allowed to bite through both 'lips'; when its jaws are firmly locked, the insect's thorax and abdomen are broken off, leaving the head and jaws as a neat staple. Similarly, stitches of plant and animal materials are used to bring the edges of wounds together.

Wound dressings are also ancient. Traditionally, Amerindians applied botanical substances to injuries; recently botanists have begun to examine what the active principles might be. The earliest-known example of medical writing is said to be a Sumerian recipe for a beer poultice dressing that was inscribed around 2100 B.C. on the clay Nippur tablet, which is now in the University Museum, Philadelphia.

Surgery also features in the famous Babylonian Code of Hammurabi of ca 1700 B.C. Incised on a tall black stone that is now in the Louvre, it describes draconian punishments for surgical 'malpractice.' If a surgeon harmed a free man's slave, he had to replace the slave; if the patient who was harmed was a free man, the surgeon's hand was to be cut off.

In ancient Egypt, some surgeons were members of the elite. The deified architect and physician Imhotep is thought to have written early surgical texts, but his life is shrouded in mystery. Hesy Ré, chief of dentists and surgeons, was identified by the wooden panels taken from his tomb. Now in the Cairo Museum, they portray him as a scribe or learned man. Other painted objects found in his tomb resemble a series of graduated cylinders.

The most complete treatises from ancient Egypt are papyrus scrolls that describe the practice of surgery. These documents are usually known by the names of the adventurers who purchased (or stole) them for taking home to Europe or America – for example, the 20-metre-long Ebers papyrus (1550 B.C.) purchased by German professor Georg Ebers in the mid-nineteenth century, and the Edwin Smith papyrus (ca 1600 B.C.), a 4½-metre scroll, which was found by Edwin Smith in 1862 and now resides in the Malloch Rare Book Room of the New York Academy of Medicine. Neither of these documents was deciphered by the men whose names they bear. Only after the 1930 translation and interpretation by James Henry Breasted of Chicago was the Edwin Smith papyrus shown to be an incomplete surgical text based on even earlier writings (ca 3000 B.C.). It describes forty-eight case histories, each with a title and instructions for diagnosis and management. It also includes a glossary of ancient terms and stated that some conditions were not to be treated.

Case 25 of the Edwin Smith Papyrus

If thou examinest a man having a dislocation in his mandible
... thou shouldst put thy thumb(s) upon the ends of the two
rami of the mandible in the inside of his mouth, (and) thy
two claws (... fingers) under his chin, (and) thou shouldst
cause them to fall back so that they rest in their places ... Thou
shouldst say concerning him: '... an ailment which I will treat.'
Thou shouldst bind it with *ymrw*, (and) honey every day until
he recovers.

– *The Edwin Smith Surgical Papyrus*, trans. J.H. Breasted (Chicago, 1930), 303–5

As a religious practice, the ancient Egyptians mummified their
dead. Mummification led to experimentation in 'surgical' procedures
such as suturing. The stitches of one embalmer on the abdomen of
a mummy have been dated to at least 1100 B.C. Breasted argued that
papyri recommended suturing for wounds. This opinion is controversial, however, because sutures in mummies are rare, and evidence
is evanescent elsewhere as a result of the organic decay. Dexterity in
removing organs through small orifices was part of the embalmer's
skill, but its impact on treatment of the living is uncertain.

Evidence for trephination by the ancient Egyptians is scant, but
they practised some operations, such as circumcision of males and
possibly also of females. Together with trephination, circumcision
is among the oldest elective procedures. Phimosis and paraphimo-
sis constituted pathological indications for the operation, but it is
unique in its additional application to the healthy, be they infants
or adults. A bas-relief on a tomb of about 2500 B.C. in Saqqara, near
Memphis, seems to represent an assembly line for circumcision; differences in posture of the two clients – one being held, the other
not – may represent the effect of anesthetic. The Hebrew religious
practice of circumcision may have arisen in Egypt, for it is described
in the eighth-century B.C. Pentateuch of the Old Testament (Genesis
17:10–14; Exodus 4:25; Leviticus 12:3) and is said to have originated

following the exodus from Egypt around 1200 B.C. (Joshua 5:2–8). Female circumcision and infibulation are still practised in African societies. Like their male equivalents, the operators of female circumcision are part of religiosocial orders rather than healers. In Western traditions, elective surgery on healthy female parts found medical indications in the late nineteenth century in the procedures of ovariotomy for psychic disorders and of clitoridectomy for sexual ambiguity (see chapters 11 and 12).

Effective pain relief has been a preoccupation of most cultures; its absence was long a barrier to elective surgery. Some substances were moderately effective analgesics. The ancient Chinese used henbane, which contains the anticholinergic drug hyoscine. The ancient Hindus practised fumigation (or 'smoking') of wounds with soothing herbs. The Greeks made use of alcohol and opium. Christ on the cross was offered (but refused) a sponge soaked in a mixture to dull his pain (Matthew 27:34).

Even small wounds could be deadly until the recent past. Ancient Greek and Roman treatises contain recipes for wound washing, dressing, and binding. Wine, beer, myrrh, and rust were thought to promote healing. According to Homer, the heroic warriors acted as surgeons for each other; they bandaged wounds with healing substances, such as rust from their spears, to prevent what the Greeks called 'suppuration,' and what we know as infection. In his book *The Healing Hand*, Guido Majno analysed the anesthetic and antibiotic properties of ancient remedies for pain relief and infection control and found that many were efficacious within our own paradigm.

Cautery – or the searing of wounds with hot metal instruments or caustic dressings – was widely practised, especially by the Arabs. The Chinese practice of *moxa*, which applied heat at sites perhaps distant from a wound, was technically speaking not a form of cautery. Heat closed vessels to staunch bleeding, and it probably created temporary sterility. Cautery with red-hot irons was standard treatment for military wounds for centuries – but unless the patient was unconscious, it was exquisitely painful.

Fractures and dislocations resulted from athletics and warfare. Many references in the Hippocratic writings describe an evolving

science of orthopedics, which used mechanical apparatuses, posi-
tioning, ropes, and gravity for reducing fractures and dislocations.
Some Hippocratic texts, especially the *Oath*, seem to frown on specific uses of the knife, such as 'cutting for stone.' But others state
that abscesses should be incised and drained, while thoracentesis
for empyema (pus in the chest) was clearly described by Hippocrates (*Diseases II*, 47).

Greek and Hindu surgical instruments further extend our knowledge of early practices. Fibulae were safety-pin-like devices for wound
closure: both sides of a wound were transfixed with a needle (fib-
ula), around which thread was wrapped to approximate the edges.
Syringes were introduced by the Greeks for draining abscesses rather
than for injection. They were based on the principle of the piston,
supposedly invented by a barber in Alexandria around 280 B.C. The
Greek word for syringe, *pyulcos*, meant 'pus-puller,' and the earliest
reference is in the first-century A.D. treatise *Pneumatics* by Hero of
Alexandria. The Romans improved on surgical instruments, fashion-
ing tools from copper alloy. Unlike their Egyptian precursors, they
devised dental procedures with special forceps for tooth pulling or
filling, and they modelled false teeth in bone and gold for wealthy
clients.

One of the best sources on ancient Roman surgery was the work of
Celsus. His treatise *De medicina* describes a wide variety of procedures,
including lithotomy, hernia repair, eye operations, and decircumci-
sion, the last to be undertaken for aesthetic reasons. Scholars debate
whether or not he was a doctor or an encyclopedist.

Medieval Surgery

During the Christian-dominated Middle Ages in Europe, disease
was seen as divine punishment; care was welcomed, but efforts to
cure might be tantamount to hubris. Healing was an act of God or
one of his holy agents. The patron saints of medicine, pharmacy,
and surgery were the twin healers Cosmas and Damian, who supposedly had been martyred early in the fourth century A.D. (see figure
10.1) During their lives and after, they were reported to have effected miraculous cures, including the transplantation of a gangrenous

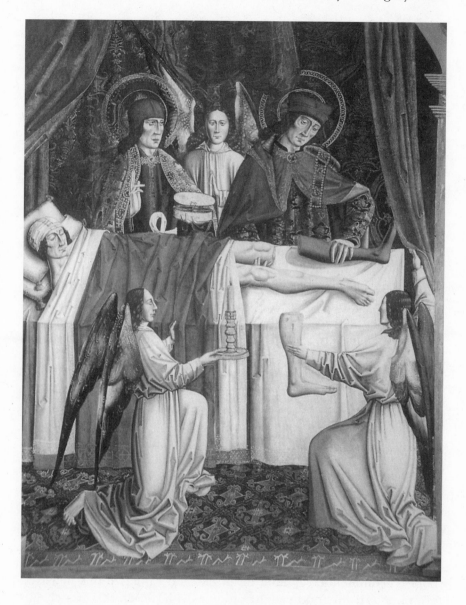

10.1   Medical saints Cosmas and Damian in the oft-depicted scene of the miraculous transplantation of a leg from a cadaver donor. Painting by Alonso de Sedano (fl. 1496), Spanish. Wellcome Institute Library, London

limb with a donor leg from a cadaver. Medical schools, hospices, and fraternities, including a Paris college of surgery, were named for these saints.

Religious conviction notwithstanding, surgical activities continued to deal with trauma. In twelfth-century Salerno, Italy, fresh wounds were thought to fare well if thick white or yellow pus could be made to appear. This pus was later called 'laudable' because it heralded healing. The unlaudable variety of pus was thin (serous), pink or red, seeped slowly from the wound, and was associated with spreading inflammation, cellulitis, and gangrene. Like their Greco-Roman precursors, medieval warriors cared for one another on the battlefield; the kit carried into the fourteenth-century battle of Crécy included tiny boxes packed with spiderweb to cover wounds.

In the later Middle Ages, a few surgeons rose to prominence through their teaching and writings. The works of the eleventh-century Andalusian surgeon Abu al-Qasim al-Zahrawi (Abulcasis or Albucasis) on bloodletting, cautery, operations, and instruments were translated into Latin in 1137. The 1300 *Chirurgia* of Henri de Mondeville emphasized anatomy and described techniques to dress wounds, relieve pain, and staunch bleeding, including the use of a tight band on a limb that was about to be amputated. De Mondeville taught that wounds could heal without suppuration. The *Chirurgia magna* (Great Surgery) of Guy de Chauliac, which appeared in 1363, also recognized the importance of anatomy, as it dealt with wounds, fractures, tumours, sores, hernias, ulcers, and cataracts. De Chauliac accepted the theory of laudable pus and devised poultices to encourage its formation. His ideas dominated surgical practice for the next two hundred years; the 1478 French translation was one of the earliest medical books to be printed with movable type.

The advent of gunpowder prompted further experimentation on wound management. In 1514 Giovanni de Vigo, surgeon to the pope, recommended boiling oil of elder to cauterize this new type of wound. His method caught on quickly; however, the French surgeon Ambroise Paré discovered quite by accident that the method was superfluous.

Paré's Accidental Discovery

My oil ran out and I had to apply a salve made of egg-white, rose-oil, and turpentine. The next night I slept badly, plagued by the thought that I would find the men dead whose wounds I had failed to burn, so I got up early to visit them. To my great surprise, those treated with salve felt little pain, showed no inflammation or swelling, and had passed the night rather calmly – while the ones on whom seething oil had been used lay in high fever with aches, swelling and inflammation around the wound.

> – Ambroise Paré, recalling the 1536 siege of Turin,
> cited in K. Haeger and R.Y. Calne, *The Illustrated History of Surgery*,
> 2nd ed. (Chicago: Harold Starke, 2000), 108

Paré wrote on many topics (see chapter 11). Later editions of his works and other early modern treatises on surgery often contained a 'wounds man' and commentary, illustrating how to manage each injury. Technical details were given for amputation, reduction of fractures, and elective procedures such as trephination. To ensure a wide dissemination of his ideas, Paré wrote in the vernacular rather than in Latin. His humility is said to be revealed in his most famous saying: 'I bandage them, but God heals them.' Paré questioned the long-held belief about laudable pus, but he recommended cautery for other problems, including amputation, and his illustrated treatise on instruments described thirty-eight types of cautery irons.

Surgical instruments were sometimes made in the shape of animal heads and named for the creatures they represented. Animal designs are found in Paré, but they originated much earlier. They were a characteristic of the surgical tools of the ancient Hindu tradition of Susruta, the author of *Samhita*, a treatise of unknown antiquity (800 B.C. to 400 A.D.). More than an aesthetic ornamentation, the designs derive from mythology and appealed to spiritual powers for healing.

Early Modern Operations

Several elective procedures were improved in early modern times, including amputation, cataract surgery, hernia repair, lithotomy, and plastic repair of skin. In amputation, the limb tourniquet was displaced by Paré's recommendation of ligatures for large vessels, but this new technique demanded time, knowledge of anatomy, a relatively clear field, and willing assistants. It was not widely accepted until the early seventeenth century after Fabry von Hilden (Fabricius Hildanus) described the releasing tourniquet, in which a stick twisted into the band could tighten or release pressure as needed. Other tourniquets were devised by Johannes Scultetus and J.L. Petit, who used screw-clamps.

Lentine cataracts had been 'couched' (from the French *coucher*, to lie down) in ancient India and Rome, according to both Susruta and Celsus. This procedure involved introducing a needle into the eye at the edge of the cornea to push the clouded lens down and out of the way. A 1559 illuminated manuscript, discovered in the twentieth century, reveals that its author, Caspar Stromayr of Lindau, was an accomplished cataract coucher and herniotomist. The 1583 work of the German surgeon George Bartisch also described both the couching of cataract and removal of the globe of the eye. In 1638 cataract surgery and lens clouding were related to the theory of vision established by René Descartes (see figure 10.2). Extraction of the lens itself was described in 1753 by Jacques Daviel.

Cutting for bladder stones, or perineal lithotomy, had also been mentioned by Celsus (see figure 10.3). Various approaches and instruments for the procedure were recommended by a special class of wandering lithotomists and barber surgeons. Its rise in popularity in the early modern period led some to postulate an epidemic of bladder concretions for dietary and environmental reasons.

In the Renaissance, certain plastic procedures were revived, including correction of harelip deformity and rhinoplasty (repair of the nose). The latter had been known to the Hindu surgeon Susruta, and it was rediscovered and revised by the Italian surgeon Gaspare Tagliacozzi, who published an illustrated treatise demonstrating a technique to replace the nose by displacing a skin pedicle from the

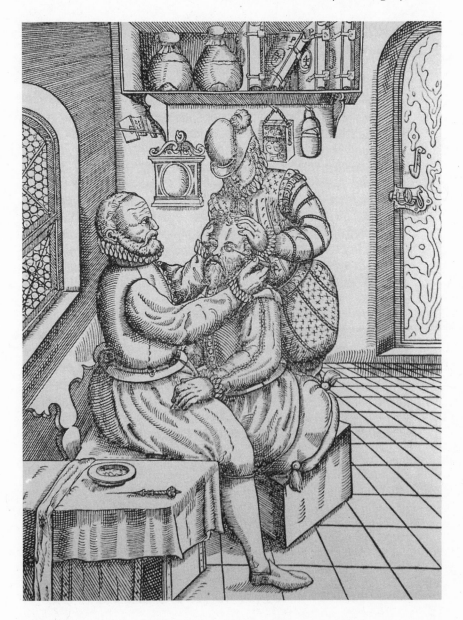

10.2   Cataract surgery in the sixteenth century. Georg Bartisch, *Ophthal-modouleia*, Dresden, 1583, facsimile

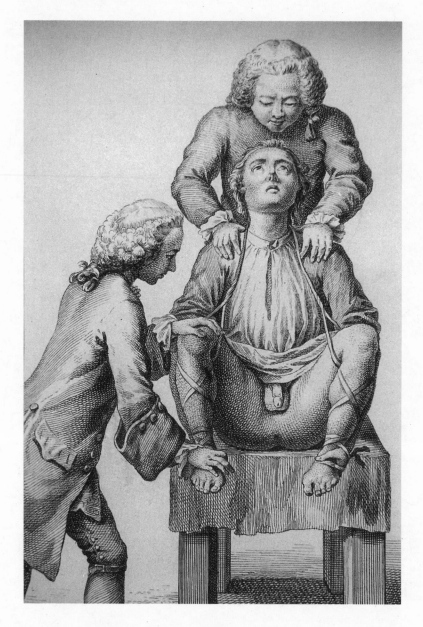

10.3   Lithotomy. Denis Diderot and Jean le Rond d'Alembert, *Encyclopédie,* planches, vol. 3, plate 12, 1772

upper arm. Operations to repair missing noses were of great importance following the European advent of syphilis (see chapter 7). In the eighteenth century, the *Encyclopédie* of Denis Diderot and Jean le Rond d'Alembert glorified the achievements of surgeons with numerous illustrations of elegant instruments wielded by equally elegant practitioners.

Professionalization of Surgery and Medicine

With these surgical innovations, the professional separation of European surgeons from physicians was firmly entrenched and surgeons began to organize. Previously surgeons had been part of the barber class; often illiterate and traditionally inferior to physicians, they derived income from shaving, cutting hair, and drawing teeth. Minor operations were incidental. Barber-surgeons learned their trade by apprenticeship, unlike the doctors who read Greek or Latin (usually Galen) at universities and rarely saw patients until after they had graduated. Many famous surgeons, including Paré, Stromayr, and Bartisch, had been trained by barbers; their humble origins hindered their acceptance in learned places.

In 1518 the internist doctors of England formed the Royal College of Physicians to control licensing and the practice of medicine. Soon after, in 1540, barber-surgeons were granted a charter by Henry VIII to form their own guild. The charter protected their right to practise and granted them autonomy over licensing and discipline. Similarly, in other countries, the incorporation of surgeons took place separately from physicians (see table 10.1). By the late eighteenth century, surgeons comprised a range of practitioners, from the village barber to an aristocratic elite, but their practical apprenticeship training continued. These professional organizations created a hierarchy and an environment in which specialties would develop. In twentieth-century North America, the centuries-old separation of the two disciplines is still reflected in separate professional bodies: for example, the American College of Surgeons founded in 1913 and in Canada the two main branches of the Royal College of Physicians and Surgeons, both founded in 1920.

By the eighteenth century, physicians were mocked for being

Table 10.1
Professional organizations for surgery

1260	Confrérie de St Côme et St Damien, Paris
1505	Seal of Cause granted to Barbers and Surgeons of Edinburgh (future Royal College)
1521	Licence by examination of the surgeon-in-chief, Portugal
1540	United Company of Barber Surgeons, London
1599	Faculty of Physicians and Surgeons of Glasgow (future Royal College)
1694	Revival of Collège St Côme, Paris
1715	Accademia Lancisiana di Roma
1731	Académie de chirurgie, Paris
1736	School of Surgery, precursor of Royal Academy of Surgery, Copenhagen
1760	Royal College of Surgery, Barcelona
1787	Royal College of Surgery of San Carlos, Madrid
1800	Royal College of Surgery, London
1920	Royal College of Physicians and Surgeons of Canada
1927	Royal Australasian College of Surgeons

impractical, bookish, and ineffectual. Their university-based education was considered stagnant: tradition dictated the textbooks, and ambivalence about anatomy reigned. Surgeons, on the other hand, maintained separate schools, where they taught by apprenticeship on living patients and by dissection of cadavers. Some began to conduct experiments, and a special dynasty of surgical innovators began in London.

William Cheselden was an anatomist-turned-surgeon who studied bones and devised new methods for lithotomy and for iridectomy to create an artificial pupil for blindness. His student, the Scottish-born surgeon John Hunter, was also an excellent anatomist who investigated inflammation and gunshot wounds. In London, Hunter ran a surgical practice and a private school of anatomy; he served King George III and the British army, rising to the position of Surgeon General. But Hunter is said to have hated performing operations because of the pain that they caused patients. His lectures were heard by many who went on to distinguished careers, for example, Astley Cooper, another skilled anatomist, who wrote on fractures, breast disease, and hernias and experimented with vascular procedures on dogs. After studying with Hunter and in Edinburgh, Phillip Syng Physick returned to Philadelphia, where he cultivated surgical innovation and served a distinguished clientele that included presidents and their families.

In eighteenth-century France, surgeons rejected the university establishment, which had been allied with the monarchy. Following the revolution, they were central to the revived Paris medical faculty, which emphasized dissection and adopted hospital-based methods of instruction for all students (see chapter 9). French surgeons rose to even greater prominence during the Napoleonic Wars. Particularly notable was Dominique-Jean Larrey, who was decorated by the emperor for his dexterity as an operator and for his invention of a 'flying ambulance' to carry the injured from the battlefield. In September 1812, at the two-day battle of Borodino near Moscow, Larrey is said to have performed two hundred amputations – one every sixteen minutes. His 75 per cent success rate was said to owe much to the anesthetic and hemostatic effects of the Russian cold.

In the early nineteenth century, a new interest in physiology was kindled, and scholars were receptive to its study by surgical methods (see chapter 3). Experimental surgery explored the inner workings of animals, but it could also lead to new operations for sick humans. Surgery became a tool of scientific inquiry, but the operations were still extremely painful (see figure 10.4).

The Advent of Anesthesia

To relieve pain during surgical procedures, alcohol, opium, and bleeding had been used for centuries. Prior to manipulating dislocations, Philip Syng Physick recommended heavy bleeding in the vertical position until the patient fainted; but this approach was dangerous. The best relief for a person undergoing surgery was rapid loss of consciousness, caused either by the analgesia or by the procedure itself. Surgeons strove for accuracy and speed.

Anesthetic gases had a protracted prehistory, but they eventually transformed practice. The earliest advocates were neither surgeons nor physicians; they were chemists and dentists with remarkable personalities. Nitrous oxide ('laughing gas') was known in the late eighteenth century and was used at social gatherings ('frolics') to produce rapid, nonsensical inebriation (like glue sniffing in our own time). In 1799 the English chemist Humphrey Davy experimented with a combination of nitrous oxide and oxygen in both animals and humans; he suggested that it might allay surgical pain.

Nitrous oxide was also used by the dentist Horace Wells in late

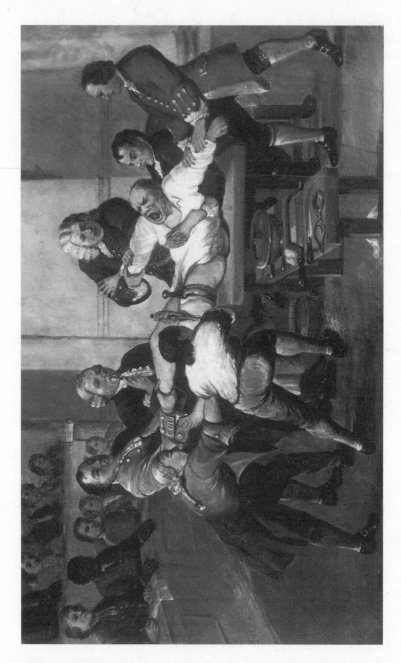

10.4 A pre-anesthetic amputation at St Thomas's Hospital, Southwark. Artist unknown. Late eighteenth century. Hunterian Museum. Royal College of Surgeons, London

---

A Vignette: Mastectomy before Chloroform

Next day, my master, the surgeon, examined Ailie. There was no doubt it must kill her, and soon. It could be removed – it might never return ... she should have it done. She curtsied ... and said, 'When?' 'Tomorrow,' said the kind surgeon ...

The operating theatre is crowded; much talk and fun ... In comes Ailie: one look at her quiets and abates the eager students ... Ailie stepped up on a seat, and laid herself on the table ... shut her eyes ... and took my hand. The operation was at once begun; it was necessarily slow; and chloroform – one of God's best gifts to his suffering children – was then unknown. The surgeon did his work. The pale face showed its pain, but was still and silent ...

It is over, she is dressed, steps gently and decently down from the table ... then turning to the surgeon and the students, she curtsies, – and in a low voice begs their pardon if she has behaved ill. The students – all of us – wept like children.

– Physician-writer John Brown, *Rab and His Friends and
Other Papers and Essays* (1862; reprint London, 1926), 24–8

1844. Wells conducted public demonstrations of 'painless tooth extraction,' but he was mocked with cries of 'Humbug!' when he demonstrated on a person resistant to the effects. His former business partner, dentist W.T. Morton, used ether with better results. In vexation over Morton's success, Wells became addicted to chloroform. While intoxicated, he threw vitriol at a prostitute and was tossed into a New York City jail, where he committed suicide.

Other Americans also experimented with anesthetic gases. The Georgia surgeon Crawford Long had attended ether parties while a student in Philadelphia, and in the winter of 1842 he experimented with it for eight minor operations. Negative public opinion put an end to his trials, and Long did not publish until a few years later. The chemist Charles T. Jackson of Boston conducted ether experiments on himself and suggested to Morton that he use it as an anesthetic in dentistry. Having disputed priority with S.F.B. Morse over invention of the electric telegraph and the Morse code, Jackson would later become embroiled in another priority dispute over anesthesia, in which he urged Long to stake a claim too.

Following the lead of Wells and Jackson, Morton used inhalation ether as a general anesthetic for tooth extraction. Then, on 16 October 1846, at the Massachusetts General Hospital in Boston, he administered ether while the surgeon John Collins Warren removed a tumour from the neck of a young man named Gilbert Abbott. Possibly alluding to the sad experiences of the past, Warren is said to have uttered the understatement, 'Gentlemen, this is no humbug.'

At first, Morton tried to conceal the substance until he had obtained a profitable patent. But he was forced by competition to reveal its composition. By 18 November 1846, Henry J. Bigelow had published his own experience with ether in the *Boston Medical and Surgical Journal*. The physician and man of letters Oliver Wendell Holmes suggested the word 'anesthesia' for the miraculous new invention. The famous 1882 painting by Robert Hinckley depicts the Abbott operation of 1846 and the Massachusetts General Hospital maintains the 'ether dome' operating theatre as a shrine.

The sixteenth of October 1846 is often but wrongly cited as the date of the first surgical use of anesthesia. Wells, Long, and Morton had used it for earlier operations. But a prestigious endorsement can consolidate acceptance; October 1846 marked the end of anesthesia's long prehistory. The following year, chloroform was introduced into surgical practice by the Scotsman James Young Simpson, who recommended its use in obstetrics (see chapter 11).

Controversy swirled around all forms of anesthesia in the late 1840s. The unmistakable danger of gaseous explosions contributed to the debate. But deaths due to anesthesia were slow to be recognized, partly because of the gravity of the preoperative illness of many patients. Operations on the healthy were avoided. If a person died on the table, the cause could easily be attributed to the underlying disease.

Since antiquity, cutting into the body cavities or the viscera was to court certain death from what we would call infection. Once anesthesia became accepted, longer and more complex operations were conceivable, and surgeons began to contemplate opening the sanctuaries of thorax and abdomen. They no longer had to fear the operations, but the postoperative dangers were still terrifying.

Another twenty years would pass before surgical innovation took off. Images from this two-decade period are strange: distinguished surgeons dominate the scene, dressed in elegant frock coats, their hair, moustaches, and beards blowing in the breeze, their hands bare and only nominally clean. The most famous of these images is the remarkable 1875 painting by Thomas Eakins of Samuel Gross operating – a painting that became the object of a huge public outcry in 2006 when Thomas Jefferson University Medical School proposed to sell it for $68 million (see figure 10.5). Through dint of civic pride and generous donations, it still resides in Philadelphia, shared between two great galleries. This painting has been used as evidence of America's slowness to adopt the next great achievement in the history of surgery.

Antisepsis and Asepsis

Like anesthesia, antisepsis had many precursors and pioneers. Cleanliness had always been a virtue in surgery. In 1847 Ignaz Semmelweis introduced the washing of hands and instruments in chlorine water solution to prevent childbed fever, but he did not publish until 1860 (see chapter 11). In 1867 the Scottish surgeon Joseph Lister announced the results of his experiments with carbolic acid in open fractures. By stating the opinion that wound infections were caused by bacteria, Lister based his method on the theory of the French chemist Louis Pasteur (see chapter 4).

News of Lister's principles travelled widely and quickly, but before the 1880s, when germ theory was established, opponents pointed to inconsistencies in the various methods used. At first, antiseptics were splashed into wounds or sprayed into the air to kill the germs presumed to be lurking there. But surgical wounds were supposed to be 'clean' from the outset. Preventative asepsis to avoid wound contamination by operators was introduced by Ernst von Bergmann in 1877. Rubber gloves were patented the following year. Lister initially clung to his original views, but by 1896 he too accepted the advantages of asepsis over antisepsis.

In Canada, antisepsis was promoted in the late 1860s by Thomas G. Roddick of Montreal and Archibald Edward Malloch of Hamilton. Sceptics William Canniff, William Hingston, and F.J. Shepherd con-

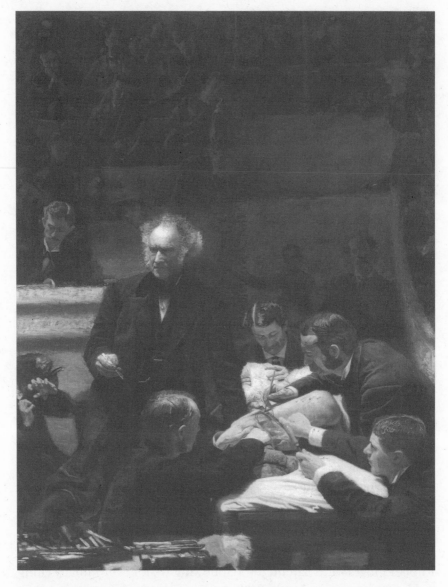

10.5   *The Gross Clinic* by Thomas Eakins, 1875, Philadelphia Museum of Art and Pennsylvania Academy of Art. Without using principles of antisepsis, the doctors operate on the thigh of an anesthetized man, while a relative cringes in horror.

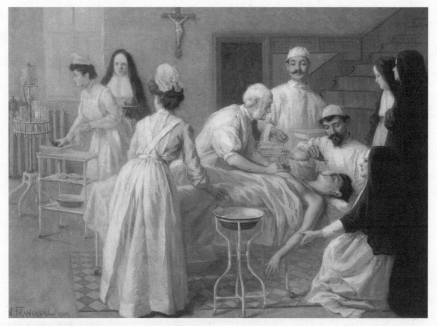

10.6   *Dr Hingston et la salle d'opération*, by F.C. Franchère, 1905. In the religious setting of the oldest hospital in Montreal, the surgeon is attended by nuns as well as the new professional nurses. He has adopted anesthesia, but his bare hands reveal his scepticism about antisepsis. Musée des Hospitalières de l'Hôtel-Dieu, Montreal

tended that antisepsis appeared to help wound healing because it drew attention to the good old rules of cleanliness (see figure 10.6).

A Montreal Operation with Antiseptic Spray

Dr Roddick assisted [Dr Fenwick] and I looked on. After the operation was over I inquired why they had sprayed the wall instead of the patient – the spray had been going all the time, but it was not turned on the patient – the fact was that it had been forgotten; however the patient did well.

– F.J. Shepherd, cited in W.B. Howell, *F.J. Shepherd* (Toronto, 1934), 108

Surgical Optimism and Its Heroes, 1870–1970

After opposition to anesthesia and antisepsis faded away, a period of unbounded optimism ensued – the 'Century of the Surgeon.' New achievements were described in military terms of 'victory' and 'conquest,' and some people imagined that all obstacles to surgical endeavour would eventually be eliminated. No medical heroes have enjoyed greater prestige than the surgeons of the late nineteenth and early twentieth centuries, surgeons who devised daring and previously inconceivable responses to internal pathology. The instruments and procedures that they invented still bear their names, and the list of their contributions flows like a litany of legendary exploits.

The German, Hermann von Helmholtz, invented the ophthalmoscope in 1851. It led to improvements in operative ophthalmology, especially the procedures for iridectomy and strabismus that had been devised by his countryman A. von Graefe. Also in Germany, Ludwig Rehn drew attention to surgery for bladder tumours; in 1896, he was the first to operate successfully on a beating human heart when he closed a stab wound in the right ventricle of a young gardener who had been attacked while strolling by the river. Theodor Billroth of Vienna embraced aseptic principles and championed gastric and biliary surgery in the 1870s and 1880s; his operating theatre was crowded with students and admirers. The American senator John S. Bobbs is said to have performed the first gall bladder operation in 1867 in Indianapolis. Another American, Charles MacBurney, also specialized in intestinal surgery, and his 1889 description of acute appendicitis led to eponymic use of his name. Frederick Treves of London put surgery for appendicitis on the map with an operation on Edward VII only days before his coronation in 1902. The cocaine- and morphine-using William Halsted, at the urging of W.H. Welch, joined with Osler and Kelly as a founder of Johns Hopkins medical school (see chapter 6). Halsted's radical mastectomy, devised in 1890, was intended to remove not only the cancerous breast but also all potential sites of local recurrence (see below).

This new ability to alter internal structures further promoted the anatomical definition of disease (see chapter 4). For example, surgery for appendicitis relied on disease concepts that were less than a century old: peritonitis had been described by Laennec in 1802, while its cause in a ruptured appendix had been suggested in 1812 by James Parkinson. Prior to anesthesia and antisepsis, only a handful of surgeons, such as Willard Parker of New York City, had dared to operate on the belly; their interventions, like the thoracentesis of Hippocrates, were confined to draining abscesses through the abdominal wall.

The new potential for surgical solutions fostered a parallel search for corresponding anatomical problems. For example, the intriguing disease 'visceroptosis' (drooping gut syndrome) was thought to provoke numerous symptoms, including back pain. Various operations to resuspend the sagging organs could relieve the symptoms. As shown by Magdalena Biernacka (MD, Queen's 1998), medical publishing on visceroptosis began in the 1880s and declined temporarily during each of the two world wars while surgeons were otherwise occupied. Its descendant, nephropexy, still figures in the schedules of recognized procedures. Was the disease constructed to satisfy the new possibility of treating it? In other words, had the cure become its cause? And how did its decline relate to military needs?

Increasingly delicate operations were devised for problems in the most complex of organs, including the brain and the heart. Surgeons were venerated like saints. In 1909 Theodor Kocher of Switzerland became the first surgeon to win the Nobel Prize, for his work on the operations and physiology of the thyroid gland. Soon after, the French surgeon Alexis Carrel, who spent many years in America, won a Nobel Prize (1912) for his technique of vascular anastomosis, a cornerstone of transplant procedures.

In the United States, celebrated surgeons became famous: for example, J.B. Murphy of Chicago; the brothers C.H. and W.J. Mayo of Rochester, Minnesota, whose clinic boasted an early department of anesthesia; George Crile, who pioneered direct blood transfusion; neurosurgeon Harvey Cushing; and cardiac surgeon Alfred Blalock, who worked with Helen Taussig to correct the tetralogy of Fallot and other congenital heart problems. Their younger colleague C. Walton Lillehei performed the first open heart operation in 1952 using hypothermia to slow metabolism while the heart was stopped. Two years later, the first successful kidney transplant was performed by

Joseph E. Murray on Ron Herrick, the donor being Ron's twin, Richard. In 1990 Murray shared the Nobel Prize for his transplantation work.

A race between American surgeons and those elsewhere ended in 1967 when the South African surgeon Christiaan Barnard successfully transplanted a human heart. The first recipient lived only three weeks, but the media celebrated the achievement with heady excitement for much longer. Transplantations of kidney, liver, marrow, lung, and heart have now become standard treatment, while work continues with other organs, including pancreas transplant for diabetes. Tissue typing, through the genetic information of HLA (see chapter 4), has made it possible to match healthy and brain-dead donors with recipients on different continents through international organ 'banks.' Some American cities have become transplantation centres, with architectural and human infrastructures revolving around brilliant individuals such as Thomas E. Starzl of Pittsburgh, specialist in liver transplant, and Nobel laureate E. Donnall Thomas of Seattle, founder of a marrow transplant program.

Canada also has its surgical greats. William Canniff, physician, historian, and founding member of the Canadian Medical Association, authored the first Canadian textbook of surgery (1866). The country doctor Abraham Groves of Fergus, Ontario, claimed to have removed the first Canadian appendix in 1883, using a kitchen table as an operating surface. During the Spanish Civil War, Norman Bethune helped to establish one of the earliest mobile plasma transfusions units. The American-born neurosurgeon Wilder Penfield, founder of the prestigious Montreal Neurological Institute, is known for his work in cerebral localization. Innovation in the postwar rehabilitation of soldiers with spinal cord injuries was the result of an interdisciplinary collaboration between neurosurgeon E.H. (Harry) Botterell and physiatrist Albin Jousse in Toronto. Congenital abnormalities of the heart were first collected and defined by the Montrealer Maude Abbott; and both heparin and operative hypothermia were developed in Canada and applied to open-heart surgery by D.W. Gordon Murray and Wilfred G. Bigelow, both of Toronto. Later Canadian innovators include William T. Mustard, who devised procedures for congenital heart disease; Wilbert J. Keon, an expert on heart transplantation; and Robert

B. Salter, who promoted research requirements for orthopedic trainees and devised both the innominate osteotomy for congenital hip
displacement and continuous passive motion for joint healing. The
University of Western Ontario in London established a multi-organ
transplant service under the direction of internist Calvin R. Stiller,
who served as its chief from 1984 to 1996.

Wars continued to have an impact on surgery during this period.
Since the eighteenth century, the British army and navy issued strict
orders about medical and surgical provisions; their records are a useful source for historians not only on surgery and medical practices,
but also on the interface with civilians at home and abroad. The
American Civil War took place during the gap between anesthesia
and antisepsis. It is said to have been the first conflict to leave large
quantities of documentation pertaining to the epidemiology and
care of surgical patients – also much studied by historians. Reacting
to the horrors he had witnessed at the battle of Solferino in 1859,
the Swiss businessman and philanthropist Jean Dunant founded
what became the International Red Cross in 1863–4. It established
the Geneva Convention (1864) to guarantee neutrality to wounded
soldiers and their attendants. Dunant shared the 1901 Nobel Prize
for Peace. The International Red Cross received the same award for
war relief in 1917 and again in 1944, although most scholars agree
that the agency could have done more for Holocaust victims. Created
to provide neutral care for the war-wounded, the Red Cross quickly
embraced a military structure, which may have hampered its success,
as historian John Hutchinson suggested.

The brutal injuries of the First World War led to developments
in plastic surgery by Harold Gillies of New Zealand. In the Second
World War, experiments with thin skin grafts and remodelling techniques took place at several centres, including East Grinstead in England, where the team of another New Zealander, Archibald McIndoe,
included Canadian surgeon Ross Tilley and the airmen patients, who
called themselves the Guinea Pig Club. The Jewish-German refugee,
neurosurgeon Ludwig Guttman, improved spinal rehabilitation and
founded the earliest Special Olympics at Stoke Mandeville. Battlefield blood transfusion, piloted in 1917, became commonplace in the
Second World War, with the added convenience of component ther-

apy. Safe transfusion was the final breakthrough for cardiovascular surgery of peacetime (see chapter 8). Historian Roger Cooter dared to challenge the long-held 'silver-lining' notion that war is somehow good for surgical innovation: certain procedures are brought into practice because of the pressures of war; however, some will have existed before the conflict made them necessary, and the deliberate carnage created by ever more vicious technology can never be worthy of celebration.

Fading Optimism: Less is More?

The uncontested value of coronary-artery-bypass grafts has resulted in grand schemes for ready-and-waiting operating rooms staffed by teams prepared to intervene at a moment's notice. These procedures and organ transplants are enormously expensive and greatly in demand. But who will pay? With rising health-care costs and a financial recession, the buoyant optimism of mid-twentieth-century surgery began to wane. Even as new surgical techniques became cheaper and, arguably, better than before, operative responses to human ills were questioned, especially in countries with national health-care programs.

In societies with private health care, such as the United States, rich people can usually afford insurance even if they cannot afford the operation; but the two-tiered system means inadequate or no care for the poor. In Britain and Canada, taxation must cover the high costs, yet elaborate procedures are available only in major centres. To control costs, elective surgery is rationed, not by the patient's ability to pay, but by delay – a situation that generates frustration and fear. Most recently one of the hottest topics in surgical research is in the area of waiting times. Furthermore, surgery itself is criticized on several fronts, including the economics of prevention and epidemiology (see chapters 6 and 15).

Sick people and their doctors worry that arguments of cost-effectiveness and population health are a bureaucratic pretext for *not* spending money, invoked by governments with relatively poor (and declining) records in funding science. Not only does innovation in surgery and bioscience potentially save lives, they argue, it is a manifestation of a 'healthy' society that places high value on thought and creativity. The most imaginative leaps of intellectual energy include surgical solutions for previously invincible problems of sick individuals. Why suppress achievement when it can also relieve suffering?

In this context, the rise of aesthetic surgery poses an interesting case study. With roots extending back as far as Susruta and Celsus, and having its major incentives in trauma and congenital malformations, the application of plastic surgery as a private choice for cosmetic reasons raises questions about surgeons' choices and cultural values. Countries with health-care systems must decide which procedures are medically necessary (and paid for) and which are not. To take one example, reconstruction of the breast following cancer surgery is variably available in different jurisdictions; studies have shown that the trend is upward but the procedure is used less often in the elderly, the poor, and in blacks. Given this skewed demographic, is it really medically necessary? Or is it a socially constructed desire in wounded women promoted by willing and good-intentioned operators? Once again, does the cure construct the disease?

Epidemiology has also taken the wind out of surgical sails in several different ways, some more effective than others. In the 1970s, epidemiologists worried that surgery would create as many problems as it solved by weakening the gene pool. For example, pyloric stenosis affects a small proportion of neonates; if uncorrected, it leads to death in infancy. People soon realized that the offspring of those with corrected pyloric stenosis would bear an increased risk of the disease, and the operation would be in increasing demand. The implied solution – not to operate on otherwise healthy babies – was totally unacceptable. Our health-care system has yet to collapse under the resultant strain. By the early 1990s, the incidence of pyloric stenosis, though increased in some places, had actually decreased in others; epidemiological studies are now devoted to explaining why, and theories under consideration include antenatal maternal medications, infant diet, sleep position, and environmental factors.

Similarly, cost-benefit analyses challenged the effectiveness of tonsillectomy, which in the 1950s was practised on approximately one-third of all children in the United States and Canada. Although the rates have been declining in most countries, studies suggest that the procedure may still be overutilized in certain places. A Manitoba group of epidemiologists asked if higher rates of tonsillectomy could be equated with lower standards of health care. Wide geographic and national discrepancies – of up to tenfold – in the utilization of this and other procedures, such as coronary bypass and hysterectomy, have also led epidemiologists to explore how economic factors relate to indications for surgery.

Mastectomy provides another epidemiological example that gave pause to surgical practice (see figure 10.7). Known since antiquity, breast cancer still causes the death of at least 10 per cent of North American women, although the trend is downward. Operative treatments are almost as old as surgery itself, since the breast – like other appendages – can be amputated without opening body cavities. In the seventeenth and eighteenth centuries, various recommendations were made on how best to achieve the desired result quickly and safely. Several riveting accounts, like the vignette cited earlier, describe the pain of mastectomy without anesthesia.

A certain apathy governed operation for breast cancer, not only because of the undeniable pain, but also because local resection would never cure what might be systemic disease. When surgery got its big boost in the mid-nineteenth century, the notion of breast cancer as a local or surgical disease was reconsidered. Surgeons worried that they might induce metastases by cutting into or close to the tumour. They reasoned that the patient might stand a better chance if more tissue and regional nodes were also taken away. This thinking culminated in Halsted's radical mastectomy, in which the underlying chest muscle was removed. The patient's arm could swell with lymphoedema for her remaining years – a minor annoyance if her life should be preserved. Halsted's procedure was the principal surgical response to breast cancer for more than seventy years.

In the 1970s epidemiological surveys suggested that radical mastectomy may prevent local recurrence, but it could not be correlated with increased survival. The result was a gradual shift from radical mastectomies to simple mastectomy. Soon people were asking if removal of the entire breast was necessary to prolong life, especially if the disease was systemic at diagnosis. The concept of 'adjuvant' chemotherapy was introduced, or chemotherapy used together with

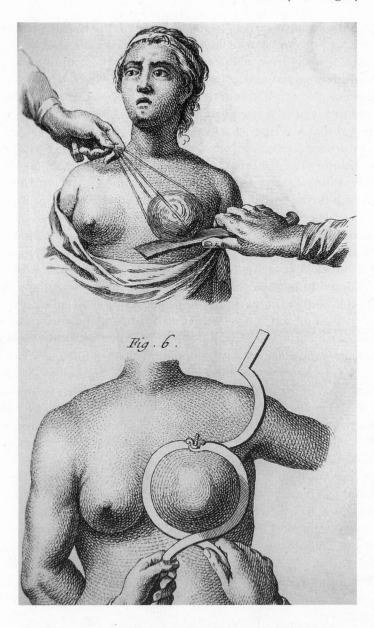

10.7   Mastectomy. Denis Diderot and Jean le Rond d'Alembert, *Encyclopédie*, planches, vol. 3, plate 29, 1772

supposedly curative surgery in the absence of disease. Surgeons were obliged to become statisticians and medical oncologists as well as technical wizards. They also looked to psychiatry to compare the psychological impact of mastectomy with the less invasive and less costly lumpectomy, which had a better cosmetic effect. Unfortunate experiences with artificial breast implants in the 1980s and 1990s again suggested that less surgery may really be more. But did the cheaper, smaller procedures have no cost in survival from cancer? So far, statistics continue to suggest that less surgery was and is better.

More rapid change in surgical practice took place in the early 1990s with the advent of laparoscopic cholecystectomy. A priority dispute over who was first to perform the operation is brewing. Erich Mühe of Germany performed the procedure in 1985, but the following year he was driven out of his professional surgical society – possibly for recklessly trying something new. Philippe Mouret of Paris also claimed to have been the first in 1987, developing it according to the methods still used today; however, he too was later prevented from operating his private clinics outside of the Assistance publique–Hôpitaux de Paris. Whoever did it first, within a short five years, the minimally invasive technique completely replaced the open cholecystectomy. It became a model for other 'keyhole' operations. Surgeons trained each other in the new skill, motivated perhaps by the safety of a less arduous procedure, patients' own appreciation of a rapid recovery, and by the economic benefit of short hospital stays. Some studies show that the rate of gall bladder removal increased as the operation became shorter and less dangerous.

The relative speed with which laparoscopic cholecystecomy replaced its predecessor contrasts markedly with the slowness of lumpectomy to replace mastectomy. Why? Is the difference due to the added attraction of new skills and instruments (present in laparoscopy and absent in lumpectomy)? Or is it because of the fear of malignant recurrence (present in breast cancer and absent in gall bladder disease)? Answers to these interesting historical questions may tell us about the conceptual and social interplay in contemporary surgery.

Finally, by the year 2000, not all life-saving operations required a surgeon. Technological advances in imaging meant that interventional radiologists, nephrologists, and cardiologists could perform some tasks that had once been the domain of surgery. Indeed, with the first edition of this book just a decade ago, robotic surgery was barely conceivable; the first telepresence operation was performed in Brussels in April 1997 – fittingly, perhaps, on a gall bladder. Now it has become a reality. When a specialist is needed on an urgent basis, location may be of no concern. Again, less is more.

Life-saving emergency operations are still of prime importance. The tradition of manual dexterity and technical innovation, which now includes telepresence, microsurgery, and laser, has not vanished. With its closer ties to medicine and consideration of economical, ethical, and epidemiological implications, surgery is perhaps more careful, more considered, more precise, and more elegant than it has ever been – even as the huge interventions of mid-century are replaced by fewer and smaller procedures.

Suggestions for Further Reading

At the bibliography website http://histmed.ca.

CHAPTER ELEVEN

Women's Medicine and Medicine's Women: History of Obstetrics, Gynecology, and Women*

If men had to have babies, they would only ever have one each.

– Diana, Princess of Wales

History seems to be about the past, but it is really about the present. Chronological lists of persons and events are not good history. Accuracy about dates and events is essential, of course, but history also contains interpretations that reflect satisfaction or discomfort with our own world. The questions asked of the past emerge from present experience. If the history is done well, then the interpretations are explicit and carefully substantiated. As a result, the same historical event can have different meanings, depending on who does the research, what is studied, when, and why (see chapter 16).

The historian-philosopher Ray Arney contrasted histories of obstetrics to illustrate differing interpretations. One scenario reconstructs the past as a series of incremental steps building progressively to culminate in our glorious present. Typifying this interpretation is the 1960 graph by Theodore Cianfranci that portrays the history of obstetrics as an exponentially increasing number of accomplishments (see figure 11.1). The units of Cianfranci's Y-axis are unidentified, but they estimate 'progress points.' Such an interpretation

---

* Learning objectives for this chapter are found on p. 455.

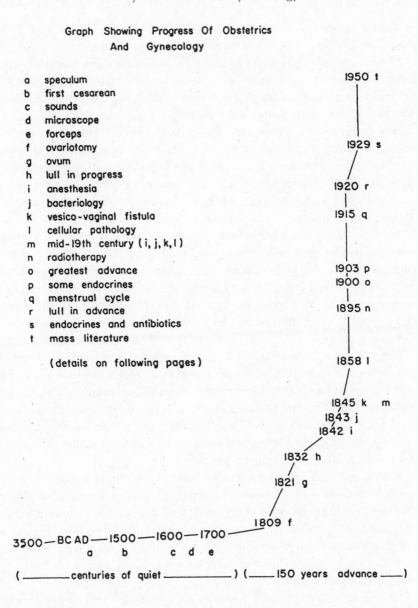

Graph Showing Progress Of Obstetrics
And   Gynecology

a   speculum
b   first cesarean
c   sounds
d   microscope
e   forceps
f   ovariotomy
g   ovum
h   lull in progress
i   anesthesia
j   bacteriology
k   vesico-vaginal fistula
l   cellular pathology
m   mid-19th century (i, j, k, l)
n   radiotherapy
o   greatest advance
p   some endocrines
q   menstrual cycle
r   lull in advance
s   endocrines and antibiotics
t   mass literature

(details on following pages)

1950 t

1929 s

1920 r

1915 q

1903 p
1900 o

1895 n

1858 l

1845 k   m
1843 j
1842 i

1832 h

1821 g

1809 f

3500—BC AD—1500—1600—1700—
        a   b   c   d   e

(_____centuries of quiet _____) (____ 150 years advance ____)

11.1   Graph displaying the progress of obstetrics and gynecology as viewed by a practitioner. Theodore Cianfranci, *A Short History of Obstetrics and Gynecology*. Springfield: Charles C. Thomas, 1960, viii

is called 'presentist,' or 'whiggish' (see chapter 16): it not only describes the past, but valorizes it in terms of the present.

Other historians reject Cianfranci's interpretation because they deplore rather than celebrate present-day obstetrics. Typifying this critical view, Arney selected the feminist philosopher Mary Daly, for whom the 'doctored diseases are increasing' and obstetrics is a 'patriarchal program' of 'gynocide.' Recognizing social construction (see chapters 4 and 7), some agree with Daly that femininity has been 'pathologized' (made sick), because doctors control the rhetoric and most doctors have been men. Hostility shines through the book titles of, for example, Brodsky, or Ehrenreich and English (for example, *Women versus Medicine* or *For Her Own Good*).

Medical students easily find arguments to refute Daly: obstetrics cannot be gynocide since maternal (and fetal) mortality has plummeted in the last century. In response, Daly might argue that improved survival is due, not to doctoring, but to better hygiene and nutrition – the McKeown hypothesis (see chapter 7). Medical students might reply that doctors welcomed better survival even if they did not provide it.

But not so fast! Cianfranci's graph also needs criticism. He awarded points for the speculum, forceps, anesthesia, and antisepsis. Yet some techniques, initially considered safe, were subsequently shown to be harmful; both forceps and anesthetic can harm babies and mothers. And twice Cianfranci marked a lull in progress, where the slope of his curve is steepest. Endorsing his present, he failed to adjust the graph accordingly, thereby revealing his bias.

Historians criticize as naive and 'internalist' the whiggish history written by those – often health-care practitioners – who seek to trace the familiar ideas of their daily work and assume that current practice needs no justification (see chapter 16). Inevitably, both histories are presentist. Even if accident or serendipity plays a role, findings in history – just like those in science – are made only when we are conscious of seeking them.

In this chapter the twin histories of obstetrics and of women in medicine will be examined from two perspectives: traditional and critical. We will explore the history of scientific investigations about femaleness and reproduction, moving on to social history examinations of this past. The chapter ends with a review of women in health care because one reason for their eventual recognition as professionals was as appropriate instruments of care for other women. We begin by examining women and their bodies as cultural phenomena.

Birthing as Women's Domain

The capacity of the female body to bear children set it apart in prehistoric societies; statues and paintings exaggerated its secondary sexual characteristics. Because bleeding could be dangerous, menstruation was mystical; its cyclic predictability signified and defined woman. Some societies viewed menstruation as a curse; remnants of that assessment survive in our language. In Orthodox Jewish culture, a postmenstrual or pastpartum woman is 'unclean' until she has taken a ritual bath (*mikveh*) (see chapter 8). The 'Churching of Women' in Christian tradition is a cognate. When women were venerated as deities, their tasks were often feminine: agriculture, procreation, birth, rebirth, and healing. In ancient Egypt, Hathor – a cow – was the earth mother nourishing the world; Isis presided over the fertile Nile and medicine; and Tauret – a hippopotamus – watched over childbirth. The Babylonian goddess Ishtar and the Greek Aphrodite were patrons of love, and the Roman goddess Juno protected mothers. Statues depicting the virginal Artemis (Diana) of Ephesus show her chest covered with breastlike eggs or egglike breasts. Her cult was absorbed into Christianity with the elevation of Mary as the Virgin mother of God.

For millennia, birthing was the exclusive domain of women. When males cared for women, special provisions were made for gender interfaces. For example, in fourteenth-century China, diagnostic dolls interposed a modest distance between doctor and patient. Well into the twentieth century, an elite Chinese woman would locate her symptoms on the doll, sparing the physician from seeing or touching her body. (The Osler Library owns a fine collection of Chinese diagnostic dolls.) Male professionals did not attend births in the West until the seventeenth and eighteenth centuries.

The Obstetrician's View: Medicine for Women

The predominance of women attendants did not prevent doctors from theorizing about conception and birth. Women and premature births were the focus of several Hippocratic treatises (*Diseases of Women I, II*, and *III; Nature of Woman; Girls; Nature of the Child; Seven Months' Child; Eight Months' Child*). These works include the notion of the wandering womb – an etiological hypothesis invoked to explain many symptoms; treatments were aimed at luring the uterus back into its proper place. Aristotle and other ancient writers held the view that the seed of the child came from the father alone to be nurtured in the mother. Other authors, including Soranus of Ephesus in the second century, described different positions in which babies emerged from the womb. This knowledge had predated writing, being handed down from midwife to midwife.

The medicalization of birth was characterized by instrumentation to prevent, terminate, hasten, or relieve deliveries. The ability to abruptly end a lengthy labour – to 'deliver' the woman from her 'travail' – distinguished those who would *intervene* (often doctors) from those who merely attended (often, but not always, midwives). In Cianfranci's graph, the vaginal speculum of the first century A.D. was the only ancient 'contribution': a three-bladed speculum, which opened with a heavy screw, was found at Pompeii, having been buried by the volcanic eruption of 79 A.D. Greco-Roman probes, sounds, hooks, and perforators, as well as knives, were used together with surgical instruments. Soranus explained how hooks were used to extract a dead child. Obstetrical forceps, which were invented in the seventeenth century, may also have been used in antiquity; they are depicted in a marble bas-relief found near Rome – a carving that may be a hoax.

Cesarean Birth

Cesarean birth also originated in antiquity, but it was reserved for when the mother was dying or already dead. This post-mortem surgery was ordered by a Roman law (*lex regia* or *lex caesaria*) to save the baby for the state. A second-century B.C. Hebrew text (Mishnah, Niddah, 5:1) suggests that Judaic antiquity also recognized Cesarean section. Islamic writings and fourteenth-century illustrations show that abdominal deliveries of dying women were known in the Middle East. The fatal operation was conducted without anesthesia, without antisepsis, and without understanding of tissue planes and suturing. In thirteenth-century Europe, the Christian church exhorted doctors to operate after maternal death to save the infant's soul by baptism. This practice continued into the nineteenth century in some places (Brittany). Early modern treatises on birthing described Cesarean section, but it was rarely used.

Vaginal Birth Too Banal for Heroes?

Asklepios, the Greek god of medicine, was taken from his slain mother's abdomen by his semi-contrite father, Apollo. Similarly, Buddha emerged from the flank of his mother, Maya. Despite the oft-repeated legend, Julius Caesar is unlikely to have been born by Cesarean section, because his mother was alive many years later. In the last scene of *Macbeth*, Shakespeare's hero Macduff reveals that he 'was from his mother's womb untimely ripp'd.'

In 1581 François Rousset published fifteen cases of abdominal delivery while the mother was still alive; however, he had never personally performed the operation, which he labelled *enfantement césarien*, citing a passage from Pliny (*Natural History* VII, 9). Legend holds that the first woman to survive abdominal delivery was the spouse of a sixteenth-century Swiss sow gelder named Nufer, who delivered his child and sewed up his wife. The first documented survival of abdominal delivery in Europe occurred in 1610, but the mother lived only a few weeks. Death so frequently followed the procedure that doctors usually opted to save a mother in obstructed labour by disposing of her child. Only in the late nineteenth century were methods devised to achieve a safer maternal outcome.

A Masterful Understatement on Cesarean Birth

This formidable operation, intended to save mother and child, has been performed during many centuries, with various success. In Britain it has never fully had the desired effect, all the mothers having died.

– John Aitken, *Principles of Midwifery*, 2nd ed. (Edinburgh, 1785), 84

Early Modern Midwifery

The advent of printing in the fifteenth century led to a flurry of 'obstetrical' literature. *Rosengarten* (1513), the earliest European obstetrical publication, was written in German by the physician Eucharius Rösslin. Purporting to be a handbook for midwives, it explained the methods and technology of delivery, including the birthing chair or stool, which took advantage of gravity for the mother's benefit while obscuring the view of the attendant. Immensely popular, *Rosengarten* appeared in more than a hundred editions and translations.

Seemingly written for midwives by either midwives or doctors, midwifery treatises are a curious genre and pose an interesting historical question: Who comprised the intended audience? Male doctors did not attend deliveries, and midwives were rarely literate. Recently, historians have suggested that these books served voyeurism of the educated elite.

One of the greatest surgeons of the sixteenth century was Ambroise Paré (see chapter 10). His treatise on women's diseases was written in the vernacular. Without claiming credit, he 'innovated' by adopting the traditional ideas of his patients, such as pessaries for prolapsed uterus and the birthing chair. He also modified instruments and reintroduced the technique of 'podalic version' once known to Soranus.

Podalic version is used to deliver a fetus in transverse lie or some other unfavourable position. An attendant locates a foot, and while others massage the mother's belly, the child is turned and delivered by gentle traction on the legs. In more than two decades of teaching, I have found that reading Paré's original description to different audiences provokes different reactions. Students in social studies crit-

Paré on Podalic Version: Good Guy or Bad?

But that she may not be wearied, or lest that her body should yield or sink down as the Chirurgian draweth the body of the infant from her ... let him cause her feet to be set against the side of the bed, and then let some of the bystanders hold her fast by the legs and shoulders. Then that the air may not enter into the womb, and that the work may be done with the more decency, her privy parts and thighs must be covered with a warm double linen cloth.

Then must the Chirurgian, having his nails closely pared and his rings (if he wear any) drawn off his fingers, and his arms naked, bare, and well anointed with oil, gently draw the flaps of the neck of the womb asunder, and then let him put his hand gently into the mouth of the womb, having first made it gentle and slippery with much oil; and when his hand is in, let him find out the form and situation of the child, whether it be one or two, or whether it be a Mole or not.

And when he findeth that he cometh naturally, with his head toward the mouth or orifice of the womb, he must lift him up gently, and so turn him that his feet may come forwards, and when he hath brought his feet forwards, he must draw one of them gently out at the neck of the womb, and then he must bind it with some broad and soft or silken band a little above the heel with an indifferent slick knot, and when he hath so bound it, he must put it up again into the womb, then he must put his hand in again, and find out the other foot, and draw it also out of the womb, and when it is out of the womb, let him draw out the other again whereunto he had before tied the one end of the band, and when he hath them both out, let him join them both close together, and so by little and little let him draw all the whole body from the womb. Also other women or Midwives may help the endeavor of the Chirurgian, by pressing the patient's belly with their hands downwards as the infant goeth out.

– Ambroise Paré, based on *Collected Works*, translation of
Thomas Johnson (1649), cited in H. Thoms, *Classical Contributions to
Obstetrics and Gynecology* (Springfield, IL: Charles C. Thomas, 1935), 102–4

icize the writing for its cold, clinical objectivity; medical and nursing students notice the frequent references to gentleness and concern for the patient's comfort.

In the seventeenth century, Antonie van Leeuwenhoek's announcement that sperm contained microscopic 'animalcules' conformed to the ancient Aristotelian views of generation. One observer (Hartsoeker, 1694) drew a tiny, balled-up, bullet-like fetus in the head of a sperm, but admitted that he had not actually seen it (see figure 11.2). Women may carry children for nine months and endure the effort of pushing them out, but most medical writers still assumed that the seed was male. If children sometimes resembled their mothers, it was the effect of gestational environment; babies were the products of their fathers. The discovery of sperm cells simply endorsed the ancient patriarchal (literally!) opinion.

Seeing Is Believing, but Imagination Comes First

Human sperm cells were seen with the earliest microscopes in the seventeenth century. The human egg is several thousand times larger, but – despite earlier postulates – it was not visualized until 1827, by K.E. von Baer. A priority dispute ensued. Once again, we learn that relative size is of little consequence. For something to be found, it must first be imagined and sought.

By the seventeenth century, the man-midwife began to serve affluent households. To avoid offending his clients' gentility, he adopted new customs, such as the modesty blanket. Why did women allow male practitioners to become involved with birthing at this time? Were the men invited? Or were they extending their market? Did they and their patients think that instruments and book learning offered something better than the midwives? Was it coincidental to the recent microscopic proof of males as progenitors? Was it because, as historian Adrian Wilson suggests, a previously homogeneous female solidarity had been split along class lines defined by wealth

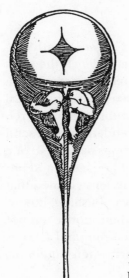

11.2   A homunculus hypothesized in a sperm cell.
From Nicolas Hartsoeker, *Essay de dioptrique*, 1694

and rising literacy? Did royal patronage play a role through the need for male witnesses to the birth of heirs? Or was this trend simply part of the increasing acceptance of doctors in all aspects of health – an early step in the medicalization of our entire culture?

Long after male physicians had entered the birthing chamber, female midwives continued to flourish. Their education, like that of surgeons (see chapter 10), was an apprenticeship separate from that of physicians. Some midwives were prominent and controversial members of their communities, for example, Jane Sharp in England, Anne Hutchinson in colonial America, and Mme Victoire Boivin of Paris. A mother of fourteen, Hutchinson is said to have given birth to a hydatidiform mole; consequently, she was accused of witchcraft, excommunicated, and banished, only to be killed during a native raid. Boivin is credited with having recognized the chorionic origin of hydatidiform mole. The notes and diaries of midwives have been recognized as valuable sources of medical and cultural history (e.g., see Fuhrer and Ulrich). But most mothers and their attendants were illiterate, and scholars must be creative in uncovering their experiences.

Forceps

The story of forceps entails several generations of a seventeenth-century English family, the Chamberlens (also Chamberlain), the most famous of whom were Peter and one of his three 'midwife' sons, Hugh. Originally from France, they discovered (or rediscovered) obstetrical forceps sometime around 1645; yet they kept the instrument secret. When a mother was in obstructed labour, the attendants would send for a Chamberlen, who would arrive with a mysterious parcel. No one was allowed to watch as the mother was relieved of her agony and her child delivered, sometimes stillborn. The Chamberlens claimed that they wanted to avoid tempting unskilled hands by publishing; however, their many offers to sell the secret imply that their motive was not patient welfare but greed. The secret soon leaked out, and forceps were rediscovered in the early eighteenth century, when numerous designs were invented for various uses.

Chamberlen on His Own Secret

'Having a better way,' translator Chamberlen wrote, 'I cannot pass without manifesting my dislike for Mauriceau's method of extracting dead or living children with hooks' (chapter 17, 270).

Chamberlen referred readers to his preface, where he wrote:

I will now take leave to offer an Apology for not publishing the Secret I mention we have to extract Children without Hooks ... which is that there being my father and two Brothers living, that practice this Art, I cannot esteem as my own to dispose of, nor publish it without injury to them; and think I have not been unserviceable to my Country, although I do but inform them that the forementionned three Persons of our Family, and my Self, can serve them in these Extremities with greater safety than others.

– 'Preface,' in F. Mauriceau, *The Diseases of Women with Child*, trans. Hugh Chamberlen (London: Darby, 1683)

Anatomy of the Uterus and Fetus

Once dissection had become respectable (see chapter 2), doctors who specialized in obstetrics began to study the structure of the gravid uterus. William Smellie of Scotland taught and practised in London during the early eighteenth century, dedicating himself to serving the poor. His illustrated treatise on midwifery described improvements to forceps and their use in breech position or in altering the presentation of the fetal head. His directions for measuring the pelvis could predict difficult deliveries.

A few years later, William Hunter became famous as a skilled teacher of anatomy in London. He and his surgeon brother, John, assembled anatomical specimens that are the nucleus for the splendid Hunterian museums of London and Glasgow. Among the most meticulous of his dissections is a delicate series, called 'the ovum,' that traced embryonic development. Hunter's *Anatomy of the Gravid Uterus* (1774) featured excellent illustrations by Jan van Rymsdyk (see figure 11.3). This atlas brought anatomy into obstetrics, but it was not devoid of interpretation. The images are cultural as well as medical documents: in the cut-off thighs and sectioned genitalia, historian Ludmilla Jordanova discerned implicit violence. With this attention, pregnancy was given its own structures, rhythms, and anatomical pathology. Shortly it would also acquire a physiology.

Soon after the discovery of auscultation, Jean Lejumeau de Kergaradec was inspired to listen to the pregnant belly. He described the fetal heartbeat and the placental 'souffle,' which is the murmur of blood in the placenta. Direct assessment of the viability of the fetus became possible with auscultation; the doctor's objective detection could bypass the mother's perception of movement (see chapter 9).

Control of Hemorrhage

The recognition of pathology in pregnancy and labour prompted a search for systematic methods to correct abnormalities. Then as now, hemorrhage and infection were the major killers of parturient women, while pain was a debilitating obstacle to intervention. Postpartum bleeding responded to ergotamine, a drug derived from *Secale cornu-*

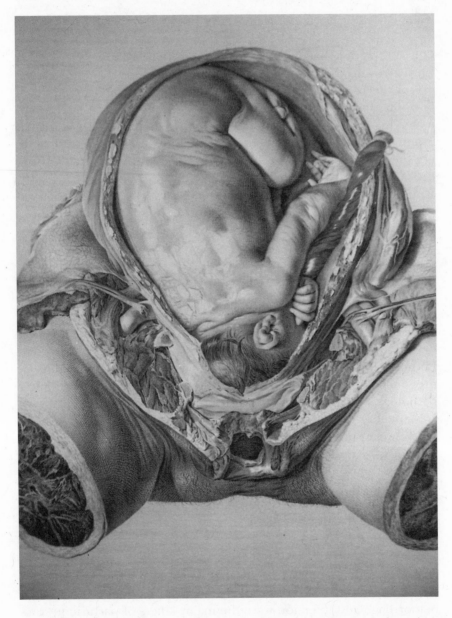

11.3   Term infant in utero. The mother died of a placental abruption.
Engraving by Jan van Rymsdyk, in William Hunter, *Atlas of the Gravid Uterus*,
1774

tum fungus of rye wheat, which causes contraction of smooth muscles in arterioles and the uterus. The German H.F. Paulizky and the American John Stearns both advocated ergot (in 1787 and 1807, respectively) for cases of delayed delivery due to ineffectual contractions, retained placenta, antepartum and postpartum hemorrhage, and even anticipated hemorrhage. Stearns also noted its side effects. But he and Paulitsky were disseminators of folk wisdom rather than innovators. As a contaminant of flour, ergot had provoked outbreaks of a disease, called St Anthony's fire, since at least the ninth century. This poisoning was characterized by widespread vasospasm, severe burning sensations, cramps, and sometimes death. Folk healers and midwives knew of the anti-bleeding benefits of ergot for many years, possibly through fortuitous observations of labour in the sick. In 1822 Stearns acknowledged an unnamed predecessor: 'I was informed of the powerful effects produced by this article, in the hands of some ignorant Scotch woman' (cited in Thoms, *Classical Contributions*, 1935, 24).

Control of Pain

The use of anesthesia in obstetrics was controversial. Early experiments with nitrous oxide were lampooned with the suggestion that shrews would become hyenas to the relief of their long-suffering husbands. Ether anesthesia was increasingly accepted in surgical practice after 1846 (see chapter 10). The following year, James Young Simpson advocated chloroform during parturition. But anesthesia for labouring mothers met staggering resistance, not only out of concern for the infant but for philosophical reasons: doctors, clerics, and others believed that labour pains had intrinsic value. They cited the Bible (Genesis 3:16) to describe women's pain as God's punishment for the 'original sin' of carnal knowledge, which, as it happened, was also the 'original cause' of labour itself. Proponents of anesthesia argued that only one member of the sinning partnership was suffering; they too cited scripture: before taking Adam's rib to create Eve, God had put Man to sleep (Genesis 2: 21–2).

The anesthesia debate was resolved for England, at least, when Queen Victoria took chloroform in 1853 and 1857 for two of her many deliveries, attended by John Snow of the Broad Street pump (see chapter 7). An image in Snow's 1858 treatise shows a refined lady, who resembles a youthful and unquestionably sentient version of the British monarch, demurely inhaling gas (see figure 11.4). Soon, educated women in Europe and North America pressured their physicians for chloroform.

Only some doctors employed anesthetic, and not every patient could afford it. The influential Charles D. Meigs of Philadelphia remained opposed. In researching a nineteenth-century rural Ontario practice, I found that women who took chloroform during labour were wives of prominent professionals – the lawyer, the minister, the newspaper editor, and the doctor himself. Did they have anesthetic because they were better informed than their poorer neighbours and knew to insist upon it? Or did their husbands provide it for them by condoning or paying for it? The record does not say. At any rate, the use of anesthesia doubled the cost of a delivery.

Other historians have shown that women became advocates of the pain relief offered by the new techniques. Various forms of general anesthesia were applied to birthing well into the mid-twentieth century, including the amnesic-analgesic 'twilight sleep' (*Dämmerschlaf*); induced by scopolamine, morphine, or other narcotics, it was first tested on five hundred women in 1906 by C.J. Gauss of Freiburg, Germany.

These systemic methods were eventually displaced in two ways. First, regional or 'local' anesthesia was less risky for the child and less intrusive for the mother. Second, natural or prepared childbirth emphasized education over medication for pain (see below).

Gradually anesthetists extended their mandate from putting people to sleep to reviving them. The field of neonatology was boosted in the mid-twentieth century by New York anesthetist Virginia Apgar, who devised a quick and reliable method of assessing newborn babies. Apgar's mentors had diverted her from surgery, in which she had qualified, into anesthesia; thence she went into perinatology and the study of congenital disabilities.

Childbed Fever

By the mid-nineteenth century, hemorrhage, pain, and prolonged labour had been partly controlled by ergot, anesthetics, and forceps. But the deadly problem of childbed (or puerperal) fever remained. Now it is known to be caused by bacterial infection of the endometri-

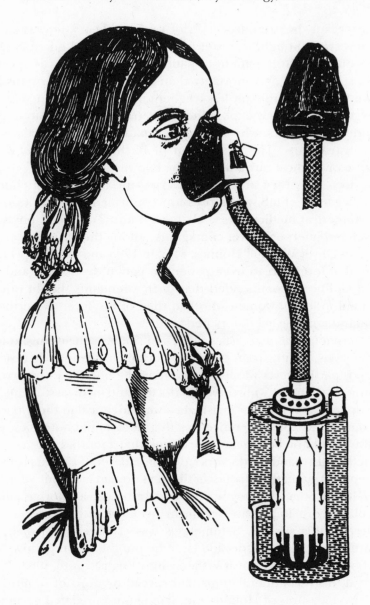

11.4   Woman who resembled the reigning monarch inhaling chloroform.
From John Snow, *On Chloroform*, 1858, 82

um, especially by streptococci. Prior to germ theory, however, child-bed fever was thought to result from environmental miasma, rather than contagion from patient to patient. In some practices, it caused greater morbidity and mortality than hemorrhage. Historians have shown that it was probably less frequent in mothers attended by mid-wives, who were rarely exposed to dangerous bacteria, than in those attended by doctors, who also tended patients with infections and used instruments. The proportion of birthing mothers who died because of medical care will never be known.

As doctors assisted at more deliveries, the incidence of childbed fever began to climb, an impression confirmed by statistics of the new numerical medicine (see chapters 4 and 7). Several physicians considered puerperal fever contagious, among them Alexander Gordon and Oliver Wendell Holmes, who, in 1795 and 1843 respectively, wrote that fever spread from patient to patient by doctors and mid-wives. Holmes recommended that birth attendants should not per-form autopsies on women who had died of the fever. Nevertheless, the dominant miasma theory persisted.

Maternal mortality statistics suggested similar conclusions to Ignaz Semmelweis, a Hungarian physician working in Vienna. He observed that postpartum fever was less frequent in the hospital wing served by midwives than in the wing served by doctors and medical students. The atmospheric conditions – miasmata – were identical in the two wings; the only noticeable difference was that doctors did autopsies, while midwives did not. Semmelweis reasoned that a morbid substance was carried on the hands of doctors from the cadaver of a dead mother to the tender, traumatized tissues of the next woman in labour. As early as 1847, he introduced a program of hand-washing in a chlorine solution and observed an impressive decline in incidence of the disease.

Despite this success, Semmelweis was criticized, ridiculed, and eventually dismissed. A decade later, he published a repetitive, rant-ing book, which was not translated into English until 1983. In the interval, his recommendations had spread by word of mouth. The effective measures of Holmes and Semmelweis predated germ theo-ry, proving, once again, that causes do not have to be known precisely in order to control their effects (see chapter 7). Incidentally, Charles Meigs of Philadelphia, who opposed anesthesia, also opposed anti-sepsis in obstetrics.

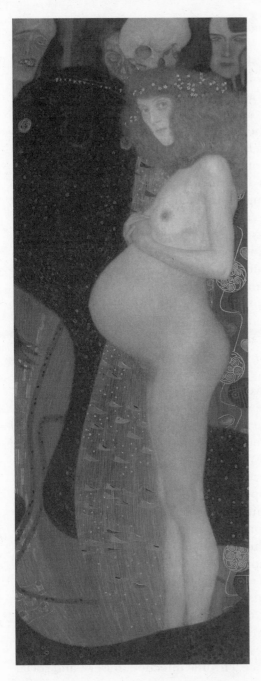

11.5 *Hope I*, by Gustav Klimt, 1903. National Gallery of Canada

Gynecological Surgery: Ovariotomy and Fistula Repair

Gynecological surgery, like all surgery, was stimulated by the mid-nineteenth-century advent of anesthesia and antisepsis. But some operations for women, such as Cesarean section and the removal of ovaries, already had a long prehistory. The first successful ovariotomy was performed in 1809 by the Kentucky doctor Ephraim McDowell. Without anesthesia, McDowell operated on a woman with a hugely swollen belly and severe abdominal pain to remove her ten-kilogram ovary. The woman outlived her doctor by many years. McDowell operated on others, later using alcohol and laudanum for pain relief. Cleanliness was his only precaution, and he later admitted that he had not expected his patients to live.

McDowell relieved desperate patients willing to be experimental subjects. By the end of the nineteenth century, however, ovariotomy had become an antidote for many female ailments, including mental illness (see chapter 12). Despite negative impressions from this distance, doctors who performed ovariotomies claimed that they served the best interests of women, and they called upon colleagues to sympathize with the tyranny of female biology. Many were venerated by their patients.

Problems of the uterus have always been recognized, but hysterectomy and amputation of the cervix were scarcely attempted before 1800, and only through the vagina. An abdominal approach was introduced for uterine cancer in 1878 by W.A. Freund of Germany. By 1900 the Austrian Ernst Wertheim had invented radical extirpation combined with oophorectomy and node dissection. James Young Simpson once labelled this operation 'utterly unjustifiable,' but soon it became standard treatment for cervical cancer, fibroid tumours, and prolapse. These conditions were also used as a pretext for surgical birth control. The 'Pap smear,' a cytological test for early diagnosis, was devised by George Papanicolaou in 1928; it reduced the need for radical hysterectomy. The benefits of the Pap smear have yet to be assessed in controlled trials, but its utility is assumed in trials conducted on how to encourage acceptance.

In the mid-nineteenth century, the American surgeon J. Marion Sims worked on repairing vesicovaginal fistula – a sequela of childbirth – producing incontinence, chronic infection, misery, and social ostracism. Between 1845 and 1857, he experimented with various techniques, relying on the lateral position for surgery and his inventions of a speculum, silver-wire sutures, and a self-retaining catheter. Sims also wrote a physiological description of vaginismus and developed a 'uterine guillotine' to amputate the cervix. His procedures cured morbid conditions that had been overlooked, partly because they were not necessarily life-threatening. At his death, he was warmly eulogized, and in 1894 a statue was erected in New York City through donations from admirers in Europe and America. But in the 1970s, scholars challenged Sims's ethics: he had perfected his techniques by repeated operations on slaves. The subsequent 'yes, but' contortions of his professional descendants make interesting reading – and provide yet another fitting subject for the Heroes and Villains game (see chapter 1).

Howard A. Kelly, one of the clinical founders of Johns Hopkins medical school, improved on techniques for vesicovaginal repair, hysterectomy, and oophorectomy, and he invented the air cystoscope. Kelly also contributed to gastrointestinal and urological surgery; he displayed some gender-related ambivalence about the status of gynecological surgery (see quotation in box).

Gender Identity and Professional Identity

The vital question which now affects gynecology is this, is she destined to live a spinster all her days? For we see her on one hand courted by her obstetrical ancestor, who seeks to draw her ... into an unholy, unfruitful alliance, destined to rob her of her virility, to be rocked into innocuous desuetude for the rest of her days in the obstetric cradle, sucking the withered ancestral finger in the vain hope of nourishment (with apology for mixed metaphor). On the other hand, we see her wooed by a vigorous, manly suitor, General Surgery, seeking to allure her from her autonomy into his own house, under his own name, obliterating her identity.

– Howard Kelly, cited in F.H. Garrison, *Introduction to the History of Medicine*, 3rd ed. (Philadelphia: Saunders, 1922), 652

Attitudes to women were invariably bound up in medical responses to their problems; appropriate treatment had to be consonant with societal expectations. For example, controversy swirled around sex alteration, widely publicized following the Christine Jorgensen case of the early 1950s. People asked, Should a man become a woman even if he could? Now sex change is accepted treatment for a previously unknown disease created by the possibility and permissibility of safe operations. Similarly, recent statistics show wide geographic variation in the frequency of hysterectomy even within the same jurisdictions, something Marc Keirse impishly described as the externally 'wandering womb' (*Birth* 20 [1993]: 159–61). The criteria depend more on attitude than on biology. As with tonsillectomy, higher rates of surgery may hint at lower standards (see chapter 10).

Physiology of Pregnancy and Delivery

Just as pregnancy acquired a physiology, labour and delivery also became objects of physiological investigation by researchers, such as John Braxton Hicks of London. Gradually, physical and chemical definitions were given to normal labour; problems could be anticipated before they became emergencies. These insights led to the practice, which some deplore, of placing electrodes on the bellies of labouring women and on the fetal head. The expressed motive was not to strip women of control but to minimize the faint yet real possibility of something going wrong before it could be fixed. Controlled studies on the benefits of monitoring are lacking – just as they are for Pap smears; some cite economic pressures as a reason for the ubiquity of this practice.

The hormones of the menstrual cycle and pregnancy are a twentieth-century concept. Their discovery recalls the lag between visualization of the sperm and that of the egg, and reflects the ancient idea that femaleness was the absence of something male. Testicular hormones had been postulated in 1775 by the French physician Théophile Bordeu. Animal experimentation, as early as 1845, by the German physiologist A.A. Berthold, suggested that transplanting male gonads could reverse the effects of castration. But ovarian hormones were not postulated until 1923 in the work of American physiologists E.A. Doisy and E. Allen. The pituitary gonadotrophins with effects on pregnancy and the menstrual cycle were described simultaneously in the late 1920s by several investigators, including S.S. Aschheim and B. Zondek, who developed a pregnancy test in 1928. Canadian Henry Friesen discovered prolactin in the late 1960s.

Pregnancy tests are now so routine that it is difficult to recall the guesswork, delay, and mystery in decoding subtle signs in the past – absent menses, sore breasts, darkened nipples, a bluish cervix, morning sickness, the inevitably growing womb, and quickening.

Assisting and Preventing Conception

Modern techniques are now applied not only to birthing but to conception. Laws and national inquiries in many countries appeared in response to controversies over access to diagnostic tests for fertility – tubal patency, ovulation, cervical competence, and fetal dates – and over assisted reproduction techniques, such as in vitro fertilization and surrogate motherhood. Available in the United States since 1981, assisted reproduction is subject to a 1992 Act requiring the annual publication of success rates through the Centers for Disease Control. The United Kingdom's 1990 Human Fertilization and Embryology Act was reviewed through an official inquiry in 2004 and amended in 2008. Elsewhere in the European Union, practices vary from country to country. In Canada, a Royal Commission on Reproductive Technologies, chaired by Vancouver geneticist Patricia Baird, reported in 1993, but several attempts to introduce legislation met with failure. In Australia, each state arranges legislation on this matter: some have no laws, others have laws from 1983.

Understanding the chemical cycles of women has been the sine qua non of contemporary birth control. Many attempted to synthesize an oral contraceptive; credit is generally given to the Austrian-born American chemist Carl Djerassi, who synthesized norethindrone, a progesterone analogue, while working for industry. Approved in 1960, the Pill played a role in the women's movement, in the sexual revolution of the 1960s and 1970s, and in patterns of AIDS and other STDs. Yet recent World Health Organization statistics reveal that birth control is unevenly distributed; and despite the wonderful new technologies, limiting births is correlated best with the education of women and improvement of child health.

OBGYN as Leader

Obstetrics and gynecology were the first specialties to apply evidence-based medicine (EBM; see chapters 5 and 14). In 1979 Archie L. Cochrane awarded the 'wooden spoon' to obstetrics as the specialty *least* influenced by randomized controlled trials (RCT). Since the early 1980s, Oxford's Iain Chalmers, with Murray Enkin and Marc Keirse, applied EBM principles to obstetrics. Their critical apprais-al of RCTs established confidence in some practices, raised doubt about others, and defined evidential lacunae for some surprisingly widespread interventions. As a result, perinatal medicine led the evi-dence-based-medicine movement in what has become the Cochrane Collaboration. Perhaps this discipline accepted the challenge earlier than others for historical reasons: mortality statistics led Semmelweis to his insights; his successors also respect numbers.

In one other area, obstetrics was prescient. Quick to adopt the laparoscope for diagnosis around 1970, gynecologists soon applied it to pelvic operations well before general surgeons began using it in the mid-1980s (see chapter 10). Perhaps they listened more carefully to their patients's preferences for minimal surgery.

The Feminist View: Criticism of Traditional Medical Ideas

So far, this history has tended to conform to the exponentially rising portrayal of Cianfranci. A similar perspective was endorsed by histo-rian Edward Shorter in his successful book *A History of Women's Bodies.* It tells how women could not contemplate liberation to vote or work until they were given control over their own biology. Shorter may be right about the timing, but feminists criticized his book: women and society at large were also instrumental in these changes; and far from being helpful, medical practitioners often opposed women's libera-tion. Now we will slice this history from a different angle to illustrate the dichotomy in interpretations introduced at the beginning of this chapter.

Women in Health Care

The main actors in modern medicine were men; and until well into the twentieth century, they did not readily welcome female colleagues. The proscriptions against women may have been more severe in the nineteenth century than in the distant past. According to the sixth-century medical writer Aetius of Amida, a woman doctor practised in Athens in the fifth century B.C. – Aspasia, the mistress of Pericles. Female physicians also were known in Rome. In the medieval school of Salerno, Trotula di Ruggiero (also Dame Trot) was a well-respected professor, physician, and midwife who is identified with an anonymous treatise on childbearing. With the advent of male midwifery in the early modern period, women faded from medicine and obstetrics, especially in the cities. But in rural areas and in the New World, midwives were still the primary accoucheurs.

Women have always wanted to study and practise medicine. Ironically, the nineteenth-century social values that thwarted their desires eventually provided an opening – through perceived inadequacies in male care of women. Man as midwife had frequently been the subject of ridicule. For example, in the eighteenth century, Mary Toft staged herself giving birth to a litter of rabbits and convinced several prominent doctors of her claims, much to their later embarrassment. Victorian society had particular difficulty reconciling woman being attended by men, especially on matters involving genitalia. To avoid offending sensibilities, doctors conducting an internal examination were taught not to look on a patient's nakedness but to gaze into her eyes or off into space.

Nursing

Women were traditionally the main caregivers for illness, as family members and as nuns in hospitals, where they cared for bodies and souls. In the early nineteenth century, women entered the professional workforce, first as teachers and later as nurses. At mid-century, driven by singular zeal and with few prior examples, Florence Nightingale improved the care given to soldiers in the Crimean War. She intended that nursing would complement medicine, but she built the profession on the 'womanly' virtues of cleanliness, patience, order, and service. Her legacy has been challenged by feminist historians, who decry the subservient, selfless position Nightingale's (always female) nurses were expected to adopt in deference to their (always male) superiors. From its inception, Victorian sexism was embedded in nursing. But from this moment on, a new professional pathway joined the orders of nursing nuns.

Nurses trained at hospitals until the mid-twentieth century, when some schools allied with universities. They were expected to work – often very long hours under stressful conditions, even as students; labour historians have shown that they constituted a vital resource to hospitals. Student nurses endured strict personal discipline in residences – rituals were built around their uniforms, their time was regulated, and they could not marry. Within hospital hierarchies, physicians were constructed as fathers or the heads of families, with nurses as subservient wives, while patients and students were children. Nurses in Britain and some other European countries were also trained in midwifery, with its centuries-long tradition of female practice. Those in North America were not; male doctors there had already consolidated control over birthing. Consequently, professional nurse training bore marked differences from nation to nation.

Nurses enabled the dissemination of technology in hospitals through teaching and in ensuring patient compliance. True to their origins, trained nurses also served the military in dangerous times of war. Many were killed. Nurses also accepted isolated work in remote areas, where they often replaced non-existent doctors by prescribing, suturing, and setting bones. Some people see these outpost nurses as the foremothers of today's nurse practitioners, who (with midwives) still face problems of acceptance by physicians. The letters and diaries of these nurses have become the focus of a burgeoning literature. As hospital schools closed, a flurry of writing took place resulting in excellent institutional histories, motivated by nostalgia and the tidiness of remembering.

Women Doctors

If nursing was not acceptable to a young woman interested in medicine, she had few other options. Some women hid their sex in order to become doctors, but how many did so cannot be determined. Dr James Miranda Barry, a medical graduate of Edinburgh, was a British military officer and surgeon who was appointed inspector of hospitals in 1857 (see figure 11.6). Her sex was not discovered until she was laid out for her funeral in 1865. She is said to have performed the first Cesarean section in the British Empire shortly after 1816. Because she travelled with the British army, she was the first woman to practise in several countries, including England, Canada, and South Africa. Barry met Florence Nightingale in the Crimea. The Lady with the Lamp was furious because the doctor kept her standing in the sun while 'he/she' chastised her from horseback. Nightingale's opinion of proper female delicacy of women is encapsulated in her account of their meeting.

Florence Nightingale on James Barry

(He) kept me standing in the midst of quite a crowd of soldiers, commissariat servants, camp followers etc. etc. every one of whom behaved like a gentleman, during the scolding I received, while (she) behaved like a brute. After (she) was dead, I was told that (he) was a woman. I should say (she) was the most hardened creature I ever met.

– Cited in C. Hacker, *The Indomitable Lady Doctors*
(Toronto: Clarke Irwin, 1974), 10

Prominent women began to insist that the best doctors for maternal and child care ought to be other women. These same activists supported the temperance and suffrage movements. After 1850, medical schools slowly began to consider female students in response to this perceived need to care for their own. Nevertheless, as historian Thomas Bonner wrote, women wanting medical education were forced to travel 'to the ends of the earth.' In 1849 Elizabeth Blackwell became the first openly female person to graduate from a Western medical school in modern times; she studied at Geneva College in rural New York State. Blackwell's sister Emily also became a physician at Cleveland. Together they helped the Berlin-born midwife Marie

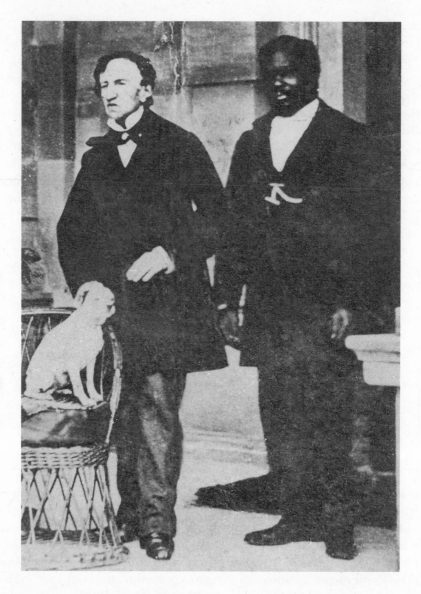

11.6 James Miranda Barry with her servant and dog in Jamaica, 1856. Widely thought to have been the first woman to practise Western medicine in Canada, Barry is said to have spent her life disguised as a man. Courtesy of RAMC Historical Museum, Aldershot, UK

Zakrzewska to qualify in 1856. Elizabeth Blackwell and Elizabeth Garrett Anderson, who had studied in Paris, were the only women known to practise in England before 1877. Two other American women graduated in Europe in 1871: Mary Putnam Jacobi at Paris and Susan Dimock at Zurich. Many of these doctors opened hospitals specializing in women and children.

But soon doors that had opened only a crack began to shut tightly. Consequently segregated schools for women's training were founded in Philadelphia (1850) and in New York City (1863, opened by the Blackwell sisters). When the medical school of Johns Hopkins University opened in 1893, it was obligated to offer 10 per cent of its places to women because of the unwelcome but intransigent condition of a key (lady) donor, Mary Garrett. Similar stories of struggle are now being told about the medical education of blacks, Jews, and other minorities (see chapter 6).

Sometimes, medical training came with narrow expectations if not stipulations for subsequent practice. Emily Stowe, one of Canada's first woman physicians, was denied education in Toronto and graduated from a segregated college in New York City in 1867. But with her formal credentials, she was refused (or did not seek) a licence to practise until 1880. In 1883, her daughter, Augusta Stowe-Gullen of Toronto, became the first woman to graduate from a Canadian medical school. Gullen's alma mater admitted no other women medical students for another quarter-century, referring all female applicants to segregated schools. Stowe-Gullen's achievement marked a watershed in higher education for women: shortly before, Mount Allison University had granted the first undergraduate degrees to Canadian women in 1875 and 1882. Stowe and her daughter were outspoken advocates of temperance, education, and votes for females, and they confined their practices to women and children.

Canada's earliest school for the professional education of women opened on 8 June 1883 in Kingston, Ontario, after a failed attempt at integrating women students into Queen's University. The Women's Medical College held classes in the City Hall; its first three graduates were Elizabeth Smith-Shortt, Alice McGillivray, and Elizabeth Beatty. McGillivray became a professor of obstetrics and later devoted her career to women and children in Hamilton, Ontario. Beatty became a missionary, and Smith-Shortt was a prominent force in Kingston society. Approximately forty women graduated as doctors in the eleven years that the college was in operation. However, a rival institution had scrambled to open in Toronto (in October 1883), and Women's Medical College eventually closed because of the competition. Many early women doctors left home to become missionaries; some historians suggest that the forces were centrifugal as well as philanthropic, owing to hostility from male colleagues. The first woman to lead an academic medical department in Canada was obstetrician Elinor F.E. Black at the University of Manitoba in 1952. Since the mid-nineteenth century, women had served as medical deans in the United States, but no Canadian woman had been chosen until 1999, when both Dalhousie and the University of Western Ontario took the plunge.

Birth Control

Female physicians concentrated on women, babies, and birthing, but they also promoted public health. Appalling conditions in hospitals were their special focus. Similarly, women doctors supported the attack on patent nostrums composed mostly of alcohol, opium, or water, and promising to cure everything. Many unsuspecting clients became addicted to these useless products and avoided medical care. The advent of medical statistics revealed inequities in the quality of obstetrical care; various campaigns aimed to improve women's health, and frontier nurse-midwife facilities were established.

Inability to control conception predicated female existence. Historian Judith Leavitt used an American woman's diary to show how for the majority of her twenty-two years of married life, she was either pregnant or nursing. In 1873 a Catholic theologian at Louvain recommended sterile-cycle sex for contraception; this 'rhythm method,' together with abstention and coitus interruptus, encompassed birth control. All other methods – including douching, sponges, condoms, caps, diaphragms, and abortion – were not only frowned upon, they were illegal in Europe and North America. The 1873 U.S. Comstock Law or its 1892 Canadian equivalent meant that disseminating contraceptives was an obscenity liable to prison.

Women were instrumental in the birth-control movement. Science may have provided the mechanism for these techniques, but medical professionals – including women doctors – rarely helped to make them available. Some champions of this cause were jailed or prosecuted for their efforts: American nurse Margaret Sanger, British paleobotanist Marie Stopes, and Canadian volunteer Dorothea Palmer.

An advocate of free love, Sanger fled the United States for England when she was charged, but returned in 1915 to face trial in a high-profile bid to garner support for her movement; charges were dropped. A year later she and her sister were convicted for running an information clinic. The feisty Marie Stopes also started free clinics and wrote manuals: *Married Love* and *Wise Parenthood.* Often threatened with prosecution, she successfully sued a man who wrote that she should be imprisoned, but that decision was overturned by the House of Lords. Less is known about Palmer, who was tried for working with A.R. Kaufman, a male philanthropist and manufacturer of rubber footwear in Kitchener, Ontario; he was not charged. After a nineteen-day trial, Palmer was acquitted on 17 March 1937; it was the first Canadian case to use the defence issue of the 'public good.' The many witnesses for Palmer's defence included the Toronto psychiatrist Brock Chisholm, who would become the first Director General of the World Health Organization (see chapter 15).

Owing to the efforts of women like these, free centres for birth control information were set up in Brooklyn, New York (1916), London, UK (1921), Vancouver (1923), Kitchener (1930), and Hamilton (1932). Two Canadian women doctors made the unusual choice of promoting birth control – Elizabeth Bagshaw and Helen MacMurchy. A 1901 Toronto graduate, MacMurchy was the first woman to intern at Toronto General Hospital and one of the first to hold a high-level bureaucratic post. She supported birth-control education by authoring pamphlets on family planning and concerned herself with infant mortality and mother-child welfare. Historical scrutiny, however, reveals that MacMurchy's main concerns were the poor and 'feeble minded,' and it has exposed her links to the now-discredited eugenics movement (see chapter 13).

Although oral contraceptives were approved in the United States in 1960, restrictions involving entire states or marital status meant that a decade passed before they were freely available to all Americans. The

United Kingdom approved them quickly. Delays in other countries owed more to social factors than biological testing. In 1969, through the international efforts of Protestant church representations and citizen activists, the 1892 Canadian law was changed to allow the Pill. (In the same year, homosexual acts between two consenting persons over the age of twenty-one were decriminalized, a process that took until 2003 for the entire United States.) Oral contraceptives and condoms were illegal in Ireland until 1980, following many high-profile protests. In Japan, approval of the Pill did not come until 1999, owing in part to decades of pressure against it by physicians.

Abortion is another controversial issue. Forbidden by the Hippocratic oath, it was practised in some Greco-Roman circles. In parts of Europe, the fetus was not considered alive until the mother felt quickening; a long-standing English tradition of tolerating abortion stemmed from this notion. Early nineteenth-century legislation against abortion was prompted by safety concerns over untrained providers. Accessible in the United Kingdom since 1967, abortion is still illegal in both Ireland and Northern Ireland. In the United States, choice has been guaranteed since the *Roe versus Wade* decision of 1973. But it is hotly contested by many politicians, leading to regional disparities. In Canada the law governing abortions was struck down in 1988 for being against the Charter of Rights and Freedoms.

Abortion may be legal, but physicians and volunteers working in clinics have been shot and sometimes killed by the 'justifiable homicide' movement. The dead include Drs David Gunn in 1993 and John Britten in 1994, both of Pensacola, Florida, in 1998 Barnett Stepian of Amherst, New York, and in 2009 George Tiller of Wichita, Kansas. Clinic security guards were also killed in the United States and Australia. In Canada, doctors were shot and injured: Garson Romalis of Vancouver in 1994, Hugh Short of Hamilton in 1996, and Jack Fainman of Winnipeg in 1997. Arson, bombings, and anthrax threats against clinics accumulated in this wave of anti-abortion violence, also called single-issue terrorism. Only some of the perpetrators have been arrested.

In other societies, however, the procedure has not carried the stigma it bears in sectors of North America. For example, Amerindians used efficient methods involving natural dilators of the uterine cervix. Modern techniques have become increasingly safe, but the controversy is not about maternal safety. It revolves around the ethics of killing the fetus. Religious views of abortion as a sin inevitably influence laws. This same philosophy restricted American funding for research involving human embryonic stem cells, until the March 2009 executive order of President Obama. In the last forty years, the Canadian physician Henry Morgentaler was prosecuted and acquitted many times for establishing abortion clinics in several provinces. When the University of Western Ontario awarded him an honorary doctorate in 2005, it reaped a barrage of petitions, rallies, and threats. Personal philosophy determines whether he is viewed as a criminal or a saint.

Control over female biology has indeed resulted in change: fertility rates have fallen, and women study, work, and vote. But the battle against sexism is not over. Women still comprise less than half the workforce, suffer more unemployment, and are paid less for work of equal value. In a world of nearly 7 billion people where thousands of children starve every year, some jurisdictions fret over declining birth rates. Fears that have a basis in xenophobia and nationalism are expressed as moral dilemmas. Women bear the brunt.

Back to Midwives

Over the years, hospital delivery and interventions have become the norm in developed countries. In 1989 some parts of United States and Canada were reporting more than 25 per cent of deliveries by Cesarean section, the highest rate in the world. Without rejecting the benefit of modern obstetrics, some questioned how much of it is needed. Does every birth need to be medicalized? Increasingly vocal women resented the intrusion into what should be a joyful and healthy event.

The natural birth movement originated in the 1950s with 'innovations' that evoke a prehistoric past: the positions found in non-industrialized societies; the assistance of family members; and home birth. Pioneers included British obstetrician Grantly Dick-Read, author of *Childbirth without Fear* (1944 and still in print), and his French counterpart Fernand Lamaze, who adapted a Russian method of 'psy-

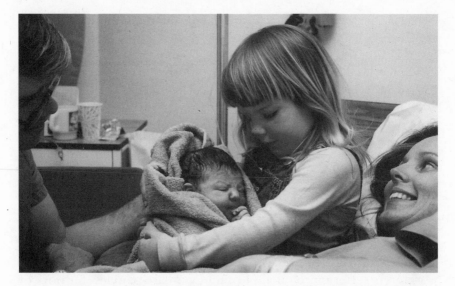

11.7   The happy results of a family-centred birth. Photograph by Eleanor
Enkin, Hamilton

choprophylaxis' as childbirth preparation. These techniques were
embraced by women and midwives, but were often ignored in academic settings. They were pioneered in Canada in the mid-1960s
by obstetrician Murray Enkin of McMaster University, who allowed
fathers to attend deliveries. In the United States, Robert A. Bradley
drew upon similar ideas for his method of 'husband-coached childbirth,' described in his 1965 book (still in print). Special settings, like
those endorsed by French accoucheurs Frédérick Leboyer or Michel
Odent, aim to mollify birth trauma with dimly lit rooms, warm-water
baths, and music – private procedures that, in France at least, com-
mand high fees. These doctors were often criticized by their peers for
using alternative methods. Not all promoters were medically trained;
for example, anthropologist Sheila Kitzinger of Britain is well known
internationally for her birthing advice.

Proponents of family-centred home delivery maintain that it is at
least as safe as the hospital: it avoids drug-resistant organisms and
provides psychological benefits (see figure 11.7). They also willingly

shared their work with midwives. In Britain, where nurse-midwives were already part of the establishment, the methods found favour quickly.

But the ancient profession of midwifery had to be rebuilt in North America. Once again, the medical profession was unhelpful. Education in midwifery had begun at the Pennsylvania Hospital in 1765, but most North American midwives had studied in other countries, such as England or the Netherlands. The American College of Nurse Midwives was founded in 1955; Columbia Presbyterian Hospital in New York City welcomed them from that year. But opposition from American family physicians and other groups made it difficult for midwives to find professional insurance coverage until 1993. By the late 1990s midwifery had become a regulated profession with opportunities for training and examination. Nevertheless, it is still illegal in some states.

Similarly, Canada was among only a few World Health Organization member countries that did not regulate midwifery until recently. As in the United States, the decisions are made in each province. Over the opposition of many obstetricians, several provinces launched task forces to study the issue: Ontario (1987), Alberta (1988 and 1994), Manitoba (1988 and 1993), British Columbia (1993), and Saskatchewan (1996). Midwifery training began in Sudbury, Hamilton, and Toronto in 1993, and the first cohort graduated in 1996. This change relied on public perception of the personal, psychological, and medical benefits of home delivery and was further prompted by the perceived economic advantages of shifting care to lesser-paid professionals. But whether we like it or not, state-funded birthing will continue to be medicalized to some extent. Governments wishing to avoid responsibility for disasters find solace in medical expertise.

Childbearing is far safer than it was a century ago, but the technological fix has not solved all the dilemmas. By creating a multiplicity of options, it generated new ethical problems. As for women doctors, feminist historians find that they abandoned the goals of their predecessors who were commited to dealing with the social and biological needs of women and children. Women who choose medicine today are said to become plain ordinary doctors, undifferentiated from and just as conservative as their male peers.

Women's medicine and medicine's women are now faced with the exciting challenge of integrating two historically rich traditions into a coherent and effective whole.

Suggestions for Further Reading

At the bibliography website http://histmed.ca.

CHAPTER TWELVE

Wrestling with Demons: History of Psychiatry*

No one who, like me, conjures up the most evil of those half-tamed demons that inhabit the human breast, and seeks to wrestle with them, can expect to come through the struggle unscathed.

– Sigmund Freud, *Dora* (1905), in *Standard Edition*, vol. 7, 109

Mental illnesses are unique because they continue to be defined by assessment of the patient's symptoms or behaviours, rather than by physical, chemical, or anatomical tests. Many themes presented earlier come into play in this chapter. They include the long-standing importance of a life force in explaining the functions of living beings (see chapter 3) and the tension between two pairs of rival disease concepts: first, disease from the outside versus disease from within; and second, disease of the individual versus disease of the group (see chapter 4).

The mind has often been equated with a vital spirit. Just as Galen's concept of a life force resonated for Christian theologians who saw it as the soul, vitalism has had explanatory power in psychological theories of illness. Vitalism makes a comeback in psychosomatic theories that link physical ailment to prior emotional suffering. As a result, mental illness relates to physiological or holistic concepts when it is diagnosed by observation of the disturbed relationship between a body and its environment.

*Learning objectives for this chapter are found on pp. 455–6.

But mental illness also relates to ontological concepts when its cause implicates discrete changes inside the body provoked by external agents, be they demons or chemical derangements. Much recent research builds on a commitment to this latter view by analysing external triggers and why or how various drugs accomplish their helpful effects.

The word 'psychiatry,' derived from two Greek words meaning 'soul' (or 'mind') and 'healer,' is relatively new: it was coined by the German physician Johann Christian Reil, and used in English less than two centuries ago. The word 'psychiatry' implies that these conditions are of the *psyche*, not the *soma*. By definition, then, psychiatric disease is disorder of mind, not body, with respect to its cause and manifestations. Mental illnesses may display alterations in the body, but they are not identified by them. Rather, they are distinguished by changes in behaviour, perception, thought, or affect. Yet in contrast and throughout history, mental diseases were usually considered to be the product of unseen *physical* causes, such as diet, poisonings, occult infections, or structural and biochemical change.

Prior to the integration of anatomy with bedside medicine, the classification of all diseases, or nosology, was based on the study of patients' symptoms (see chapter 4). As physical pathology grew, some diseases once thought to be of the mind were reclassified as diseases of the brain, the nerves, or the metabolism: epilepsy, tertiary syphilis, tetanus, congenital mental deficiency, cretinism, and deafness. They now appear in the psychiatric literature only because of associated symptoms, such as depression and anxiety. Psychiatric disorders are ailments that are 'left over'; they cannot yet be sorted into an anatomical or physiological realm.

Classification of disease in modern psychiatry remains in a state of subjective symptomatology akin to eighteenth-century nosology. Notwithstanding the exciting discoveries of many scientists, no blood tests, biopsies, ultrasounds, scans, or electrodynamic studies can objectively confirm a psychiatric diagnosis.

Themes in the History of Psychiatry

First, the tension between the physical and psychological causes of mental disease has been apparent throughout the history of mental illness. Until recently, neurology, as the study of brain and nerves, was indistinguishable from psychiatry. Disorders of the mind were assumed to be of the brain; premortem detection of specific lesions was beyond the capacity of doctors. Indeed well into the twentieth century, practitioners often specialized in both neurology and psychiatry. Only with the advent of anatomical definitions, and especially imaging, did the neurosciences begin their distinct rise (see chapter 3). The dichotomy between physical and psychological causes of mental illness has increased, and a debate over their relative importance pervades psychiatry today.

Second, 'normal' behaviour is socially and culturally determined; therefore, behaviours that are labelled 'abnormal,' 'mad,' or 'insane' can also be socially determined. Actions considered normal in one culture may be unacceptable in another; examples include incest, cannibalism, killing, genital mutilation, predicting the future, and political dissent. As a result, the mental state that leads an individual to socially unacceptable actions can be viewed variously as criminal, sinful, or sick. Psychiatric diagnoses can and have been socially constructed; as a result, psychiatry is vulnerable to abuse as an instrument of social control. The judiciary exploits the subjective nature of psychiatric diagnosis when expert witnesses are selected to contradict each other in court over questions of sanity. Additionally, the recognition and the experience of mental illness varies from culture to culture; our concern in this chapter, as elsewhere in this book, is psychiatric history in the West. (For histories of other medicines, see online resources at http://histmed.ca).

Finally, mental illness has carried a stigma, deriving from the patient's apparent unreliability, unpredictability, tendency to violence, and perceived responsibility for the illness. Unlike most bodily ailments, mental disorders can sometimes be feigned. Homer's Odysseus, the biblical King David, and other ancient heroes pretended to be mad to achieve specific ends. This common knowledge tends to imply that all persons who behave unacceptably may have consciously chosen behaviours that they could or should be able to control or prevent.

Historical Overview

Madness has been recognized since the earliest times, but it was not always a problem for doctors. In antiquity, it was identified by wide-ranging symptoms, including convulsions, crying, laughing, screams, violence, emotional pain, and the inability to learn or remember. In Hellenic and Judeo-Christian traditions, people so afflicted were sometimes taken for prophets; examples include the Trojan princess Cassandra and the Christian saint John the Baptist. A few ancient writers cited psychological or emotional causes to explain the behaviour, but most found physical explanations residing in naturalistic and material theories of the humours. For example, in Hippocratic writings, epilepsy was the result of phlegm obstructed in the brain; depression was due to an accumulation of black bile – hence the term 'melancholia' (from Greek, *melanos* [black], *khole* [bile]); Afflictions of women, both physical and mental, were attributed to a wandering womb (*hystera*) – the origin of the term 'hysteria,' invented at a much later time (see chapter 11). 'Hypochondria,' now restricted to excessive worry about illness, originally referred to any symptom, usually pain, situated under (*hypo*) the ribs (*chondros* [cartilage]), that is, in the upper abdomen; the term was indifferent to the perceived cause, be it physical or mental.

In the second century A.D., Aretaeus of Cappadocia, who vividly described diabetes and other physical ailments, defined 'mania' as delirium without fever, distinguishing it from 'phrenitis,' which was delirium with fever. He also recognized that periods of mania, or fury, could alternate with periods of depression (*Chronic Diseases I*, v, vi). Emphasizing the perceived physical causes for these conditions, treatments were also physical, including diets, baths, ointments, drugs, and rest. Greek and Roman societies created laws to protect families from dangers posed by the insane, who were feared, shunned, prayed over, and mostly left alone.

The first institutions for the care of the insane were the ninth- and tenth-century *mauristans* in the Islamic cities of Baghdad, Cairo, Fez, and Damascus. Muslim societies believed that the insane were divinely inspired rather than demonically possessed; words to describe them were *majnoon* (veiled) or *majthoob* (pulled, by the grace of God). Because mad people were holy, emphasis was placed on providing comfortable accommodation rather than treatment or confinement. *Mauristans* are said to have been luxurious, but restraints were used to control violent outbursts.

The first European mental institutions appeared in places that had felt Islamic influence, especially fourteenth-century Spain at Granada, Valencia, Zaragoza, Seville, Barcelona, and Toledo. A Spanish shepherd-turned-merchant, who had suffered a psychotic episode, founded an order of hospitaliers, later named after him as the Order of St John of God; he was buried in Granada and canonized in 1690. Like their Middle Eastern predecessors, these widespread institutions functioned as hospices for decent care, not cure, of people suffering from all ailments, physical and mental (see chapter 9).

Citing literary sources, some scholars have suggested that medieval doctors conceived of emotional causes for mental disturbances and consequently sought emotional cures (Alexander and Selesnick, 52). In the late Middle Ages and Renaissance, social control of deviance became a major preoccupation. Persons given to unusual behaviour were thought to have let down their moral guard and been possessed by demons. 'Treatments' resembled persecutions and included beating, whipping, expulsion, and execution. Care of the mentally disturbed was the responsibility of each community, and patients were lucky if they were simply neglected. Some communities in northern Europe are said to have hired sailors to remove the unruly – hence the origin of 'ship of fools,' a metaphor for the human condition in sixteenth-century Germany. Over a period of three centuries, unknown numbers of unconventional women were burned as witches by perpetrators who feared epidemics of madness – perpetrators who themselves have been portrayed, more recently, as victims of mass hysteria. Those whose distress did not threaten their survival or that of others managed alone, doubting that help could come from medicine.

Mind and Medicine

What physic, what chirurgery, what wealth, favour, authority can relieve, bear out, assuage or expel a troubled conscience? A quiet mind cureth all.

– Robert Burton, *Anatomy of Melancholy* (1651), pt 3, 4.2.4

Hospitals founded to provide humane care gradually became horrifying places of incarceration. The Charité de Senlis, in France, run by the order of St John of God, forbade restraints and punitive therapies, but such lenience was the exception. Ostensibly to protect society, criminals, beggars, prostitutes, the poor, the chronically ill, and some mad people were held indefinitely in squalid, rat-infested places and subjected to punitive 'treatments,' designed to shock or humiliate them into behaving 'rationally.' The administrators of these so-called hospitals in France, Germany, and Britain enjoyed absolute power over the occupants and immunity from the courts and police.

By the eighteenth century, St Mary of Bethlehem Hospital in London, built in 1247, had become the fearful 'Bedlam.' In his series of engravings, *The Rake's Progress*, William Hogarth depicted Bedlam as the miserable and deserving end of a wanton bon vivant. Custodial rather than medical, these institutions employed few doctors and ignored physical health. Their seemingly less-than-human occupants became objects of paid entertainment; however, the oft-repeated claim that 96,000 annual spectators paid a penny apiece to stroll the wards of Bedlam is probably a gross exaggeration (Patricia Alldridge, in Bynum, Porter, and Shepherd, vol. 2). At Bethlehem hospital four generations of the Monro family occupied the post of director; John Monro's 1766 case book has recently been published by J. Andrews and A. Scull, shedding some light on the matter. Scholars now try to discern how much (or little) superintendents focused on diagnosis and care of patients.

Asylum reform spread over the Western world at the end of the eighteenth century. 'Asylum' implies a safe place for seclusion, care, and restoration. The movement was fostered by Benjamin Rush in Philadelphia, William Tuke in England (who was a Quaker and not a physician), and Christian Reil in Germany. In France after the revolution, Philippe Pinel was appointed director of two Paris hospitals – the Bicêtre for men and the Salpêtrière for women, where he implemented a figurative 'unchaining' of the insane (see figure 12.1). Influenced by English writers, he argued that many patients were sick from emotional or 'moral' causes, and their treatment should be based on emotional or 'moral' principles. Unchaining is an appropriate metaphor for Pinel's work, and it has been portrayed many times in medical art, although the precise moment probably

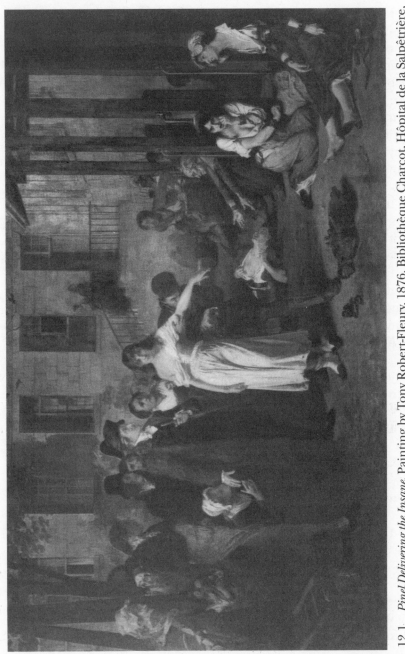

12.1   *Pinel Delivering the Insane.* Painting by Tony Robert-Fleury, 1876. Bibliothèque Charcot, Hôpital de la Salpêtrière, Paris

never took place in the literal sense. Controls were not abandoned. Patients continued to be confined, and their violence was subdued by modified straitjackets and other forms of coercion, such as hydrotherapy (baths). However, tending to diminish the gothic horrors ascribed to this past is R.J. Esther's analysis of the use of restraints in a late nineteenth-century American state hospital: they were applied about 10 per cent of the time, at a rate similar to that of Esther's time of writing (1997).

Asylums gathered many people with like symptoms and gave physicians an opportunity to observe patterns of mental illness. Their goals were to protect and to 'console and classify.' In conjunction with the scientific zeitgeist, classification of insanity (also called alienation, or vesania) became the cutting edge of research into mental disturbances. William Cullen of Edinburgh created a category called neurosis – a Latinization of the word for nervousness. He reasoned that functional conditions resulted from a highly sensitive reaction to outside stimuli mediated by the nerves. Within this physiological category of neurosis, he situated the older concepts of melancholia, hysteria, hypochondria, and sexual deviation. In France, Pinel and his student Jean-Étienne-Dominique Esquirol also devised classifications; they distinguished between mental retardation, cretinism, senility, melancholia, and a category called monomania, in which the descriptions of neuroses used today could be grouped (see figure 12.2). These doctors were known as 'alienists' – specialists in diseases that alienated patients from reality.

As explained in chapters 4 and 9, all disease concepts became increasingly anatomical during the nineteenth century. In conjunction with the asylum movement, scientists were forging links between physical changes in the nervous system and certain behavioural disorders. Gradually, organic correlatives were found for conditions that could no longer be thought of as diseases of the mind: epilepsy, tertiary syphilis, vasculitis, allergy, and stroke. Rigorous anatomical localization of specific changes in the nervous system led to the growth of the related but separate discipline of neurology. The anatomo-physiological explanations that had characterized Cullen's approach gave way to purely functional explanations. The category of neurosis persisted, but lack of physical findings led to its 'denervation.' 'Psy-

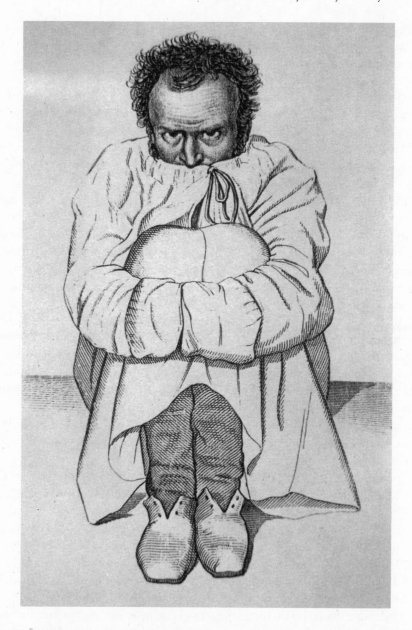

12.2   *Mania Succeeded by Dementia.* Engraving by Ambroise Tardieu, in J.E.D. Esquirol, *Les maladies mentales*, vol. 2, 1838

chosis' became the mid-nineteenth-century term for serious alienation or complete disorientation. 'Neurosis,' or 'monomania,' was
reserved for alienation in only one dimension.

Psychiatry dealt with what was 'left over' when the neurological disorders were removed. Reil's new word 'psychiatry' (like ped*iatrics* and
pod*iatry*) referred to 'healing' of the soul, unlike most other medical
designations, which end with the suffix '-ology' (= words or theory
about). The etymological choice is telling: the newborn psychiatry of
the early nineteenth century was confidently optimistic that it would
not only care but cure.

Asylum architecture was designed to demonstrate the imposing
stature, power, and authority of the promising new profession. Historians have used architectural designs as a vital source for the aspirations of various societies. Unlike the ancient hospitals in Europe,
which slid more or less into becoming warehouses for the insane,
asylums in North America were purpose-built through the well-intentioned principles of the asylum movement.

In the United States several institutions were founded on the basis
of dignified care: the Maclean Hospital in Massachusetts (1811), the
Hartford Retreat in Connecticut (1822), Brattleboro Retreat in Ver-
mont (1834), and the Pennsylvania Hospital for the Insane (1841).
They were deeply influenced by Quaker ideals and the European
concepts of moral therapy; William Tuke's York Retreat served as a
model. Reformer Dorothea Dix, who had herself suffered a 'nervous breakdown,' and physician Thomas Kirkbride of Philadelphia
worked to implement these plans on a broad scale.

In Canada, the first dedicated-use asylum was completed in 1850
at 999 Queen Street West, Toronto (see figure 12.3). It was quickly
filled to capacity with over 500 patients brought from other hospitals,
attics, basements, barns, and shelters. In Hamilton the 1875 asylum,
built to house 200 patients, accommodated more than 1,300 by late
1914; during the same period, the London asylum grew from 120
beds to 1,130. The superintendents, Joseph Workman at Toronto and
Richard Maurice Bucke at London, became known for their practice
based, like those of asylum keepers elsewhere, on the principles of
moral restraint.

The word 'asylum,' which still conjures up notions of safety and

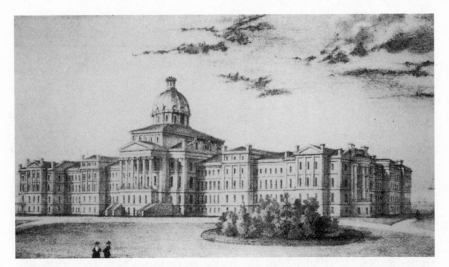

12.3   Design for the Provincial Lunatic Asylum, Toronto, ca. 1854. From Henry Hurd, *The Institutional Care of the Insane in the United States and Canada.* 4 vols. Baltimore: Johns Hopkins University Press, 1916–17, vol. 1

shelter in a political sense, gradually took on the stigma of mental illness, and various other terms were used to describe the institution (see table 12.1). Strangely, rather than abolishing the negative stereotype, the stigma would eventually attach itself to the new name and another would be chosen. For the Toronto asylum, the address itself also became synonymous with madness and was changed, in the 1970s, to 1001 Queen Street West in an attempt to obliterate its negative associations. Typifying the experience in many places, other Ontario institutions experienced rapid expansion.

As these institutions kept careful records, recent study of their practices and their directors has launched a veritable boom in historical writing because they reveal so much about society as well as medicine (see Suggestions for Further Reading). Some take the life and works of an individual asylum keeper as a window on practices in a time and place: Kirkbride, Monro, Workman, Bucke, Cotton, and many others have been examined in this way. More recently scholars, such as Kerry Davies, Ellen Dwyer, and Geoffrey Reaume, have used remarkable sources produced by patients to uncover personal experiences and the nature of life inside.

Table 12.1
Successive name changes in various Ontario hospitals for mental illness, 1850–2000

Lunatic Hospital
Lunatic Asylum
Asylum for the Insane
Insane Asylum
Sanatorium
Ontario Hospital
Mental Health Centre
Psychiatric Hospital
Regional Centre
Retreat
Developmental Centre
Continuing Care Centre

Historians are divided over whether or not the asylum keepers were heroes or villains. In the more traditional histories, they are portrayed as heroes because they attempted to improve conditions, sought better understanding of psychiatric disturbances, adopted the ideals of moral cause and moral treatment, and tried to find cures. Despite the medical, verbal, and architectural trappings, however, asylums continued to be places of confinement, where diagnoses often incorporated prejudicial notions of class, gender, and race. Some new therapies were worse than useless; they were eventually shown to be harmful. Yet these therapies were not designed to hurt patients deliberately. Why did they once seem to be rational, justifiable, and effective? The answer lies in the generally accepted concepts of mental disease in the nineteenth and twentieth centuries, and possibly also in the frequency of spontaneous remissions, now estimated to be 30 per cent. Natural remissions of illness would suggest effectiveness of treatment through the logical fallacy of *post hoc ergo propter hoc* (one thing occurring before another makes it *seem* to be the cause).

By the late nineteenth century, psychiatry was losing professional credibility. Anesthesia, antisepsis, germ theory, and public health had fostered effective interventions for other human problems and had generated great optimism for surgeons, internists, obstetricians, and their patients. Psychiatrists, on the other hand, had yet to make equivalent discoveries – discoveries that could explain, predict, cure, or prevent. One Canadian scholar (Dowbiggin) cited this borderline professional despair as a reason why psychiatrists clung passionately and stubbornly to etiological theories of heredity, degeneracy, and self-abuse – hypotheses that tended to blame patients, rather than medicine, for their incurability – hypotheses that latter fed the eugenics movment.

Notwithstanding the moral cause and moral treatment hypothesis, psychiatric disorders were increasingly perceived to be disorders of the brain, not of the 'soul.' If mental processes resided in the brain, then physical and physiological treatments seemed to be justified. Johannes B. Friedreich took a strongly somatist approach to mental disorders; Wilhelm Griesinger combined physical and emotional therapies. Jean-Martin Charcot, a French neurologist, studied hysteria and its modification through hypnotism, but some contemporaries and historians have demonstrated that his desire to find hysteria prompted his patients to reproduce it for him.

Sophisticated observation of the mentally ill continued with the longitudinal study of case histories and autopsies; modifications to the classification schemes were made. In 1899 Emil Kraepelin defined the two major psychoses as manic depression and dementia praecox, subdividing the latter into hebephrenia, catatonia, and paranoia. Two years later, dementia praecox was named 'schizophrenia' by Paul Eugen Bleuler. With considerable modification, these categories are still in use.

Twentieth-Century Psychiatry

At the beginning of this century, psychiatric research expanded in three different directions, all of which continue: psychoanalysis, psychosomatics, and psychobiology.

Psychoanalysis

Psychoanalysis had precursors but did not receive medical approbation until the work of Sigmund Freud. A Viennese Jew, Freud began his career as a physician interested in physical and neurological disturbances. During 1885–6, he spent a few months in Paris with Charcot and Pierre Janet, where his interests turned from neuropathology to psychopathology. But as Freud himself later claimed, it was through the 'teachings' of his own patients, most of whom were wealthy and neurotic, that he was led to his theories of the unconscious.

The ideas expressed in Freud's extensive publications have become cultural icons: the interpretation of dreams, the unconscious, the ego and the id, the importance of childhood experience, sexual conflict, the hydraulic theory of neurotic defence mechanisms, repression, fixations (anal, oral, and genital), fantasy, wish fulfilment, symbols (phallic and otherwise), catharsis, free association, analysis, and complexes named for mythic figures of antiquity. Critics claim that Freud's work applied only to himself or to upper-middle-class males in turn-of-the-century Europe, and that its ethnocentric and andro-centric concepts, such as penis envy, made it irrelevant to others. Yet whether Freud is lauded or deplored, medicine, psychiatry, and Western culture in general were irreversibly altered. The rapid dissemination of his thought testified to a perceived need for the articulation of non-physical etiologies.

Freud first began publishing in the 1890s. His ideas met with some opposition, but he and his collaborators, Carl Jung and Alfred Adler, found supporters almost immediately. His influential book *The Interpretation of Dreams* was published in 1900; the first international congress on psychoanalysis was held in Salzburg in 1908; and by 1911 the American Psychoanalytic Association had been founded.

An important boost to psychoanalytic theories of disease came during both world wars, when psychiatrists interpreted the debility of soldiers exposed to the stress of war: 'healthy' soldiers accepted the constant threat of killing and being killed without incapacitating distress or fear. Unlike other specialties and possibly due to the influence of Jung, psychoanalysis sometimes welcomed the leadership of women: for example, Karen Horney, Anna Freud (daughter of Sigmund), Melanie Klein, and the Canadian Grace Baker.

The ideas of Freud and Kraepelin came to the United States through the Swiss-born Adolf Meyer of Johns Hopkins University; he insisted on careful record keeping and influenced two generations of psychiatrists as his trainees and in his role with national associations. Two of the eight founders of the American Psychoanalytic Association were from Toronto: Welsh-born Ernest Jones and Canadian-born

John T. MacCurdy. Jones first learned of Freud in 1903. He brought analysis to Toronto in 1908, when he began working for the dean and first professor of psychiatry, Charles Kirk Clarke; the prestigious psychiatric institute bears his name. Jones was charged with sexual misconduct several times, but he was never convicted. Perhaps the accusations were an occupational hazard of zealous application of the new psychoanalytic theory in a disbelieving society. Jones was one of Freud's many biographers, and his personal acquaintance with the master lent an authority to his opinions that has only recently been questioned by new historians free of filial devotion. Because Canadian analysts participated in the American organizations, the Canadian Psychoanalytic Society was not formed until 1952.

Theoretical rifts in psychoanalysis developed. But Freud's ideas have been an important prototype, if not the basis of all psychotherapy – which is treatment by talking, without drugs or other physical modalities. Reflecting the biases of its creators, psychotherapy is generally thought to help the educated, middle- or upper-class neurotic and to be of little benefit to the uneducated, the poor, or the psychotic. Rifts among analysts are reflected in the medico-historical study of Freud, in which his life, his patients, and the evolution of his theories are debated with passion. Restrictions on access to his papers have led to media scandals (see Malcolm 1985; Gelfand and Kerr 1992).

In the last two decades Freud has virtually disappeared from medical school curricula, although his ideas are visible elsewhere. Some medical historians, like Edward Shorter, find this to be a just turn of events away from a brief aberrant moment, when emotional rather than physical causes came to the fore, when deluded doctors invested time in the ramblings of patients rather than probing their brains with scalpels, electrodes, and drugs.

Resolving Conflicts

Fortunately, analysis is not the only way to resolve inner conflicts. Life itself still remains a very effective therapist.

– Karen Horney, *Our Inner Conflicts* (New York: Norton, 1945), 240

Psychosomatics

The second direction taken by psychiatric research is the psychosomatic approach, which began in the late nineteenth century and
flourished in the 1930s with the founding of specialized journals.
Challenging the historic and artificial distinctions between mind
and body, research was conducted on the physical effects of strong
emotions. In other words, physical changes were no longer the cause
but the result of mental turmoil. The focus of inquiry shifted from
mental changes to the somatic damage caused by prolonged psychic
stimulation. Pioneers in this field included physician Harold G. Wolff
of New York, an expert on migraine and author of *Stress and Disease*
(1953); German-born physiologist James P. Henry, who served the
American space program; and the Vienna-born Montrealer Hans
Selye, who started out in endocrinology just as the adrenal hormones
became understood as a response to stress.

These scientists concentrated on the physical products of prolonged stress. Personality was classified into 'types,' following Jung,
and it was measured on newly devised scales, reflecting a spectrum
of normal rather than pathology. Certain personality types were
thought to favour certain diseases; for example, the psychic stressors
associated with 'Type A personality' were correlated with ulcer and
coronary heart disease. More recently, researchers have been turning to the effects of stress, burnout, daylight, and depression on the
immune system and on other body functions to explain disorders
such as chronic fatigue syndrome and seasonal affective disorder.

Body and Mind

As physicians, we cannot afford to lose sight of the physical
aspects of mental states, if we would try to comprehend the
nature of mental disease, and learn to treat it with success.

– Henry Maudsley, *Body and Mind* (New York: Appleton, 1870), 94

Psychobiology

The third direction taken by psychiatry in the twentieth century was to embrace radical treatments of a physical nature. The discovery of the spirochete germ that causes syphilis completed the anatomo-clinical definition of neurosyphilis; in 1917 a cause was found for viral encephalitis. The linking of these formerly 'mental' disorders to germs and organs raised expectations that physical links would eventually be found for all the rest.

Sometimes, treatments were developed in advance of a known cause. Historians have tried to explain this aspect of the psychiatric past by recalling the turn-of-the-century frustration felt by psychiatrists who cared for the mentally disabled but failed to find effective cures. The development of treatments now viewed with repugnance constitutes a fascinating but sobering collection of clinical vignettes and imaginative reasoning.

Ovariotomy, or the removal of ovaries, was one of the earliest gynecological operations, originating in the early nineteenth century before the advent of anesthesia (see chapter 11). In 1872, an American surgeon Robert Battey, recommended that it be used on the normal ovaries of women with a wide variety of conditions ranging from insanity to menstrual difficulties. The technique was much promoted as a cure for hysteria by the German gynecologist Alfred Hegar. By the end of the century, the removal of normal ovaries to produce a premature menopause had become a standard treatment for mental illness in North American and European women. Critics, including some physicians, warned of its dangers and deplored the apparent lack of positive results. Others justified the intervention, claiming that women's lives were unbearable as they were subject to menstruation, childbearing, and hormonal variation. Cultural justifications for the castration of women derived both from ancient disease concepts and from Victorian discomfort with expressions of female sexuality.

Mental diseases were also treated by deliberately invoking physical disease. Noticing that symptoms of syphilis remitted when patients were febrile, the Austrian psychiatrist Julius Wagner-Jauregg instigated malarial-fever treatment for patients with tertiary syphilis. His goal was to produce a 'curative' fever; he chose malaria because it could be treated and eliminated. His achievement was hailed as a model for the future of psychiatry – organic disease treated organically. In 1927 he was awarded the Nobel Prize and is the only psychiatrist to have been so honoured. Related theories about infection as a cause rather than a treatment of mental disturbance led to drastic surgical treatments, especially those of Henry A. Cotton in New Jersey (see p. 336).

Insulin-shock therapy was discovered in a similarly fortuitous manner. From 1927 to 1933, Polish-born Manfred Sakel worked at a Berlin hospital, where he treated narcotic addicts and noted that abstention led to overexcitation. He reasoned that the overexcitation arose from hyperactivity of adrenal and thyroid glands, the hormone products of which had only recently been discovered. His insight is said to have been inspired by a clinical experience with a famous German actress who was both diabetic and addicted to narcotics: an accidental insulin coma reduced her craving for morphine. At first Sakel used insulin as addiction therapy, but when he treated an addict who was also psychotic, he saw a concomitant improvement in the mental disturbance. Between 1933 and 1935, Sakel wrote a series of papers, claiming to have found the first effective weapon against schizophrenia. Psychological and physiological explanations were developed (but never proven) to explain the regression in schizophrenic symptoms that followed insulin shock. The treatment was widely used for a short time and then abandoned in the 1940s, because of its dangers, cost, and displacement by safer ways of inducing shock.

Studies in epilepsy and psychosis led the Hungarian psychiatrist Ladislas Joseph von Meduna to the conclusion that epileptics were never psychotic (now proven wrong). He reasoned that convulsive agents might cure schizophrenia. Unaware of earlier reports, Meduna believed himself to be the first to have produced convulsions with camphor in 1933, and later with its less toxic derivative, metrazol. Reactions to these drugs were unpredictable and uncontrollable: convulsions followed at variable intervals after the adminstration, and seizures could be so powerful that bones were broken, tongues bitten, and teeth lost.

Electroconvulsive shock therapy (ECT) was developed by the Italians Lucio Bini and Ugo Cerletti, who also had been studying epilepsy. By experimenting on hogs at a slaughterhouse, they established a safe dose of electricity and administered their first electroshock treatment to a human with schizophrenia in April 1938. By 1941, curare was being used to control the violent convulsions; the more easily monitored ECT was considered safer and more effective than chemical shock therapies. Though much demonized in popular literature and film, ECT is still used today for some psychotic disorders and for refractory endogenous depression. A typical dose now might be 70 to 130 volts passed through the brain for 0.1 to 0.5 second, but much higher doses were used in the past. For example, in 1948 L.E.M. Page and R.J. Russell developed intensive shock therapy using 150 volts for a full second, followed by five shocks of 100 volts during the convulsion; the process was repeated once or twice a day. With the lower doses, a rear-guard defensive action is being mounted by psychiatrists, historians, and patients to explode myths attached to ECT. Patient-satisfaction rates are often high, but study results relate to author opinion; as with other scientific investigations, disappointing findings are not published.

The first prefrontal lobotomies were performed in 1935 by Antonio de Egas Moniz and Pedro Manuel de Almeida Lima. A Portuguese-born neurosurgeon, Egas Moniz had invented cerebral angiography in 1927; he also served for twenty years as a liberal politician. He and Lima reasoned that morbid thoughts cycled repeatedly through the brains of psychotics, and that physically interrupting the cycle might be beneficial. They had learned from American experiments on chimpanzees that after prefrontal lobotomy, animals were more manageable and less easily frustrated. By extrapolation, they predicted that obsessive persons who were refractory to shock treatment could be 'relieved' with surgery into a state of manageable indifference. Their initial report on lobotomy, published in 1936, dealt with twenty human patients: seven had been cured, they claimed, seven improved, and six showed no change.

Prefrontal lobotomy (removal of frontal lobe tissue) and its less invasive successor, leucotomy (cutting tissue tracts), were widely practised in the 1930s and 1940s. American Walter J. Freeman performed over three thousand lobotomies, staking his career on the procedure, which he claimed could be done simply through the orbit (eye socket) with a device like an ice pick. A public outcry gradually caused the medical establishment to recognize that some patients so treated had become profoundly altered, tactless individuals, devoid of character – 'zombies.' Far from being a cure, the irreversible procedure was little more than a surgical straitjacket. What was obvious by the 1970s had been nearly invisible two decades earlier. It is both humbling and instructive to notice how often doctor-written histories of psychiatry ignore the embarrassing fact that in 1949 Egas Moniz, like Wagner-Jauregg before him, was awarded the Nobel Prize.

Freud himself believed that mental processes would eventually find biophysical explanations. Indeed, some physical models of mental disease met with success, especially in genetics and psychopharmacology. In the 1960s, studies of twins with schizophrenia examined the old theories of heredity in the light of modern genetics. Also in the latter half of the twentieth century, Alzheimer's disease and other dementias moved out of the realm of psychiatry into neurology, genetics, and pharmacology.

Psychopharmacology

Most of the psychobiological interventions described above did not turn out to be the hoped-for miracle cures, but the latest incarnation of this movement is the pervasive and successful psychopharmacology. Certain drugs were known to be effective in the care of a variety of psychic conditions, if only for inducing sedation. Bromides were introduced as sedatives in the nineteenth century, and by 1928 they were so popular that they accounted for 20 per cent of all prescriptions (Alexander and Selesnick 1966, 287). But sedatives did little for major psychotic disorders. In the mid-twentieth century, asylums were still full of people who could neither support nor care for themselves. This situation changed dramatically with the advent of effective psychoactive drugs.

The first major tranquillizers were derived from *Rauwolfia serpentina*, the snakeroot plant, long known in Asia for sedative properties; its products were also used for the treatment of hypertension, despite numerous side effects. Phenothiazines were discovered as a by-product of antihistamine research and introduced in the form of chlorpromazine in 1952 by the French psychiatrists Pierre G. Deniker and Jean Delay. Notwithstanding their many side effects – hepatitis, photosensitivity, tardive dyskinesia, and reduced seizure threshold – the phenothiazines did not provoke as much drowsiness as earlier agents; they calmed agitated patients, reduced the frequency of hallucination, and partially restored disordered thought patterns. They were brought to North America in 1954 by the German-born Canadian Heinz Lehmann, who first used chlorpromazine at the Verdun Protestant Hospital in Montreal.

Other psychoactive drugs have contributed to our concepts of mental disease. Two types of mood elevators, first the monoamine oxidase (MAO) inhibitors and then the tricyclic antidepressants, were introduced in 1956–7 for the treatment of depression. Minor tranquillizers in the form of benzodiazepines, beginning with chlordiazepoxide (Librium) and then diazepam (Valium), were initially applied to depressive states. Now they are used to control anxiety, but in the 1960s they were overprescribed, especially to women.

More impressive was the effect of lithium on manic-depressive illness. In 1949 the Australian John F.J. Cade was looking for toxins in mania. His strange experiment studied the relative quantities of human urine needed to kill guinea pigs: manic urine from psychotic patients was more lethal than normal urine, but it became less lethal when mixed with lithium. After experimenting with the administration of lithium (without urine), first on guinea pigs, then on himself, he gave the drug to manic individuals with startling success. Lithium results in improvement so marked and so specific that it has been taken as proof of the organic nature of bipolar disorder. At the time of writing, studies of neuroimaging are beginning to report consistent differences in the brain function of such individuals.

The advent of phenothiazines and lithium resulted in a deinstitutionalization movement, or what historians call 'decarceration,' as the asylums emptied in the late 1960s and early 1970s. Public consternation was roused when group homes and outpatient facilities were created in ordinary neighbourhoods. Hallucinogenic drugs, such as LSD (a derivative of ergotamine and mescaline), seemed to mimic psychotic states and were employed in studies of psychosis. But in the midst of these pharmacologic successes, experience with other drugs, such as amphetamines and vitamin B3 was less certain.

The Great Canadian Schizophrenia Controversy

Beginning the mid-1950s, the team of Abram Hoffer and Humphry Osmond of Saskatchewan began to explore megadoses of vitamins in the treatment of acute schizophrenia. Their experiment was prompted by concern over the side effects of the new psychoactive drugs and by biochemical understanding of the disease. Their popular claims to success were disputed and eventually rejected by the psychiatric establishment in Canada and the United States. In 1976 they marshalled the support of Nobel laureate Linus Pauling and responded with a blistering attack on the objectivity of their critics, the questionable methods of funding in psychiatry research, and the putative value of double-blind methodology in randomized controlled trials – one of the first epistemological objections to evidence-based medicine, well before the term was coined.

In the 1990s a group of drugs came on the market to become among the most profitable pharmaceutical products of the last two decades. Called the Selective Serotonin Reuptake Inhibitors (SSRIs), they include Zoloft, Prozac, and Paxil. In a sense, they are designer drugs developed over three decades of growing understanding about chemical substances in the brain: dopamine and serotonin. First discovered to be a neurotransmitter of the brain in 1957 by Swedish neuroscientist Arvid Carlsson, dopamine was quickly found to have a role in Parkinson's disease; Carlsson also suggested it may be active in schizophrenia. As a drug, dopamine can improve mood, but it has many side effects. Other drugs seemed to improve mood by raising serotonin levels in a more stable way. In contemplating the mysterious action of psychoactive drugs that seemed to work through the serotonin system, Carlsson suggested that a drug to prevent the reuptake of serotonin might enhance its availability and prove effective in depression and anxiety. His idea rested on the further hypothesis that something might be wrong with that serotonin system in mental illness.

The earliest SSRIs were developed by Carlsson in the early 1970s, but they had many side effects and are no longer used. Indeed Prozac was patented in 1974, but not released until 1988. Furthermore, no real problem is needed in the serotonin system of the brain for these drugs to have an effect on mood and personality; they do not correct an error. As a result, they are applied to a wide array of situations that are the product of social and cultural stressors rather than biological illness. Manufacturers have been accused of actually constructing diseases, such as premenstrual dysphoric disorder, to expand the market. Nevertheless, many cite their effectiveness as a kind of 'proof' of the biological origins of mental distress. Carlsson shared the Nobel Prize in 2000 for his work on dopamine.

Irish psychiatrist David Healy was concerned about the overuse of the SSRIs and the possibility that they might lead to suicide; but he was punished for speaking out about his convictions when a job offer from University of Toronto was withdrawn in 2000. Observers suggest that the university had foreseen a threat to its pharmaceutical support should he be hired. After a vigorous protest over this infringement of academic freedom, Healy was compensated in an out-of-court settlement with a visiting professorship and an undisclosed amount of money.

Drugs are now used as a mainstay for many minor mental disturbances; they are also used for psychosis and as adjuvants to psychotherapy for other problems. Some psychiatrists now observe that their job is to provide biological methods, leaving psychic methods for psychologists. For fiscal and pharmacological reasons, most psychiatric patients are managed outside hospitals; but social critics relate the recent increase in homelessness to the closure of asylums and the inability of untreated and uncared-for psychotics to manage on their own.

Antipsychiatry Movement

Mental diseases still continue to be diagnosed 'eighteenth-century style' by observation of symptoms and behaviour. In open recognition of the subjectivity of such an approach, the American Psychiatric Association (APA) sponsored the production of the first *Diagnostic and Statistical Manual* (DSM-I, 1952). Like an annotated nosological tree, the DSM strives for standards in nomenclature and diagnosis by providing statistical analyses of many similar cases. Since 1952, and through many subsequent revisions (1968, 1980, 1987, 1994, 2000), new diseases are recognized, defined, and subdivided; others are eliminated. Decisions to establish or delete categories are taken by a panel of distinguished experts. Sensitive to the possibilities of socio-cultural bias and stigma, the DSM-IV emphasizes that no diagnosis should be made without evidence of impairment in daily life. Planning for DSM-V began in 1999; the APA predicts its release for 2012.

In parallel with this endeavour to standardize diagnosis and eliminate bias, an antipsychiatry movement emerged, motivated by the abuses of physical therapies and the failures and inaccessibility of psychoanalysis. Some find it ironic that antipsychiatry grew during the period of psychopharmacologic achievements, the merits of which the movement refuses to acknowledge. Informed by the philosophies of social criticism, including feminism and Marxism, antipsychiatry strives to delineate and prevent abuses of power. Former patients are called 'survivors,' diagnosis is viewed with scepticism, and all treatments, including psychotherapy, are seen as methods of social control, while psychiatry itself has become the enemy, if not the disease. The conflict between psychiatric power and self-determinism was vividly expressed in the acclaimed Hollywood film *One Flew Over the Cuckoo's Nest* (1975), loosely based on the novel by Ken Kesey. Like psychoanalysis, antipsychiatry writers, such as Kate Millet and Paula Caplan, have become icons of popular culture.

Antipsychiatry garnered support from knowledgeable insiders, such as Thomas Szasz, who claims that mental illness is a myth, because it does not fit the medical model. His stance exemplifies the extent to which organic-based diagnosis has permeated our world view; but it has a fundamental weakness. What, in Szasz's opinion, would happen to these 'non-diseases' if a physical basis for them were found? Would they become real diseases after all, like the many mental disorders that were quickly transmuted into neurological, metabolic, or chemical problems? For example, within a decade of EEG, epilepsy was distinguished from hysterical convulsions. Similarly, the efficacy of lithium argues for the chemical basis of bipolar disorders; and the advent of histamine-2-antagonists, Helicobacter pylori, and beta-blockers closed prolix discussions of the personalities predisposing to ulcer disease and high blood pressure. Will the advent of technological diagnosis or an effective pharmaceutical invalidate the earlier psychic observations and correlations? Does it mean that subjective accounts are delusions or fabrications? Does 'pre-organic' suffering deserve to be ignored? Or, is psychiatric wisdom no longer relevant in a reductionist medical world?

Antipsychiatry: Who Pays?

During the 1980s an Ontario antipsychiatry periodical, *Phoenix Rising,* presented full-issue reports with dramatic titles: 'Death by Psychiatry,' 'A Close Up Look at the Enemy' (i.e., psychiatrists), 'Psychiatry Kills,' and 'Abolish Forced Psychiatric Treatment.' It inspired several spinoff publications, including David Reville's personal account of six months in Kingston Psychiatric Hospital, called *Don't Spyhole Me.* Support of *Phoenix Rising* was provided by the Ontario Arts Council until late 1988, when the folly of government-funded criticism of government-funded medical endeavour was exposed. The funds were withdrawn, sending *Phoenix Rising* into an irreversible death spiral.

Feeding the antipsychiatry movement are the biases that contaminated psychiatry in the past. For example, asylums were used in the former Soviet Union to incarcerate political dissenters. In North America, hundreds of women were castrated because they could not conform to societal norms of comportment. Poor people and criminals were confined in the absence of disease and sometimes over the protests of asylum keepers. Cultural beliefs, such as the evil eye and voodoo, also have been subjected to the psychiatric analysis of a different but dominant society. Certification has been used as a means of control, and mentally disturbed individuals have been stripped of their rights and inappropriately mutilated by experimentation. Critics point out that psychiatric diagnoses become tenacious labels equating people with their diseases in a physiological sense (see chapter 4): a person *is* 'a schizophrenic,' 'a manic depressive' – whereas other branches of medicine long ago turned away from terms such as 'leper' or 'AIDS victim' in favour of 'people living with leprosy/AIDS.'

Also among the activities that informed the antipsychiatry movement are the radical physical treatments of the past; for example, Henry Cotton's commitment to the theory of infection as a cause of mental illness resulted in operations to remove sites of 'focal sepsis.' He ordered tooth-pulling, tonsillectomies, sinus draining, cervix cleaning, and abdominal surgeries; his poor supervision and disastrous mortality rates results were exposed in 1925.

Another example comes from the 'psychic driving' experiments conducted by Donald Ewen Cameron at the Allan Memorial Institute in Montreal in the mid-1950s. Cameron was born in Scotland and trained in the United States at Johns Hopkins University and in Switzerland. His first job was to organize a network of mental health clinics in Manitoba. In 1943 he was recruited to McGill by the Yale-trained neurosurgeon Wilder Penfield. Two years later he was one of three North American psychiatrists invited to Nuremberg to assess the Nazi leader Rudolf Hess. There he learned of the atrocities committed by Nazi doctors in the name of science. A medical historian, Werner Leibbrand, who was a witness for the prosecution at Nuremberg, suggested that Nazi doctors (45 per cent of all German doctors) laboured under an attitude called 'biological thought,' in which the patient had become simply an object for scientific study. Despite his trip to Nuremberg, Cameron would commit similar crimes.

In the postwar climate, Cameron and his colleagues feared the mind-control capacities of communist enemies. The aura of urgency and international importance led him to investigate ways of preventing mind control by creating it. In short, he experimented on mentally ill patients by administering so-called treatments that were not only unnecessary but damaging. Secret funding for his research came from the Canadian government and the U.S. Central Intelligence Agency.

Cameron had hoped that his institute at McGill would become the first successful centre for psychosomatic or biological psychiatry. In the mid-1950s, with his associate Hassan Azima, he developed 'psychic driving' by modifying a Russian technique of sleep treatment: patients were heavily sedated with the newly discovered tranquillizers, occasionally combined with hallucinogenic drugs and electroshock. While asleep for hours, days, or weeks, they were forced to listen to repetitive, tape-recorded, personal messages that often dwelt on their faults. The theory used to justify such torture was that the regression so induced would disrupt resistance to psychotherapy.

In 1956 Cameron announced the success of his technique. But the full story, which emerged only thirty years later, is that many of his patients were irreparably damaged by the brainwashing – stripped of their personalities, their livelihood, and their families. Cameron's relationship with Penfield cooled, and he left Montreal in 1964 to direct a laboratory in Albany, New York. He died three years later with his reputation intact, having risen to the highest prominence in psychiatry, serving at various times as president óf the Quebec Psychiatric Association, the Canadian Psychiatric Association, the American Psychiatric Association, the World Psychiatric Association, the American Psychopathological Association, and the Society for Biological Psychiatry. In 1992 the Canadian government compensated the victims of Cameron's psychic-driving experiments.

Stories like these help to explain the antipsychiatry movement, and they appeal to historians and social critics. As a result, antipsychiatry has come to pervade the field of medical history, where the debates within psychiatry itself are now championed by its historians both for and against. As described by the pro-biological-psychiatry historian Edward Shorter, 'zealot historians,' imbued with aberrant Freudian thought, peer at shameful episodes of the past through biased lenses. They and many doctors object to the use of the words 'mad,' 'madness,' and 'madhouse' to refer to the past because they are disrespectful. In contrast, historians, like Andrew Scull, remind us that Shorter's zealots strive only to use the language of the past in its context; it is still early to be claiming triumph over mental illness: 'chlorpromazine is no penicillin,' Scull once wrote. Some episodes may be unpleasant to recall, but they should not be forgotten; it would be naive to suppose that our present system is devoid of prejudice. As for the pejorative word 'mad,' it is now taken by survivors' movements and by teachers, like Geoffrey Reaume, determined to give voice to patient experience and to raise 'Mad Pride.'

In this context, it is fascinating to note how much recent history of psychiatry has been built around national endeavours, especially in oppressive regimes, such as Russia, Argentina, and African colonies. The management of the mentally ill and other vulnerable people cannot be separated from a nation's view of itself. Indeed, through the example of historians who have taken on upsetting moments in the past of mental illness, previously neglected topics in other areas have been given new edge: disability, deviance, crime, and aging.

Ambivalent Status of Psychotherapy

Important questions are raised by the definition of psychiatric diagnoses and by acceptance of therapies. Payment of fees for outpatient psychotherapy is being reconsidered in some jurisdictions, and the status from nation to nation is variable. Psychoanalysis is partially reimbursed by Canadian health insurance; most patients must pay for this expensive treatment themselves. The 'talk therapies,' including psychoanalysis, are now being subjected to evidence-based medicine analysis, and over two hundred reviews concerning psychotherapy appear in the Cochrane database.

Yet why should psychotherapy be disallowed? Too expensive? Ineffective? Inegalitarian in a society that demands equality for everyone in everything? Is it because psychotherapy tends to downplay the biological causes? And if psychotherapy is not 'covered,' will only the wealthy be able to afford it, meaning that the poor and middle classes will be increasingly directed to drugs? The status of psychotherapy funding becomes a public and political pronouncement on the physicality of mental illness.

Disease When Drugs Do Not Work

Psychiatric diagnoses rely on observation, after eliminating disorders with identifiable organic causes. A decision must be made about whether or not the behaviour, thought, and mood are appropriate or inappropriate, healthy or sick. Equating inappropriate behaviour with sickness leaves psychiatry open to the biases, described above, of culture, race, religion, politics, and class. In other words, in psychiatry more than in any other medical field, the definition of normal can be ethnocentric.

Variations occur not only between cultures, but within culture through time. Some conditions previously thought of as sicknesses have become variations of normal; for example, homosexuality. In ancient Greece, homosexuality was tolerated, even approved. In Judeo-Christian cultures, it was a sin, and, by extension, it also became a crime. In the late nineteenth century, it was retrieved from moral disapprobation (if not legal) and reconstituted as a disease by Richard von Krafft-Ebing and Henry Havelock Ellis. When I was at medical school in the early 1970s, homosexuality was still a disease, but physicians were uncomfortable with that label. As a disease, homosexuality theoretically required treatment, and if treatment was unavailable, then research should be undertaken. But homosexuality was not life threatening, it was rarely 'curable,' and few of its 'sufferers' wanted to be cured. Instead, homosexuals wished that society could be cured of its intolerance.

One way of dealing with an 'incurable' condition that does not kill its sufferers is to decide that those who have it are not sick. In 1973 homosexuality was deleted from the DSM by a non-unanimous vote of mostly male, mostly white, mostly heterosexual psychiatrists. A heated debate followed over retaining an entry for homosexuals who were uncomfortable with their sexual orientation. Now, homosexuality is recognized as a variation of normal. Changes in the cultural and sociopolitical climate have contributed to this decision.

Should the existence of diseases be decided by the votes of highly educated upper-middle-class professionals? Are physical diagnoses determined in this way, or is universal agreement implicit in their first definitions? How often were votes cast on the status of appendicitis? Diabetes? Leukemia? Epilepsy? Cancer? Arthritis? Should our recognition of psychiatry's special vulnerability and cultural subjectivity allow us to reject this method of diagnosis? My answer is no.

Psychiatry is a fascinating blend of sensitive humanitarian ideals with the latest in pharmacological and neurological research. Its goal is to help unhappy people move from chronic incapacity to contented living and self-sufficiency. Positive outcomes restore the well-being of patients and their contributions to communities. Perhaps the old ambition to effect radical cures for 'diseases,' which had yet to be delineated, has been softened to a more realistic yet worthy aim to help people adjust to themselves and their world. Unique among medical specialties, psychiatry admits and deals with its susceptibility to social construction. The successful practice of psychiatry is not hampered by acknowledging its vulnerability through an awareness of the triumphs and transgressions in its past. In history as in analysis, 'being entirely honest with oneself is a good exercise' (Freud, 15 October 1897, in *Origins of Psychoanalysis*, New York: Basic Books, 1954, 223)

Suggestions for Further Reading

At the bibliography website http://histmed.ca.

CHAPTER THIRTEEN

No Baby, No Nation:
*History of Pediatrics**

Pediatrics does not deal with miniature men and women, with reduced doses and the small class of diseases in smaller bodies, but ... has its own independent range and horizon, and gives as much to general medicine as it has received from it.

– Abraham Jacobi (1889), in P. English, 'Not
Miniature Men and Women' (1989), 254

The wisdom that infants and children were subject to certain specific diseases and problems originated in antiquity. But medical – as opposed to parental – care for children emerged in the seventeenth and eighteenth centuries, together with a marked shift in social attitudes toward children. The specialty of pediatrics (from the Greek words for 'child' and 'healer') did not come into being until the nineteenth century. The history of this specialty cannot be separated from the history of concepts of childhood; in this chapter we will briefly examine both.

Pediatrics has focused on prevention of disease and disability as much as on cure. To accomplish this goal, it was forced to wrestle with the social and economic determinants of health sooner and more effectively than all other medical endeavours.

*Learning objectives for this chapter are found on pp. 456–7.

Have All Peoples Loved Their Babies? History of Children and Childhood

With his influential book of 1960 (translated in 1962 as *Centuries of Childhood*), Philippe Ariès claimed that childhood was culturally conditioned – a social construction (see chapters 4 and 7). He meant that care for growing children satisfied social expectations. How often should babies be fed? What should they eat? How should they be dressed? At what games, where, and how often should they play? What stories may they be told? When and where should they sleep? And – the most important question for Ariès – should they be educated? If so, how? Examining evidence from the Middle Ages to the twentieth century, he found that the answers to these questions varied widely and had evolved slowly through time. He concluded that the notion of childhood as a time of innocence, play, and learning was entirely modern.

Several writers modified Ariès's arguments; some cited earlier authors who had anticipated his ideas. Lloyd De Mause (*History of Childhood*) claimed that child care was an indicator of human civilization as it moved through six positivistic stages of improvement, beginning with ancient brutality and ending with modern helping. Others simplified these rigid self-congratulatory categories to manifestations of economic realities in time and place: were children perceived to be 'financial assets,' born to increase family wealth and provide for aging parents? Or were they 'financial liabilities' whose upbringing entailed investment and debts willingly incurred? The extent to which societies embraced one or the other attitude determined the extent to which children were granted a childhood.

Many scholars now reject the idea that brutality to children ever formed part of any socially sanctioned tradition. They criticize it as an unjustified presentist projection upon a scarcely knowable past; and they point out that infanticide and abuse continue to be significant causes of child mortality in the seemingly civilized developed world of the twenty-first century. Nevertheless, all historians who write about children recognize that the length and nature of childhood has varied.

Child Care and Health in Antiquity

In antiquity, pediatrics did not form a distinct body of medical knowledge. Several historians scoured extant ancient texts to dredge up references to children. The Hippocratic Corpus (of the fifth century B.C.) includes treatises on dentition and on premature infants, while the famous *Sacred Disease* contains astute observations on child patients.

On Childhood Epilepsy

Such as are habituated to their disease have a presentiment [aura] when an attack is imminent ... Young children at first fall anywhere, because they are unfamiliar with the disease; but when they have suffered several attacks, on having the presentiment they run to their mothers or to somebody they know very well, through fear and terror at what they are suffering.

– Hippocrates, *Sacred Disease*, XV

References to children appear in the works of Celsus (first century A.D.), Soranus of Ephesus, Aretaeus, and Galen (all in the second century), and Oribasius (fourth century). Childhood diseases recognized in antiquity include *aphthae* (thought perhaps to be ulcers, thrush, or diphtheria), hydrocephalus, rickets, ophthalmia, rashes, 'epilepsy' (infantile convulsions), and *seiriasis* (possibly meningitis or dehydration). By their very scarcity, however, these citations indicate that the professional medicine of ancient Greece was generally not for kids. As if to endorse this conclusion, Mettler recalled that one of the most detailed ancient accounts of human birth is found in Aristotle's *History of Animals*. Children may have been the property of their fathers, as were their mothers and slaves; however, responsibility for their care resided with women – mothers, midwives, and wet nurses – not with doctors. And most women could not read or write.

What was baby care in antiquity? At birth, children were 'salted' with alkaline soda ash, avoiding the eyes, and then washed to remove the vernix. This practice probably arose in prehistory, and it persisted until approximately 1000 A.D. The Arabic authors preferred oil to soda ash, and later writers recommended diluted wine. Infants were 'swaddled' (bound tightly) to prevent movement, to keep them warm, and to ensure that they would grow straight. Sometimes, thus bound, they were hung on hooks to keep them out of the way. Breast milk was the food of choice. The obstetrical treatise of Soranus of Ephesus described the 'fingernail test' to assess the quality of mothers' milk: a drop should retain its form, being neither too runny nor too thick. This test was still being cited in the eighteenth-century work of William Smellie (see chapter 11). When a year old, the child would be offered gruel mixtures of honey, sprouts, barley porridge, and goat's or cow's milk. For irritability associated with teething and other ailments, infants were drugged with opium or wine.

Controversial evidence, both literary and demographic, suggests that ancient Greeks and Romans may have practised infanticide of deformed babies and some healthy females by leaving them exposed; how many newborns perished in this way is unknown. Wealthy women used paid wet nurses even in antiquity, and the practice eventually spread to all social classes, including slaves. Breastfeeding was known to be contraceptive; a slave was more 'useful' if her baby was sent away to be nursed, allowing the mother both to work and to breed another future slave. If a child fell ill, medicine would be given to the wet nurse for transmission to her charge through her milk. If wet nurses could not be found, artificial feeding preoccupied those who cared for orphaned or abandoned children. But effective compositions were elusive, and the mechanics of feeding small infants from sponges, spouts, boats, and spoons were complicated and risky. Until the twentieth century, artificial feeding usually meant disaster.

What we know of child care is derived not only from written sources but from artwork and from objects such as infant feeding vessels, catheters, cradles, clothing, shoes, amulets, and toys. Some congenital deformities, including dwarfism, club foot, and dislocated hip, can be recognized in ancient art. The Canadian pediatrician and nutritionist Theodore G.H. Drake amassed and researched an extensive collection of prints, books, and artefacts, including 250 feeding vessels, from antiquity to the present, now the property of the Royal Ontario Museum in Toronto (see Spaulding and Welch 1991).

Arabic, Medieval, and Renaissance Pediatrics

Arabic authors adopted the infant-care practices of their Greco-Roman precursors, but they also acknowledged society's responsibility for children. Perhaps because the prophet Mohammed had been an orphan, the Koran laid out provisions for children of divorced or deceased parents. It also condemned female infanticide and discrimination against women.

Again, evidence of 'pediatrics' in the Middle Ages is scant; most medical writings scarcely mention children. The tenth-century Persian, Rhazes (see chapter 4), distinguished smallpox from measles on the basis of symptoms and signs, recognizing their peculiarities in children; however, the diseases thought to afflict children had changed little since antiquity. In his *Canon*, Ibn Sina (Avicenna) compiled views of his predecessors on infant ailments. Like them, he envisaged the wet nurse as a therapeutic instrument; for example, a baby should not be bled, but the nurse could be bled or cupped on its behalf. Even female medical writers who might be expected to have had some existential familiarity with child care, including Dame Trot of Salerno and Hildegard of Bingen, refer to birthing, but say little about children.

The relative silence of medieval medics on the subject should not allow us to suppose that there was no theory of child care. This knowledge lay in oral traditions conveyed by wise (but illiterate) women to other women, beyond the sphere of learned men. The German historian Karl Sudhoff studied multiple manuscript copies of two treatises on the care of children dating from the sixth to ninth century. The authors and their intended audience are unknown, but the treatises describe practices similar to those outlined in ancient and Arabic writings (Ruhräh 1925, 22–6).

Another indicator that oral tradition played a role in child care is the special genre of pediatric poems. Shortly after the advent of printing, versified works on the care of babies and children appeared in the vernacular, rather than in Latin. The *Versehung des Leibs* (Proper Care of the Body), composed by the monk Heinrich von Louffenburg, was printed in 1491 from a 1429 manuscript held in Munich. The inspiration is said to have been a much older and much-copied Latin manuscript, the *Regimen sanitatis* of Salerno (ca 1000 A.D.). The appearance of these poems in the fifteenth century does not imply that they originated at that time. More likely, they had been chanted for generations in easy-to-remember verse before being preserved in writing, like the songs of Homer, Norse sagas, the Anglo-Saxon *Beowulf*, and nursery rhymes.

Christianity disapproved of infanticide, abortion, and contraception; the practices may have declined but did not disappear. Children continued to be sold or stolen into slavery; others were maimed to make them more effective beggars. A new cause of child death emerged during the Middle Ages – 'overlying' – the supposed fatal accident of an adult lying on a child who shared the same bed; a special device, the *arcutio*, was invented to prevent it (see figure 13.1). Scholars now doubt the realistic probability of overlying, suggesting that this 'disease' may have been invented to conceal murder.

In contrast to the silence of previous writers, among the earliest printed medical books were new works on disease in children. Paolo Bagellardo published the first treatise devoted solely to childhood diseases – *De infantium aegritudinibus ac remediis* (On diseases of children and remedies), printed in Padua in 1472. The following year, Bartholomaeus Metlinger of Augsburg produced a work in the German vernacular. A decade later, Cornelius Roelans did the same, but his book is so rare that only two copies are known to exist. Rösslin's much-reprinted midwifery treatise, *Rosengarten* (1513), also contained advice on child care (see chapter 11). The illustrated 1577 treatise of Omnibonus Ferrarius contained images of various ambitious gadgets, including a breast pump, a helmet to prevent head injury, a walker, and a toilet chair. Finally, Hieronymus Mercurialis of Padua prepared a 1584 compendium of children's diseases, liberally annotated with observations on parasitic worms and other topics. Artificial feeding continued to be an important preoccupation, and recipes were provided for broth, called 'panada,' and flour-based mixtures called 'pap.' Rather than presenting new discoveries, these

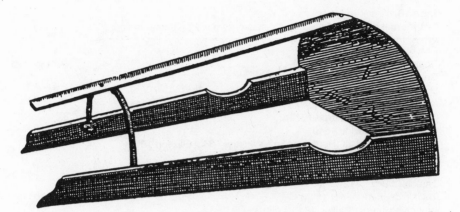

13.1   *Arcutio*, a device to prevent overlying. Inside the frame, a baby could not be accidently crushed by a parent who shared the bed. From *Philosophical Transactions* 422 (1732), opp. 223

books compiled the knowledge of the ancients, the Persians, and local women, finally bringing the child to the attention of medical practitioners.

Enlightenment: Diseases and the Discovery of Child Mortality

During the seventeenth and eighteenth centuries, two parallel processes emphasized the health status of children: first, nosology, or the definition of all diseases, including those of children; and second, the rise in medical statistics.

Nosology arose from a study of symptoms to classify and distinguish diseases as separate entities (see chapter 4). Most conditions had been recognized in antiquity, but a few new accounts of ailments peculiar to children distinguished them from other sufferers. Picking up where the tenth-century Rhazes had left off with his separation of measles and smallpox, several children's diseases were described in the seventeenth century (see table 13.1).

By 1689, Walter Harris of London had assembled many disease descriptions into a Latin treatise, which has been called the first modern textbook of acute pediatric diseases. The reputation of this book, one historian said, extended 'far beyond its merits'; yet he acknowl-

Table 13.1
'Classic' descriptions of childhood disease from the seventeenth century

Chicken pox (Chanael 1610)
Chorea (Sydenham 1686)
Cretinism (Plat[t]er 1625)
Diphtheria (Villareal 1611)
Neonatal syphilis (Guillemeau 1609)
Neonatal tetanus (Andreu 1678)
Rheumatism (Baillou 1640)
Rickets, or rachitism (Reusner 1582; Whistler 1645; Glisson 1650)
Scabies (Wurtz 1612)
Scarlet fever (Sennert 1641; Sydenham 1676)
Thrush (Wurtz 1612)
Thymic death (Plat[t]er 1614)
Whooping cough (Baillou 1640; Willis 1675)

edged the impact of the eighteen editions published over the next half-century in English, French, German, and Latin (Still 1931, 291). Harris's treatise found an English successor in Michael Underwood's 1784 work, the last edition of which appeared nearly sixty years later. Extending the nosology of the preceding century, Underwood described neonatal icterus, poliomyelitis, and congenital heart disease. In the United States, Benjamin Rush wrote a new account of the ancient cholera infantum, a form of diarrhea and vomiting that was called the 'summer complaint.' These descriptions of specific diseases invited a search for specific cures.

The second process to captivate would-be pediatricians was the shocking revelation of high mortality rates among children across Europe and North America. Because Islam and Christianity both condemned infanticide, formal provision was made for orphaned or abandoned infants. Beginning in 787 in Milan, asylums had operated throughout continental Europe, founded by bishops, priests, and other clerics, one of whom was St Vincent de Paul. But these dwellings were unlike the hospitals of today, although some, like Florence's Hospital of the Innocents, bore the name. Instead, they were warehouses rather than places of healing. Children were brought in the wagons of porters, who commanded fees for use of their regular circuits. A turnstile system was invented to provide anonymity and protect infants awaiting discovery at the asylum door. Called

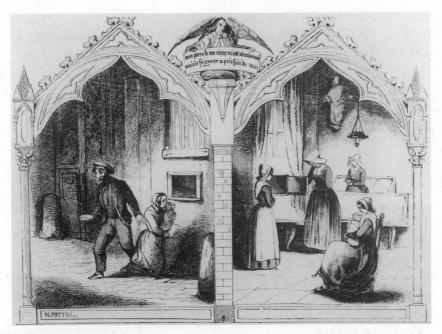

13.2   A foundling home. Outside, the parents leave their infant; inside, the nuns make ready to retrieve the babe. *Enfants trouvés: Le tour, extérieur et intérieur.* Engraving by Henri Pottin, after a seventeenth-century original. Drake Collection, Canadian Museum of Health and Medicine, Toronto

a 'tour' (turn) in both English and French, it had a small door on the outer wall which could be opened to place the child on a revolving table or shelf; a bell might ring, someone inside would open an inner door and retrieve the child; no names, no questions (see figure 13.2). Cities ran fostering systems for nurslings until they could feed themselves. Survivors were cared for, taught a trade, and eventually released, usually by the age of eight. Mothers of illegitimate infants were sometimes welcomed if they would nurse one or more of the other children with their own.

The eighteenth-century discovery of the high mortality rates in these institutions seems to have come as a horrifying surprise. Furthermore, the rates were rising. Historian Philip Gavitt demonstrated that foundling mortality in fifteenth-century Florence ranged from 12 to 60 per cent. Joan Sherwood showed that in the Inclusa of Madrid three hundred years later, the annual death rates ranged between 53 and 87 per cent of admissions, with a rising trend. Economic and cultural factors meant that admissions increased, alms declined, and the price of wheat rose; there were more mouths to feed and fewer resources to pay for wet nurses and provisions.

In Paris on the eve of the revolution, between 5,000 and 6,000 children were abandoned annually. According to Dora Weiner, these numbers had been increasing steadily throughout the eighteenth century. Whether the foundlings were placed in the various city hospices or were fostered in the countryside, about 60 per cent succumbed in their first year; another 30 per cent died before the age of five. In London, a similar picture emerged. Bills of mortality from 1730 to 1750 reveal that 75 per cent of all infants did not live to five years. The carnage did not respect class boundaries: Queen Anne bore seventeen or eighteen children, but none survived childhood. In any year, 40 per cent of all deaths were of children under five. The historian Daniel Teysseire, who analysed references to children in the *Encyclopédie* (1751–77) of Denis Diderot and Jean d'Alembert, concluded that to be a child in eighteenth-century France was to be sick. With the Industrial Revolution and the privations associated with poorly remunerated labour in factories and sweatshops, the health even of children who had not been abandoned or institutionalized began to deteriorate.

Malthus on Foundling Homes

The greatest part of this premature mortality is clearly to be attributed to these institutions, miscalled philanthropic ...

If a person wished to check population, and were not solicitous about the means, he could not propose a more effectual measure than the establishment of a sufficient number of foundling hospitals.

– T.R. Malthus, *Essay on the Principle of Population,*
bk 2, iii (1803; reprint, Cambridge, 1989), 177–9

The fate of innocent children became a matter of national pride. With a newly rising liberalism in social and political thought, the ideas of philosophers like physician John Locke and Jean-Jacques Rousseau endorsed the value of an extended period of youthful learning and play. Combined with the appalling statistics, the new numerical methods in medicine also turned medical minds to prevention. The bleak outlook shamed reformers into action. But what exactly should or could be done to save the lives of children?

The Dawn of Child Welfare

Once they fell ill of the acute illnesses that tended to plague them, children rarely survived; it had to be admitted that medicine could not save them. On the other hand, most children were born healthy; the goal should be to keep them that way. Prevention of illness had to be the best medicine. Reformers moved on several levels at once: dispensaries and hospitals; policies to promote hygiene; advice literature; medical and surgical research; and legislation.

What Mothers Want and What They Need

The mother wishes that her child be happy, as long as he is, she is right; when she is wrong in her methods, it is necessary to enlighten her.

– Jean-Jacques Rousseau, epigraph in Michael Underwood,
Traité sur les maladies des enfants (1784; trans.,
Quebec: Nouvelle Imprimerie, 1803)

Hygiene and Advice

Philanthropists tried to improve conditions in foundling homes, and they also created dispensaries for free care, in a process similar to the concurrent asylum movement for the mentally ill (see chapter 12). Unlike major cities in the rest of Europe, London had no children's hospice until after the realization of the high mortality rates. In response, the merchant Thomas Coram established London's Foundling Hospital in 1741; however, this gathering of healthy infants could not guarantee their survival. Coram and his reformers were immediately challenged on how to keep motherless children alive; once again, artificial feedings proved to be a failure. An advocate of artificial feeding ('dry nursing'), George Armstrong opened a dispensary for the free care of the ailing 'infant poor' of London in 1767. Armstrong also wrote a description of pyloric stenosis. Three years later, a rival dispensary was inaugurated under the supervision of J.C. Lettsom, who launched vitriolic attacks on Armstrong. Philanthropy had become politically correct, and physicians vied for the spotlight. From 1730 to 1810, the London bills of mortality showed a steady decline in mortality before age five from 75 to 40 per cent. Similarly, in postrevolutionary France, with the new provisions for cleanliness and accountability at child-care institutions, mortality of abandoned infants under five supposedly fell from 83 per cent in 1798 to 13.5 per cent in 1813.

The education of parents, especially the poor, became yet another arm of this multipronged attack on infant mortality. Medical experts took up the venerable practice of offering advice on how to rear healthy children. Guidelines for the London Foundling Hospital were based on the 1748 *Essay* of William Cadogan, who wrote (at first anonymously) against a tide of tradition by prescribing loose clothing (rather than swaddling), daily bathing, and maternal breastfeeding. In 1761 the Swiss hygienist Simon A. Tissot laid down rules for physical and mental health, through heating and aeration of homes, moderate diet, and exercise. Tissot was one of the first to describe the dangers of masturbation, which was much touted as a cause of somatic and moral degeneration until well into the twentieth century. Similar instructions emerged in Germany, where 'school hygiene' originated. In his 1780 treatise, Johann Peter Frank stipulated the state's obligations to care for and to educate children. Frank's work inspired the widely distributed and oft-translated *Catechism of Health* (1794) by Bernhard C. Faust. Inadvertently, or perhaps deliberately, however, the social hygiene movement tended to blame mothers and nurses for the suffering and loss of their children.

Communicating this wisdom to the often illiterate masses, especially to mothers, was not always easy. In some places, monetary rewards for the survival and number of children were established. Remnants of these programs survive today: France and Quebec maintain tax relief and price reductions for *les familles nombreuses* as part of an active pro-natalist policy. The rising literacy of women opened the door for advice literature for families – almanacs and self-help manuals – that often contained liberal doses of moral philosophy, led by John Wesley's *Primitive Physic* (1746). *Domestic Medicine* (1769) by the Scottish physician William Buchan saw multiple editions in many countries and translations into at least seven languages until its demise in 1913. Numerous imitators and 'improvements' were printed widely. Addressed to a rural elite, these 'family physician' books were novel in their emphasis on child care. Academic physicians also participated in the movement

In Germany, the distinguished liberal professor Christoph W. Hufeland published a vulgarization, *The Art of Prolonging Human Life*, just as he launched an early medical periodical. Similarly, the 1803 Quebec edition of Michael Underwood's treatise summarized his recommendations to mothers of ailing children. The practice continued with the work of Severin Lachapelle, professor of hygiene in Montreal, who wrote several advice manuals for the general public and translated the popular *Practical Home Physician* of the Chicago professor Henry M. Lyman. Recommendations could vary widely, and some confident pronouncements on neonatal feeding now seem peculiar – for example, the early introduction of egg, or the withholding of banana. With modifications in specifics, this tradition continued with the popular mid-twentieth-century manual of Dr Spock (see below) and its numerous descendants.

Medical and Surgical Advances

Anatomical research on childhood diseases led to surgical and medical solutions for long-standing problems. Even the fetus began to attract attention when in 1827 Hufeland wrote a treatise on diseases in utero. The life-saving method of tracheotomy for diphtheria, first suggested by several authors in the early seventeenth century, was promoted by Pierre Bretonneau in 1826. Chief among these impressive achievements was Jenner's discovery, published in 1798, that cowpox could protect people from smallpox (see chapter 7).

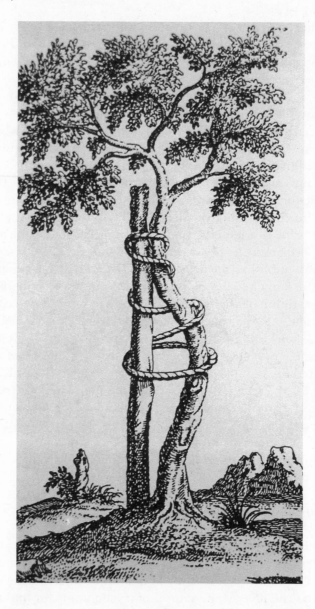

13.3 The tethered tree symbolizing the goals of orthopedics. From Nicolas Andry, *Orthopedia, or the Art of Correcting and Preventing Deformities in Children,* vol. 1, 1743, opp. 211

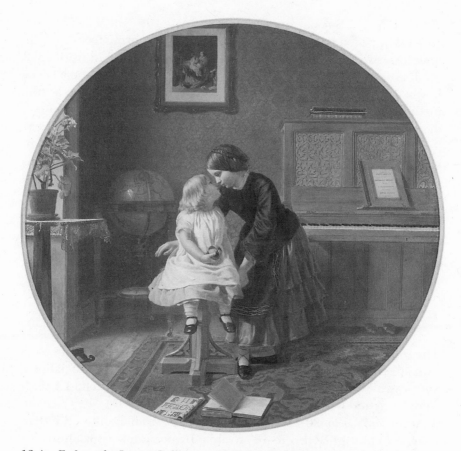

13.4 *Enfance*, by James Collinson, 1855. National Gallery of Canada

Chronic ailments also received attention. In 1741 Nicolas Andry introduced the word *orthopédie* (derived from the Greek for 'straight' and 'child'). His treatise described procedures for the correction of club foot and hip disorders (see figure 13.3). But not all his recommendations were surgical: he also prescribed for tics, chlorosis (anemia), rashes, nail problems, pimples, warts, lisping, and stuttering. Deaf children were taught to communicate through the efforts of Thomas H. Gallaudet in the United States and J.M.G. Itard in France.

Finally, medicine and surgery had something to offer sick or disabled children. Special hospitals were created for the specific *treat-ment* (as opposed to warehousing) of children suffering from specific diseases. Paris opened the Hôpital des Enfants Malades in April 1802 on the site of a much older orphanage; now merged with the Necker hospital, it claims to be the world's oldest pediatric hospital in a truly medical sense. Infants with neonatal syphilis were transferred imme-diately to a special venereal hospital at Vaugirard, where they were 'treated,' in the ancient tradition – through wet nurses taking mercu-ry, sometimes for their own syphilitic afflictions, sometimes not (see chapter 7). Children's hospitals also appeared in Germany (1840s), London (1852), New York (1854), Philadelphia (1855), Edinburgh (1860), Chicago (1865), Boston (1869, after an 1846 precursor had closed), and Toronto (1875). Physicians hoped that these hospitals would provide treatment, as well as human resources for further research. Since most inpatients were poor and uneducated, reform-ers also envisaged the hospital as a locus of moral training.

Professionalization of Pediatrics

The following decades saw the professionalization of pediatrics as its own specialty, defined by professorships, departments, associations, and journals. Many new periodicals devoted solely to child health were launched between the 1790s and 1920s (for a list, see Garrison and Abt 1965, 125–30). A chair in pediatrics was inaugurated in Par-is in 1879 and in Berlin in 1894, while professional associations for pediatrics were founded in Germany (1883), Russia (1885), and the United States (1888). The American specialty board was created in 1933, its Canadian equivalent in 1937, with certification being grant-ed in 1942 by 'grandfathering' and in 1946 by examination.

Convinced that social solutions could be found for biological prob-lems, many pediatricians maintained links to political liberalism. The first president of the American Pediatric Society, Abraham Jacobi, had left his native Germany after the right-wing revolution of 1848. As the pediatrician and historian Peter C. English argues, Jacobi's vision of pediatrics was predicated on his concept of social interven-tion to disrupt the continuing high mortality in foundling homes (which was still 75 per cent or greater). Jacobi thought that the main killers of children, especially diarrhea and respiratory illness, could be eradicated only by attacking the underlying problems of poverty and housing.

The arrival of the new professional bodies followed hard upon Koch's 1882 discovery of the mycobacterium tuberculosis and the concomitant realization that the notorious killer, consumption, could be spread through cow's milk. Pediatricians finally were able to devise safer methods of artificial feeding of motherless babies through application of innovations in nutrition and sterilization. The technology of the rubber nipple (U.S. patent, 1845) had been a boon to artificial feeding, while pasteurization, developed by Louis Pasteur in 1864, promised to improve its safety. At the end of the nineteenth century, keeping newborns healthy seemed to be an attainable goal.

At the turn of the century, public hygienists became increasingly preoccupied with childhood mortality. Dispensaries for advice and well-baby care were set up in all major cities, beginning with Paris (1892) and New York (1893) (see figure 13.5). Similarly, milk depots were created to provide a steady, affordable supply of clean milk. The municipal milk station that opened at Rochester, New York, in 1897 claimed to be the first in North America. Success was measured by annual reviews of mortality. Montreal was reputed to have one of the highest rates of infant mortality in North America, and its *Gouttes de lait* clinics were opened in 1901 to offer safe milk services in French and English. The system quickly grew to twenty-eight depots by 1915. In cities and rural areas, public health nurses instructed mothers in the principles of hygiene and infant feeding. Between 1905 and 1911, international conferences on the provision of milk were held in Paris, Brussels, and Berlin, but discussion extended to all causes of infant death.

With improved hygiene, mortality rates began to fall; however, prior to antibiotics and vaccines against other childhood diseases, the life-saving power of hygiene alone was limited. In their study of the United States around 1900, Preston and Haines demonstrated that child mortality remained as high as 20 per cent. In Canada, some decline in mortality may have been more apparent than real, as it coincided with increased reliability in recording of births. It is impor-

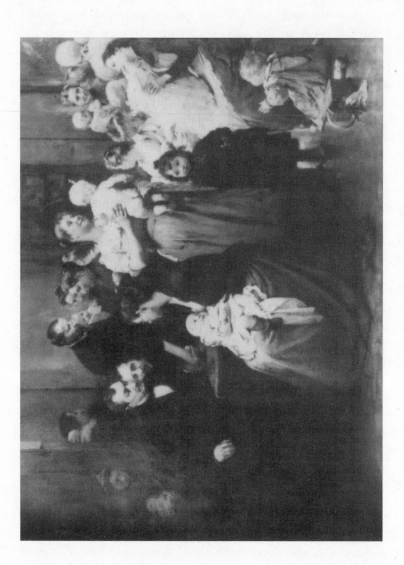

13.5   At a clinic in a poor suburb of Paris, doctors dispense advice and milk to mothers who are eager to keep their babies healthy. *Goutte de lait de Belleville*, detail from a triptych by Henri Geoffroy, Musée de l'Assistance Publique, Paris

tant to remember that early success may also have been due to a general willingness to let children live (see 'Social Pediatrics,' below).

Medicalizing Growth

In the early twentieth century, several exciting discoveries meant that what had once been the domain of wise women and entrepreneurs now became the purview of doctors, scientists, and industrial giants (see figure 13.6). These discoveries included germ theory, vaccines, diphtheria toxoid, hormones, genetics, vitamins, and antibiotics. One by one, the scourges of childhood were dramatically reduced, if not eliminated: measles, diphtheria, mumps, whooping cough, scarlatina, and rheumatic fever with its associated heart and kidney complications. An epidemic of poliomyelitis in the early 1950s was stemmed by the advent of Salk and Sabin vaccines; experts now predict the global eradication of this disease (see chapter 7). Even congenital abnormalities, including heart disease and hip displacement, which had once condemned children to chronic dependency if not early death, could now be repaired, allowing them to reach maturity as productive members of society. Many surgeons made important contributions to these endeavours (see chapter 10). Childhood disability, especially mental retardation, was taken on as an issue for prevention; concerted efforts were mounted to eliminate medical causes of this problem through neonatal screening and vaccination: congenital syphilis, Rh hemolytic disease of the newborn, kernicterus, measles, Hemophilus influenzae type B meningitis, congenital hypothyroidism, phenylketonuria, and congenital rubella syndrome. After half a century of concerted effort, these causes have been markedly reduced, but they constituted only about 16 per cent of cases in 1950. Critics believe that this serious concern is ignored and underfunded.

Subspecialization

Pediatrics began to divide into various subspecialties, defined by child age. Neonatology arose out of specific achievements in the mid-1950s. New York anesthetist Virginia Apgar developed her sim-

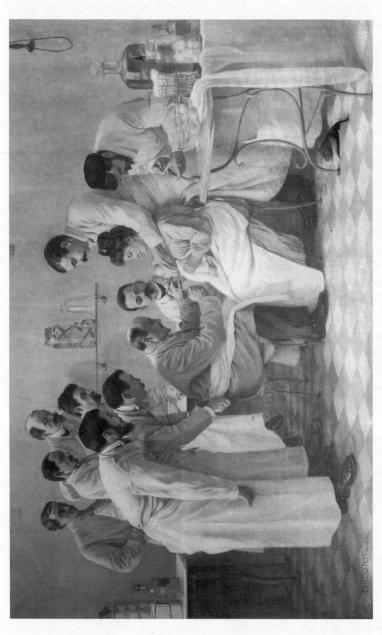

13.6   Surrounded by concerned adults, a child with diphtheria is being intubated by a physician, who may be a partisan in the debate on intubation versus tracheotomy. Lines in the tableau converge on the infant's throat. *Le tubage*, attributed to G. Chicotot, early twentieth century, Musée de l'Assistance Publique, Paris

ple score for rapidly assessing the status of the newborn (see chapter 11). In 1958 phototherapy was introduced for newborn jaundice, drastically reducing the sequelae of a very common problem. The role of surfactant in the respiratory distress syndrome of premature babies was discovered by Mary Ellen Avery and Jere Mead in 1959; it prompted the technological advances that have made it possible to save the lives of infants at only twenty-six weeks of gestation or less.

Keeping the emphasis on prevention, physicians soon became aware of the danger of maternal smoking, drinking, and drug use. By 1963, immunological prevention of erythroblastosis foetalis in children not yet conceived could be accomplished by administration of rhesus antibodies to the Rh-negative mother (see chapter 8).

Genetics and Eugenics

No baby; no nation.

– Helen MacMurchy, *The Canadian Mothers' Book*,
The Little Blue Book Mothers' series, no. 1
(Ottawa: Department of Health, 1927), 8

From its inception, the social hygiene movement was intimately connected to the aspirations of developed nations. Children were the future; their welfare reflected that of the state. The new possibilities for saving infant lives raised a deeper question: Should all lives be saved? Or, put differently, should all citizens become parents?

The word 'eugenics' had been coined in 1883 by the British physiologist Francis Galton to signify 'ideal breeding.' On the one hand, science could identify and prevent inherited disorders; on the other, dominant races and ideologies could use this knowledge for political ends in defining 'superiority' (see chapter 15). The philosophy of eugenics lent scientific approbation to that project. In 1902 A.E. Garrod demonstrated that Mendelian laws governed the inheritance of alcaptonuria, making it the first human disorder to be identified as 'genetic.' Soon a succession of congenital abnormalities were linked to genetics (see chapter 4). Situating these complex problems in the

structure of DNA informs genetic counselling and invites research
into new biotechnologies to prevent or control them. In the past,
however, nations and physicians resorted to more drastic measures
for producing 'ideal' genetics.

Eugenicists were neither 'monsters' nor 'simple-minded reaction-
aries'; they 'saw themselves as progressives who were seeking to wed
science, medicine, and social welfare' (A. McLaren, *Our Own Master Race*, Toronto: McClelland and Stewart, 1990, 166). Some, like
Charles Davenport, who was director of Cold Spring Harbor laboratory, were attracted to eugenics from scientific work on heredity. Davenport studied the presumed degenerative effects of 'race crossing'
(miscegenation). Enthusiastic bureaucrats and educators, like Canadian physician Helen MacMurchy, also subscribed to an ideal that was
white, middle class, and Protestant (see chapter 11). Their initiatives
were packaged appealingly in the form of 'help' for the 'helpless,'
and centred on issues of immigration, education, and sterilization of
the 'feeble-minded.' The apparent reasonableness of these solutions
in promoting what are now seen as offensive infringements of civil lib-
erties is a sobering reminder of the difficulty in identifying all the subtle complexities of any process of intervention before it takes place.

Vitamins and Nutrition

Among the most intriguing of twentieth-century scientific achievements from a pediatric perspective is the discovery of vitamins. Since
antiquity, manipulation of milk, food, and feeding practices had been
the mainstay of therapy for children. With the concept of vitamins,
a number of vague, apparently infectious illnesses were transformed
into specific dietary deficiencies, which could now be identified and
prevented by science.

Long before Vitamin C had been imagined, its deficiency disease,
scurvy, was known to be the result of poor diet. In the sixteenth century, Jacques Cartier was shown how to prevent it by aboriginal people, who gave him a recipe for a special tea (see chapter 5). In 1753
the English sea captain James Lind described the antiscorbutic properties of orange juice (though boiled); the practice of carrying cit-
rus fruits is said to be the origin of the British epithet 'limey.' These

diseases are exceptions. Many other conditions, now known to result from dietary deficiencies, could not be distinguished from infections. Like epidemics of influenza or measles, deficiencies occurred as 'outbreaks' in specific populations, localized by time and place. Following the advent of germ theory, avid researchers went looking for the bacterial causes of pellagra and rickets, and discovered instead that these 'epidemics' were nutritional rather than infectious.

In 1896 the Dutch physician Christiaan Eijkman noticed that pigeons fed on supposedly 'better quality' polished rice developed a paralytic disease resembling human beriberi, which resolved with a 'poor quality' whole-rice diet. In 1901 his colleague G. Grijns hypothesized that the rice hull contained an anti-beriberi substance. Similarly, the American Joseph Goldberger working in the southern states demonstrated that pellagra was a dietary deficiency by experiments on prisoners in exchange for pardons. But these results were not believed. In 1916, a frustrated Goldberger tried to transmit pellagra to himself and his associates by inoculating and ingesting secretions and blood from human sufferers. The failure of their experiment was taken as evidence of the non-infectious nature of the disease, but some still refused to abandon the infectious theory.

Chemical research on vitamins ultimately provided specific causes and treatments for previously vague diseases with widespread effects. The word 'vitamin' (from 'vita' [life] and 'amine' [a chemical unit]) was coined in 1912 by the Polish biochemist Kazimierz Funk to express the new theory of accessory foodstuffs. Frederick Gowland Hopkins also thought of vitamins as nutritional catalysts related to hormones. He studied synthetic diets and milk feeding in rats.

Over the next fifty years, individual vitamins were recognized, named, isolated, and synthesized (see table 13.2). Once the biochemical concept was in place, the length of time from recognition to isolation or purification of each vitamin was greatly decreased. For example, in the case of thiamine (B_1), thirty years would elapse; however, the time shrank to less than two years for riboflavin (B_2) and vitamin K (given its name by Henrik Dam for its role in 'Koagulation'). Reflecting the heady atmosphere created by this research, Nobel Prizes were awarded quickly: Hopkins and Eijkman (1929); Whipple (shared, 1934); Szent-Györgyi (1937); Dam (1943).

Table 13.2
Milestones in vitamin history

	Named or postulated by	Year*	Purified or isolated by	Year*	Structure or synthesis discovered
A	Bloch	1924	Karrer	1931–7	1937
B$_1$	Eijkman and Grijns	1896	Jansen	1926	1936
B$_2$	BMRC/Warburg	1927/1932	Kuhn	1933	1935
B$_3$	Goldberger/Voegtlin	1914–15	Funk/Subbarow	1914/1937	1867
B$_6$	György	1936	Keresztesy et al.	1938	1938
B$_{12}$	Whipple	1922	Rickes et al.	1948	1955
C	Funk	1911	Szent-Györgyi	1928	1933
D	Mellanby (chemistry)	1918	Pappenheimer	1921	1936
	Huldschinsky (light)	1919	Angus	1931	
E	Evans et al.	1922–3	Evans et al.	1936	1938
K	Dam	1934	Dam	1939	1939

* Years indicate either date of research or publication.
Sources: *Goodman and Gilman's Pharmacological Basis of Therapeutics* (New York: McGraw-Hill, 1996, and earlier editions); Roman J. Kutsky, *Handbook of Vitamins and Minerals and Hormones*, 2nd ed. (New York: Van Nostrand Reinhold 1980).

The chemical reduction of infant food to component parts of vitamins, proteins, fats, and carbohydrates simply added to the rising authority of doctors. Now the composition of breast milk could be closely approximated with 'infant formula.' Emphasis on sterility and strict schedules prevailed, as medical experts explained how babies could be fed artificially in answer to the anxieties of mothers and the financial aspirations of industry. Motherless children were to benefit, but the impact of this achievement spread to the healthy infants of ordinary women, who trusted science to ensure that their babies would have enough good-quality milk. Ironically, the milk substitutes could never match the immunological value of breast milk; and the rubber nipple, once lauded for saving infants from choking and starving, is now the subject of toxicological warnings.

As historians Rima Apple and Katherine Arnup have shown, doctors continued to advocate maternal nursing, even as they provided more information on artificial feeding. But the bottles won. By the early 1970s, less than one-third of North American children were breastfed. Worried about this trend, the La Leche League (founded in 1956) and health-care professionals actively promoted a return to natural methods; they feared that breastfeeding would continue to decline as women lost familiarity with it. Once again, a shift in cultural values, combined with increased scepticism over scientific expertise, helped the activists to reverse the trend and foster the late twentieth-century revival in breastfeeding. Nevertheless, industry is criticized for continuing to promote its more expensive and less effective formula feedings in developing nations.

Breasts, Bovines, and Babies

Breast milk is for babies; cow's milk is for calves ... Breast milk is best because it doesn't have to be warmed, you can take it on picnics, the cat can't get at it, and it comes in such cute containers.

– Alan Brown, physician at Toronto's Hospital for Sick Children, cited in K. Arnup, *Education for Motherhood: Child-Rearing Advice for Canadian Mothers* (Toronto: University of Toronto Press, 1994), 97

Experts' Advice to Parents: Dr Blatz and Dr Spock

Behavioural and psychological research moved into the vacuum created by the conquest of the biological killers in developed countries. Child study and adolescent medicine became separate new fields with a special emphasis on behavioural and psychological well-being. The sociologist Sydney Halpern suggests that the trend to emphasize the psychological over the biological in academic pediatrics was influenced by government funding agencies.

As early as 1924, the physician-psychologist William Blatz headed a child-study centre at the University of Toronto, where he developed a relatively permissive approach to childrearing. Among many other activities, Blatz directed his controversial research on the Dionne quintuplets, whose nursery became a 'laboratory' for the analysis of nature versus nurture in child development (see figure 13.7). The project was terminated by the Ontario government in 1938 under pressure from the family. Nevertheless, the public had become aware of the promise of science in the rearing of healthy children.

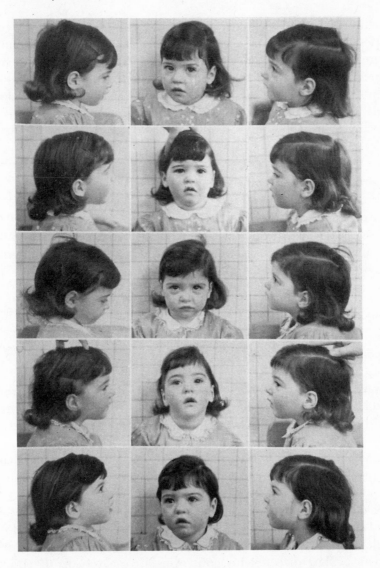

13.7   *Biological Study of the Dionne Quintuplets.* The composite image reflects the investigators' concerns in their study of nature versus nurture, but it also speaks eloquently of the now unacceptable 'scientific' incursions made into the lives of these five children and their family. From J.W. MacArthur and Norma Ford, in Blatz et al:, 1937, frontispiece

The advice manual for parents written by the New York pediatrician Benjamin Spock became the world's third-largest-selling book, after editions of the Bible and Shakespeare. A Yale graduate, Spock held professorships at the Mayo Clinic and at Case Western Reserve University. In simple words and short sentences, his *Baby and Child Care* (1946) brought Freudian theory to average Americans, by emphasizing the child's need for love and by relaxing the rigid standards for feeding, toilet training, clothing, and play that had prevailed in previous decades. You cannot spoil a child by cuddling. Spock bolstered parents' confidence with understandable information; he appealed to common sense and reassured the innate parental desire to please children while guiding their physical, emotional, and moral growth. The first edition of 1946 sold more than half a million copies in ten months.

In the mid-1960s, Spock was shocked by the Vietnam War and its wanton destruction of the very youth he had helped to raise. Becoming an outspoken advocate for disarmament and peace, he was arrested several times for participating in protests. In 1968 he was actually convicted for conspiracy to resist the draft and fined $5,000. Many Americans then turned against the aging pediatrician, angered by his adoption of an antigovernment stance seemingly in favour of communism. They claimed that his emphasis on love over discipline had caused an entire generation to be permissive and selfish; they also blamed Spock for the hippie movement, with its sexual, political, and social revolution.

Spock denied that his work had made such an extraordinary impact. He pointed to similar cultural turmoil in countries where his work was unknown, and he contrasted the upheaval in America with its absence in other nations where his book was equally successful. He also changed his position on some matters such as circumcision. Scholars are reluctant to accept Spock's modest assessment of his own influence, even as they criticize dated aspects of his ideas. Indeed, he is now blamed for an estimated 50,000 sudden infant deaths (SIDS) through his widely followed recommendation that babies sleep on their stomachs to avoid inhalation pneumonia; only in the 1990s was sleep position shown to be associated with SIDS, a disease that had been recognized only in 1969, twenty years after his book first appeared. This information is often used to show the enormous power of advice literature.

Never shy about publicity, the nonagenarian pediatrician participated in a September 1992 press conference to advocate breastfeeding and warn of the dangers of whole milk in early and later life. True to form, he succeeded in angering dairy farmers and business interests across North America. Still a bestseller, *Baby and Child Care* was translated into thirty-nine languages; total sales now exceed 50 million copies. The eighth edition appeared in 2004, six years after the author's death.

Social Pediatrics

After the social hygiene movement, more infants survived to become adults, but the statistics still betray class-based and geographic imbalance. The realization that social provisions define child health did not come equally to all nations – even within each nation. As Preston and Haines have shown, American children of densely populated areas and those disadvantaged by poverty, race, or abandonment, did not enjoy the same life expectancy as their more privileged peers. But some poor children were healthy. Gradually pediatricians began to re-evaluate the benefits of childrearing practices once deemed primitive such as swaddling, discovering what had been known by mothers all along.

Child Labour, Experimentation, and Abuse

Laws against infanticide, like those against murder, have long been on the books of Western nations, but they were enforced only sporadically; convicted mothers rarely paid the full penalty, especially if they were single and poverty stricken. Legislation to protect children is vulnerable to interpretation through prevailing social attitudes about their value to society. Child labour laws are similar.

In the early nineteenth century, young children were recruited into the labour force, in dismal conditions so vividly portrayed in the novels of Charles Dickens. By the 1830s, Britain had enacted laws against child labour in factories. In North America, the economy was based on agricultural work, and industrialization came later; as a result, legislation to protect children in factories and mines on that continent was not passed until the 1870s and 1880s. But these laws did not apply equally to all children. London orphans, supposedly barred from work, grew more numerous and desperate. The preacher-physician Thomas J. Barnardo founded homes across Britain, but in 1868 he began to export these children to families or labour situations in Australia and Canada. The trickle became a torrent, leading to the emigration of a total of 80,000 British Home children – at least 20,000 of whom were 'Barnardo boys' or 'girls' – before the practice was abolished in 1925. Many destitute children may have been spared a short life on the London streets; but as Joy Parr has shown, most became workers rather than adoptees. At least one-third of the exported youth were not orphans; and as many as 10 per cent, usually from disadvantaged groups, were sent in a form of 'philanthropic abduction,' against the wishes or without the knowledge of their parents. Measures were taken to ensure the well-being of the children in care, and their wages were carefully collected; however, Barnardo's system also reduced the costs of caring for waifs in the home country, assuaging the financial interests of the banks and agencies directly involved. Special circumstances have always provided new justifications for keeping children at work rather than at school. Child labour continues to be a problem of global significance: UNICEF estimates 158 million children aged 5 to 14 years are engaged in work.

'Baby farms' also illustrate ambivalence in the application of laws to protect children. Homes for unwed mothers and their children served a 'black market' for adoption. Late nineteenth-century legislation to curb the practice was not enforced, and many baby farms operated illegally under the guise of private hospitals. For example, the lax hygienic standards, cruelty, and high (but unreported) mortality rates of the Ideal Maternity Home in Nova Scotia were notorious among locals between 1925 and 1945; however, they did not receive wider attention until the 1988 report of investigative journalist Bette Cahill, entitled *Butterbox Babies* – a grim allusion to the makeshift coffins remembered by former employees of the home.

Medicine, too, has witnessed an evolution in legislative attitudes surrounding children as experimental subjects. For several centuries, it strove to help children by investigating the diseases peculiar to them. Jenner's smallpox vaccine was tested on an eight-year-old boy, who was then challenged with active smallpox to prove the point (see chapter 7). Other nineteenth-century trials – on measles prevention, for example – entailed inoculating blood from active cases into child subjects in the almshouses and orphanages of great cities. As Susan E. Lederer and her colleagues have shown, institutionalized children were similarly used in research on other vaccines, infections, and nutritional diseases – to their great good fortune, it was thought, when the experiments were a success.

But not all experiments met with success; they could also cause pain and suffering. In 1970 public outrage greeted the discovery that, for fifteen years, children with severe mental retardation had been deliberately infected with 'inevitable' hepatitis at the Willowbrook State School of New York, supposedly with parental consent. The result was legislation to control biomedical research (U.S., 1974; Canada, 1978) and the subsequent laying down of guidelines and codes of conduct for the ethical use of all human subjects, especially children.

As everyone is now aware, child abuse can also happen at home or school, and in any social setting. This dangerous and prevalent problem was recognized as a medical concern only recently. First proposed in the 1860s by the French forensic doctor Ambroise Tardieu, it was largely forgotten at a time when no technology allowed observers to second-guess the parent's story. On another level, matters of privacy and attitudes to what was right for children were different. In 1946, American radiologist John Caffey drew attention to specific radiographic changes in the long bones of six children who presented with subdural hematomas; in 1974 he outlined the elements of 'shaken baby syndrome.' Not one to shrink from ugly truths, Caffey also demonstrated that a large thymus shadow in an infant was a normal finding, helping to end the medically abusive practice of thymic radiation for non-existent disease. Caffey's colleague from Denver, Charles Henry Kempe, developed a series of criteria to identify the 'battered child syndrome' (*JAMA* 181 [1962]: 17–24).

Irradiation of the thymus ... is an irrational procedure at all ages.

Most mistakes I've seen were not because one didn't know some disease, but because he didn't know he was looking at normal.

– John Caffey (1945 and 1974), cited in
M.T. Jacobs et al., Radiology 210 (1999): 11–16

'Child Abuse' became a Medical Subject Heading (MeSH) in 1964, and 'Shaken Baby Syndrome' in 2002. In 2004, a busy clinic in Arizona reported that active screening for domestic violence detected children at risk in up to 15 per cent of the population and at least seven times more frequently than without the screening (Wahl et al., *BMC Medicine* 2 [2004]: 25). Doctors are now trained in vigilance.

Recently, a Toronto pathologist was found to have zealously over-read the signs of child abuse, leading to several wrongful convictions of child murder; his mistakes have been ascribed to a toxic mix of confidence and inexperience. Caffey's comment on errors is apt. In France in late 2008, two doctors were convicted of failing to prevent the murder of a five-year-old child by his parents; they were given suspended sentences and fines for having accepted the mother's story without properly examining the boy.

The late recognition and greater public awareness of child abuse does not imply any recent increase in the crime. Rather it reflects a cultural shift away from tolerating any form of corporal punishment in childhood and a new willingness to accept state intrusion into the domestic environment on behalf of the child. Since 1979, when Sweden outlawed any form of violence by adults on children, school spanking has declined. Most members of the European Union have also banned spanking in any form. One of only four hold-outs, Britain is considering changing its 140-year-old law that allows parents to administer 'reasonable chastisement'; the last attempt in 2004, was resoundingly defeated. Canada has adopted a middling position, allowing light slapping of children between ages two and twelve years, but not with objects and not on the head. The United States stands alone (with Somalia) as being one of two nations that have failed to ratify a 1990 UN convention on children's rights, guaranteeing protection from all forms of violence both physical and mental.

These changes in attitude result in a marked change in medical perception – as to what constitutes a disease, a treatment, and the doctor's role.

Pediatrics and the Wider World

With control of infectious diseases and diarrhea, infant mortality rates in developed countries fell dramatically during the twentieth century, from roughly 150 deaths per 1,000 live births in 1900, to 26.6 in 1954 and to 13.1 in 1979. Pediatricians gradually turned to the health of children elsewhere. Typifying these endeavours are the contributions of Cicely Williams in child nutrition and Dr Brock Chisholm first director-general of the World Health Organization (WHO). The pediatricians' reflex to prevent disease made them public health activists on a global scale (see chapter 15).

WHO statistics indicate that the problem of child mortality may have been lessened but is far from solved. Each year more than a million children die of malaria, while 9 million more children under age five succumb to pneumonia, neonatal tetanus, diarrhea, measles, and HIV, aggravated by malnutrition and pollution. Since the causes of these diseases are social as well as biological, effective control inevitably entails delicate interference with cultural practices relating to gender, race, religion, and tradition. Solutions to these child killers will also aggravate the problem of overpopulation, invoking the spectre of malnutrition and starvation. As a result, contraception continues to be an important issue. Birth-control methods have been developed as a lucrative product of industry – just like the infant formulas before them. But recent studies suggest that the limitation of birth rate is better correlated with the education of girls than with the provision of drugs or devices (see chapter 11).

The leadership of Chisholm, Williams, and others led pediatricians the world over to face a stark irony: efforts to save individual children from treatable, infectious illnesses pale when compared

Table 13.3
Estimates of percentage of children living in poverty

	1980s	1990s	ca 2000
Australia	15.5	10.9	11.6
Canada	15.8 ·	12.8	13.6
Denmark	4.0	1.8	2.4
United Kingdom	9.7	17.4	16.2
United States	25.1	22.3	21.7

Source: OECD, in Peter Whiteford and Willem Adema, 'Reducing Child Poverty. What Works Best?' OECD, *Social Employment and Migration Working Papers*, no. 51 (2007), 14.

with the thousands who continue to die annually from starvation and filth, or the millions who stand to die from a war that might exterminate the entire species. Long schooled in prevention, pediatricians were aware that no medicine could help a nuclear disaster, and they supported the founding of the International Physicians for the Prevention of Nuclear War and similar organizations (see chapter 15).

Children without advocates – orphans and 'delinquents' – continue to be abused, especially those who are in 'havens' or are wards of the state. We realize with horror that money cannot begin to compensate the harm done to children in times of war. In 2004, the United Nations released a Truth and Reconciliation report for the children of Sierra Leone. Abuses also occurred in the name of 'helping'; in 2006, Canada committed to a financial package and a Truth and Reconciliation Commission to help repair the damage to First Nations, Métis, and Inuit children in the residential schools.

Even with loving care, children in poverty are disadvantaged physically, intellectually, and emotionally. For decades now governments in rich countries have promised to tackle child poverty; rates are mostly flat and highest in nations that spend the least on social welfare (see table 13.3). The uneven distribution of the problem depends on region and race. Progress is slow. Reports suggest that since 2000 rates fell in Britain but rose almost everywhere else. As the figures for child poverty climb, the problems of global health hit closer to home. In 2000, the members of the WHO recognized the role of poverty in health and unanimously adopted the Millennium

Declaration "to free our fellow men, women and children from the abject and dehumanizing conditions of extreme poverty, to which more than a billion of them are currently subjected." The goal was to eliminate extreme poverty by 2015. Here too, progress is slow.

Pediatricians continue to be experts in prevention, but there has always been a tension between reasonable intervention and unacceptable intrusion into the private lives of individuals and other cultures. Some methods, once touted as medical salvations, have been abandoned as shameful exploitations or regrettable mistakes, while others remain entrenched in law. In the midst of a process, it is sometimes impossible to discern the right way. With their focus on prevention and on the social (as well as biological) determinants of health, pediatricians have not only influenced the rest of medicine; they have created a model for enhancing survival of all life on the planet.

Suggestions for Further Reading

At the bibliography website http://histmed.ca.

CHAPTER FOURTEEN

A Many-Faceted Gem:
The Decline and Rebirth
of Family Medicine*

Never could I see myself listening all day with a stethoscope to chest sounds, or looking down throats or up rectums ... General practice [is] one of the most difficult fields of medicine because a competent general practitioner must be one of the most expert diagnosticians. He not only must know when he can help, but what is just as important, he must be quick to recognize a situation that is beyond him and refer such a seriously ill patient to more expert care than he can give.

– W. Victor Johnston, *Before the Age of Miracles* (1972), 8–9

Historians of family medicine often begin by commenting with surprise on how little has been written on their subject. After all, they contend, general practice is the oldest medical activity, predating the formation of any specialty; by rights, then, it should have the longest tradition of documentation. But two good reasons account for this apparent neglect.

First, general or family practice is *not* ancient; it is among the newest of specialties. As medical and surgical specialties developed in the early twentieth century, doctors who did everything – the *omni-practiciens*, as they are tellingly called in French – began to fade into nostalgia, becoming the stuff of legend or backwardness. The rise of family medicine was a postwar phenomenon.

*Learning objectives for this chapter are found on p. 457.

Second, history of medicine – indeed all history – underwent a shift in focus after 1950. Historians used to be preoccupied with medical elites, academic issues, and the vast intellectual and technological transformations of science. General practitioners did not qualify for their attention. Only in the middle of the twentieth century did historians turn to 'everyday life.' Rather than fixing their sights on pivotal moments with lasting effects, they began to explore the context of the ordinary and of continuity – history of the *longue durée*. Given this double caveat – that family medicine is new and that historians tended to ignore the ordinary and the continuous – it is scarcely surprising that a synthetic history of family medicine has yet to be written.

In this chapter, we will briefly examine the prehistory of family medicine – what is known of the life and work of ordinary doctors of the past. Then we will explore the social, political, economic, and intellectual forces underlying the professionalization of family medicine in the third quarter of the twentieth century. Finally, we will examine the influence of this discipline on other specialties.

Prehistory of General Practice

After the advent of man-midwifery in the seventeenth and eighteenth centuries and the conceptual melding of surgery and medicine in the early nineteenth, there followed a century during which most doctors were 'general' practitioners; they did surgery and midwifery, and they looked after young and old alike (see chapters 10, 11, and 13). Only professors and researchers could claim to be specialists, but some resented the label. The rules governing practice were dictated by legislation in each country and reflected societal expectations. From the late eighteenth century on, doctors in Canada, for example, were licensed by credentials and/or examination in the triple disciplines of medicine, surgery, and midwifery.

Our knowledge of general practitioners (GPs) has increased with the shift in historical focus from the exceptional to the ordinary and with the advent of computer technology. In projects covering a long period and numerous interactions, volumes of data must be assimilated and manipulated to produce reliable statements about practice, its stability, and its gradual change. Recent scholarship has unveiled the more distant past of general practice in a variety of ways.

One approach involves the examination of community records pertaining to health, illness, birth, and mortality in specific places and times. Using records of dispensaries, hospitals, and religious and philanthropic organizations, historian Hilary Marland traced the medical facilities in two contrasting towns in nineteenth-century England. She found a variety of practices, ranging from pluralistic 'self-help' to 'institutional' care. Similarly, Estes and Goodman, who set out to commemorate the centennial of a hospital in Portsmouth, New Hampshire, discovered a wealth of sources pertaining to the town, and they extended their research to cover three and a half centuries of births, diseases, mortality, and practitioners – both 'regular' and 'irregular.' Their achievement serves to represent an ordinary American town, since few municipalities have preserved equally rich sources. Future studies on regions and climates will undoubtedly reveal patterns of disease and practice that differ from those of Portsmouth.

Another approach has been to analyse groups of practitioners in a specific period or place. Fine studies of this type exist for both Britain and France. The historian Irvine Loudon first examined the nature of medical practice in Britain between 1750 and 1850, attending to its relationship with pharmacy, surgery, and obstetrics. His sources included parliamentary papers, medical periodicals, professional archives, and the personal records of individual practitioners. He found that the status of general practice rose following the Apothecaries Act of 1815, which, despite its name, had little to do with pharmacy; it was a preliminary attempt to create national standards for practice and for regional licensing bodies. The Apothecaries Act resulted in a conscious movement to organize general practice, but GPs had to wait another century before they acquired full autonomy over accreditation. Anne Digby picked up the topic at 1850; relying on similarly diverse sources, she traced the aspirations of general practitioners until the beginning of the National Health Service. Loudon returned to the subject with John Horder and Charles Webster and followed the evolution of family medicine from 1948 to 1997.

Using a similar approach for his work on peri-revolutionary France, the historian Matthew Ramsey scoured the archives in scores of *départements*, medical faculties, and professional bodies for records pertaining to health and medicine in order to construct a complex picture of diverse practitioners. He showed that in 1770 the boundaries of practice were diffuse: 'officially' trained doctors worked beside, and in competition with, a wide range of folk healers, mountebanks, empirics, druggists, and 'witches.' By 1830, legislation and custom had considerably altered the scene; a single profession of certified practitioners had come to the fore, clearly distinguished from their competitors and theoretically capable of all types of medical work. Similar studies of later periods have been conducted by Gelfand, Léonard, and Weisz. Weisz's study of specialization in Britain, France, and the United States provides an interesting corollary with information on general practice. Other historians have studied groups of regular doctors and their alternative competitors to uncover patterns in identity, work, and income.

The extent to which practice was regulated through legislation indicates the extent to which the general public was willing to grant autonomy to formally trained physicians. In the United States, the medical profession was impressively successful in retaining control over licensing and practice. The American Medical Association was formed in 1847 as a monopolistic lobby against homeopathists and other 'irregulars' (see chapter 6). By contrast, European countries and Canada were relatively more tolerant of alternative health care – not, as Connor has shown, because physicians welcomed it, but because they failed to convince their governments to ban the competition. For example, a homeopathic representative sat on the council of the Ontario College of Physicians until 1967.

A variation on the doctor-based approach to the history of general medicine is the study of individual practitioners. Some doctors actually wrote their own histories, diaries, or autobiographies. These documents provided diverting reading for generations of physicians, but they were ignored or at least mistrusted by historians because of the potential distortions embedded in any subjective writing. Now, however, scholars understand that these classic and antiquarian tales reveal issues that were significant for doctor and patient, even if they seem to be of little consequence to their successors. A number of these first-hand records have recently appeared, based on documents or interviews or recollections (see table 14.1). Often published pri-

Table 14.1
Some first-hand accounts of general practice

Period	Place	Author*
Britain		
1606–35	Stratford	Lane
1690s	London	Cook
1780–1870	Yorkshire	Marland
1790–1990	Yorkshire	Hainsworth
1800–2000	Cornwall	Pocock
1818–73	Scotland	Pairman
1826–9	Newcastle	Johnson
1880–1987	Edinburgh	Jellinek
1882–1925	Lancashire/London	Mair
1870–1952	Edinburgh	Ashworth
Canada		
1826–76	Prince Edward Island	Shephard
1832–42	British Columbia	Tolmie
1849–89	Ontario	Duffin
1871–1930	Ontario	Groves
1885–1965	SW Quebec	Geggie
1893	Labrador	Curwen
1907–12	Saskatchewan	MacLean
1912–38	Labrador	Rompkey
1920–70	Cape Breton, Nova Scotia	Mullally
1929–31	N. Alberta	Jackson
1930s	SW Newfoundland	Rusted
1933–47	Yukon	Duncan
1935	Aklavik	Urquhart
1924–54	Ontario	Johnston
United States		
1623–1983	New Hampshire	Estes
1650–1750	New England	Berman
1798–1803	rural New York	Ackerman
1822–55	Ohio & Indiana	McDonell
1830–70	Kentucky & South	Stowe
1852–1900	Wisconsin	Leavitt
1881–1927	Corning, New York	McNamara
1880s	Wisconsin	Coombs
1894–1930s	Kansas	Hertzler
1897–1926	Boston	Crenner
1930–1982	Wyoming	Wilmoth
1934–35	Minnesota	Haddy et al.
Mid-20th C	North Carolina	Crellin
1940–90	S. Illinois	Mitchell

*For full references see Suggestions for Further Reading for chapter 14 at the bibliography website http://histmed.ca.

vately, they open fascinating vistas on medical life of the past especially in remote areas – indeed, with few exceptions they extol rural life.
When groups of these sources are analysed, the triad of medicine,
surgery, and midwifery typified the work, while the gap between the
theoretical training of medical school and the realities of practice
was a common complaint.

Ordinary medical practice can also be explored through medical daybooks and hospital records. Here, especially, microcomputers help to exploit the historical potential in the records that chart
doctors' daily lives. To analyse the practice of the Ontario physician
James Miles Langstaff, I transcribed information contained in forty
years of daybooks and accounts into a database program to build a
profile of his patients, their diseases, his diagnostic and therapeutic
methods, the journals he read, and the money he earned. The results
showed how his practice changed through time.

A Doctor Remembers

My first introduction to the tragedy of diseases ... A long line
of teams came slowly down that road. Driving the lead team
... was my father ... In the bed of the farm wagon were three
oblong boxes ... As days wore on I learned that the wagon had
borne the coffins containing the bodies of three of my play-
mates. Five more followed in quick succession. Eight of the
nine children in that one family died of diphtheria in ten days.
There remained only a baby of nine months. The mother took
to carrying this child constantly even while she did the farm
housework. Clutched to her mother's breast, this child seemed
inordinately wide-eyed as though affected by the silent grief
which surrounded her ...

Prayers for protection literally filled the air in those days
of doom. There was no appeal to the science of medicine because there was none.

– A.E. Hertzler, *The Horse and Buggy Doctor*
(New York and London: Harper, 1938), 1–2

The average medical practice of the late nineteenth and early twentieth centuries was challenging and diverse. Most patients were seen on house calls, although doctors also kept offices in their homes. As Hertzler so vividly reminds us, infectious diseases, including diphtheria, chest problems, diarrhea, postpartum fever, and scarlet fever, dominated the diagnostic spectrum. Doctors were also called to deliveries, often using forceps at the request of women attendants. They performed small operations, such as extracting teeth, lancing abscesses, suturing wounds, and reducing fractures and dislocations. On rare occasions, they undertook major operations, including amputations, mastectomies, and repair of congenital abnormalities such as club foot and hare lip. Operating on a kitchen table in Fergus, Ontario, in 1883, the intrepid Abraham Groves is said to have been the first in North America to remove an appendix (see chapter 10). Groves had already performed a vaginal hysterectomy, an ovariotomy, and a small transfusion. Of his long travels to make house calls, he wrote, 'One had time when driving alone to go over every aspect of the case, and I found the time so spent far from wasted' (*All in a Day's Work*, Toronto: Macmillan, 1934, 5).

General Practice in Fiction

A list similar to table 14.1 could be made from the stirring fiction of several physician-writers who drew on their own experience. They include John Brown (Scottish), Anton Chekhov (Russian), Oliver Wendell Holmes (American), Tobias Smollett (English), and William Carlos Williams (American).

Nonphysician writers also created memorable vignettes of general practice. Among the most celebrated are the doctor stories in George Eliot's *Middlemarch* and Gustave Flaubert's *Madame Bovary.*

For more examples, consult the online database *Literature, Arts and Medicine* at its website, http://litmed.med.nyu.edu/

Work on billing records suggests that nineteenth-century doctors rarely expected to be paid in full. When Haddy and colleagues compared the finances of a mid-1930s American physician with those of a general practice sixty years later, they found that the number of surgical procedures had declined and the most common diagnoses of the 1930s had almost vanished because of vaccines and antibiotics. This change through time is apparent even within individual practices. Langstaff's prescribing habits altered more slowly but in concert with the changes described for major centres. Country doctors also adopted the new technologies for diagnosis and treatment, such as anesthesia, antisepsis, thermometers, and electrical machines. In the 1880s Langstaff's surgical practice seemed to wane, perhaps in competition with (or through relieved recognition of) specialists in nearby Toronto.

Despite rarely having time off work and, even less often, enjoying full payment, rural doctors usually managed to live comfortably and enjoy the respect of their communities. By the turn of the century, however, doubts about competence had tarnished the image of the kindly GP and respect began to wane.

Specialists versus Generalists

The rapid increase of knowledge has made concentration in work a necessity; specialism is here, and here to stay ... The desire for expert knowledge is ... now so great that there is a grave danger lest the family doctor should become ... a relic of the past.

– William Osler, *Boston Medical and Surgical Journal* 126 (1892): 457–9, esp. 457

'I'm Just a GP': The Threat to General Practice

The threat to general practice was manifested first by declining numbers in specific geographic regions and by criticisms of incompetence. At the end of the nineteenth century, specialists were increasingly numerous in urban areas. General practice became the equivalent of rural practice and was characterized by culture-based assumptions about the 'modern city' and the 'backward country.' Optimistic trust in science meant that specialists were thought to be more effective than their humble rural colleagues because they were perceived to be more 'scientific.' Before the telephone, the automobile, highways, and air transportation, availability preserved a role for GPs – people in isolated areas had to be satisfied with one doctor for all their needs. But with shrinking distances and more trainees, some GPs began to predict the eventual demise of their metier with 'doleful misgivings' upon 'looking into the gloom' (Hattie, *CMAJ* 22 [1930]: 548).

In the more populated centres of the United States, France, and Great Britain, the proportion of general practitioners began to decline. Sociologist William G. Rothstein showed that from 1930 to 1962, the number of GPs in the United States fell in both absolute and relative terms from 90 to 37 per 100,000 population, or from 71 per cent of all doctors to only 27 per cent. In Canada and Australia, with their huge distances and vast areas of low population, specialty practice was both impractical and unprofitable; specialists there concentrated in cities, but the overall numbers of GPs remained proportionately higher. However, by 1948, more than two-thirds of Toronto graduates planned to seek specialty training, although at least three-quarters eventually found themselves in general practice. That outcome was perceived to be a second choice for (presumably) second-rate doctors.

A Vignette from Vancouver Island

When [the city of] Victoria was young ... you did not have a special doctor for each part. Dr. Helmcken attended to all our ailments ... You began to get better the moment you heard [him] coming up the stairs. He did have the most horrible medicines ... Once I knelt on a needle which broke into my knee ... The Doctor cut slits in my knee and wiggled his fingers around inside it for three hours hunting for the pieces of the needle ... [He] said, 'Yell, lassie, yell! It will let the pain out.' I did yell, but the pain stayed in.

– Emily Carr, *The Book of Small* (London and
Oxford: Oxford University Press, 1942), 199–200

By the mid-1940s, general practice was experiencing a massive identity crisis, which constituted yet another threat. With few mechanisms for maintaining and guaranteeing standards, competence could be questioned. The public and the profession alike were aware that some doctors were more conscientious than others. Made to feel like second-class citizens, many GPs seemed almost resigned to the inevitable disappearance of their way of life. But the more optimistic formed professional associations, touting the undeniable merits of their enterprise: hard work, diagnostic challenge, diversity, continuity, and comprehensive care. Calls for the recognition of general practice as a specialty in its own right became more insistent and frequent.

In delineating the early twentieth-century competition between obstetricians and GPs in the United States, Charlotte Borst observed a fundamental irony: GPs, who had once been the very doctors arguing for physician-assisted births 'would, in the end, find themselves eliminated from the birthing room' by their specialist competitors (1995, 130). Historian David Adams found a similar development in the 1945 attempt of a hospital in Cincinnati, Ohio, to limit privileges for tonsillectomy to specialists in Ear, Nose, and Throat (ENT). Increasing in numbers, the ENT specialists knew that the incidence of medically unmanageable tonsillitis was stable or was likely to decline with the promise of antibiotics: more doctors, fewer procedures. They perceived the operating GP as a financial threat, but they cloaked their opposition in the morally superior issue of patient safety. The posturing failed. The GPs formed their own association, and the resultant uproar caused the hospital to rescind its decision. The organizational momentum of these GPs spilled well beyond the borders of the city to both the state and the nation. As postwar incursions on the scope and profitability of their work grew ever more hostile, GPs became angry, and they mobilized.

Professionalization of General Practice

Stanley R. Truman wrote of the sense of 'despair and discouragement' that pervaded the first meeting of the GP section of the AMA

> As the diamond with its many facets is the finest of gems, so
> ... the family physician with his multiple viewpoints should be
> inferior to no other.
>
> – W. Victor Johnston (1948), cited in D. Woods, *Strength in Study:*
> *An Informal History of the College of Family Physicians of Canada*
> (Toronto: College of Family

meeting in San Francisco in 1946. He rose to tell how he and his
colleagues in Oakland, just like those in Cincinnati, had fought off
the attempt by specialists to limit their hospital privileges by forming
their own incorporated association. The idea caught like wildfire and
the mood of the meeting immediately improved. By 1947 the American Academy of General Practice had been formed; its first meeting
took place that June in Atlantic City in the presence of approximately
two hundred GPs. In 1948 it established headquarters in Kansas City
to escape the 'Chicago dictatorship' of the AMA, although the second meeting was held there in conjunction with that of the AMA.
The 1949 meeting, fittingly, was in Cincinnati, where Dr Truman
remembered a record turnout of members who crowded the rooms
and 'so overwhelmed speakers with their eagerness and enthusiasm
that word spread around the country that nothing like this had ever
been seen or heard of before' (*The History of the Founding of the Ameri-*
can Academy of General Practice, St Louis: Warren H. Green and AAGP,
1969, 59). How many of us come away from professional meetings
with that kind of exaltation?

In Britain, the Royal College of General Practitioners was founded
in 1952 almost as a self-defence measure in reaction to the extraordinary demands placed on GPs with the introduction of the new health
insurance system. Its first meeting was held in the great hall of the
British Medical Association House in 1953; the first president was
William Pickles, a GP from the Yorkshire Dales with an interest in
epidemiology.

The Canadian College of General Practitioners (CCGP, later
CCF[amily]P) was inaugurated in 1954 at a salmon luncheon in Van-

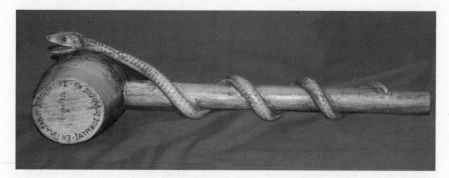

14.1   Gavel representing the snake and the staff of Asklepios, made of wood from the tree under which Hippocrates supposedly taught. Presented to the Canadian College of Family Physicians by the physicians of Cos.

couver; its permanent home would be Toronto. W. Victor Johnston, a GP from Lucknow, Ontario (pop. 1,100), was appointed the first executive director, a post he occupied for a decade. To mark the occasion, the Hippocratic society of physicians on the Greek island of Cos presented the new college with a gavel, entwined with the serpent of Asklepios and carved in wood taken 'from the plane tree under which Hippocrates taught' (see figure 14.1). The CCGP immediately sought advice and support from its slightly older siblings in the United States and Great Britain; in turn, it mentored similar groups in other countries. This national body emerged within the age of jet travel, easily linking it to events elsewhere in the world.

The newly formed professional associations immediately went to work on several fronts. They countered the charge of incompetence in two ways: first, through workshops for the training and continuing education of their colleagues; second, by demanding the right to certify their own trainees. They also sought recognition within hospitals and medical schools. As they reminded their critics, ambulatory care comprised the bulk of practice after graduation – even for specialists; medical education should somehow reflect that fact. The initiative immediately raised the morale of the much-maligned GPs, who seemed to revel in their annual (and soon to be tax-deductible) meetings. But achieving their goals took some time.

Opposition from specialists was a major obstacle to GP goals. Truman described a tense meeting with the *JAMA* editor Morris Fishbein, who was alarmed by the growing membership and charged the GPs with having 'employed a high pressure executive at a fantastic salary.' The ice was broken when the new AAGP president was introduced as the 'Republican Truman.' Fishbein was convinced the AMA could offer everything necessary, but he had to admit that the AAGP requirement of postgraduate work was original. Early organizers in Canada recall a similarly frosty reception by the executive of the Royal College of Physicians and Surgeons of Canada (RCPSC), which had been founded in 1929 to certify specialists. The two bodies held a joint meeting in 1960 in an attempt to mend fences, but friction persisted for some time.

Specialists, who dominated undergraduate medical education, were loath to yield structural or curricular space. Hospitals were slightly more receptive, and GPs continued to find admitting and practice privileges through departments of obstetrics, pediatrics, and psychiatry, where they performed routine tasks for lower fees than the specialists. The Canadian government sponsored pilot projects to develop GP training in Calgary, Alberta, and in London, Ontario. By 1960 thirty-three Canadian hospitals offered postgraduate work in general practice, although certification and academic departments had yet to be established.

Political differences, either actual or perceived, no doubt played a role. Specialists, who were well trained, older, and better paid, tended to be conservative, while the young physicians, medical students, and interns more commonly leaned to the left. During the war, younger medics in Canada had been intrigued by the decentralized community health-care initiatives and *feldsher* system of their Russian ally, and they willingly contemplated similar arrangements for home. These idealistic doctors, who worried less about money or prestige and more about public welfare, joined with the tired, rural practitioners to promote general practice issues. They also supported the simultaneous struggle for universal health care (see chapter 6) and called for collaboration with nurse practitioners, social workers, rehabilitationists, and other health care providers. But in the Cold

War of the following decades, their zeal was characterized as naive, amateurish, and dangerous. This multiplicity of political perspectives within the Canadian medical profession constitutes a striking difference between it and its neighbour to the south.

Once the Canadian specialist group finally became resigned to the tenacity of the generalists, it tried to 'hug them to death' by promoting certification in general medicine as a branch of the RCPSC. The GPs firmly resisted this new threat, viewing the right to certify their own as a necessary prerequisite for autonomy; they kept their own College. Further impediments arose in 1963 with the formation of the Fédération des médecins omnipracticiens du Québec (FMOQ), which promoted the political and economic interests of Quebec GPs but opposed certification.

The process to professionalize family medicine was happening on a global scale. Seeking strength in numbers, professional colleges and associations for general practice began to unite in a movement that transcended national boundaries. In 1964 Montreal was selected to host the first international conference of general practice. This meeting was the beginning of what in 1972 came to be called the World Organization of National Colleges, Academies, and Academic Associations of General Practitioners/Family Physicians (WONCA). It has held triennial meetings since 1980. These early meetings inspired the GPs to go home and keep fighting.

Canadian residencies began in 1966. The CCFP viewed the achievement as a major victory; certificates of examination were first awarded in 1969. Forty years later, these professional bodies seem to have forgotten the initial mistrust; they maintain cordial relations and reciprocate on many levels. Also in 1969, family medicine was recognized as the twentieth American 'specialty.'

Having solved the residency problem, the GPs moved on to tackle the last frontier: medical schools. Some universities had already nodded in the direction of general medicine. For example, non-specialists were employed as lesser mortals in specialty programs; students could receive credit for preceptorships in private offices; and general practice units were created within existing departments of epidemiology and public health.

Table 14.2
Some milestones in general/family practice

	Professional association	Specialty training	'Family' medicine
United States	1947	1969	1971
Britain	1952	1965	no
Canada	1954	1966	1967
Australia	1958	1973	no
Singapore	1971	1972	1975
New Zealand	1973	1977	no

The family residency at McMaster University was the first program launched by the fledgling school in 1967. The following year, the University of Western Ontario lured the GP guru Ian R. McWhinney from Britain to be the first professor. McMaster also pioneered outreach training in northern and rural settings. Other universities soon followed suit. In 1976 the government used grants to raise the percentage of medical schools with general practice departments above the 67 per cent level reached in that year. By 1979 all sixteen medical schools in Canada had departments of family medicine.

British and American medical schools soon moved in the same direction; the professional associations were active in encouraging the change (see table 14.2). The first American department of family medicine was part of the newly founded Penn State College of Medicine in Hershey, Pennsylvania, which opened its doors to students in 1967. By 1969, when family medicine became the twentieth specialty in the United States, many schools created departments. The first English chair in family medicine was established in Manchester in 1972.

The presence of an academic department and residencies did not guarantee the visibility of general practice in the undergraduate curriculum, which was still dominated by specialists. Curriculum time is a form of currency in medical education. In 1983, according to Rothstein, only 56 per cent of American and Canadian schools required family practice rotations in the final year of training. Its presence was even less visible in the more junior years. Renaming helped.

What's in a Name?

The American founders of the Board of Family Medicine have found it necessary to repudiate the name 'general practice' because of its associations with a type of practice which is deplored in academic circles ... 'Family medicine' as a name for our discipline and 'family physicians' for its members are both descriptive and dignified. Most of us, however, would recoil from a formal change of name and would be content, I think, to let evolution take its course.

– Ian R. McWhinney, 'General Practice as an
Academic Discipline,' *Lancet* 287, no. 7434 (1966): 419

The Advent of 'Family Medicine'

Irvine Loudon has traced the use of the words 'general practice' back to 1809, but he warned that seeking the expression in the more distant past is hopelessly anachronistic. When used in the eighteenth and nineteenth centuries, the term 'general practice' referred not to the work of the family doctor or the *omnipracticien*, but to the usual or customary course of action for all clinicians, medical or surgical, specialists or not. The older usage resurfaced in the late twentieth century, when 'general internal medicine' and the 'general internist' came along to threaten GPs on the issue of primary care. In contrast, the term 'family physician' rarely appeared in nineteenth-century medical literature. Instead, it was used in the titles of 'self-help' medical encyclopedias and other forms of advice literature for people who wished either to demystify or to avoid their doctor. In her study of the popular literature of France, historian Martha Hildreth found that the new sciences of disease meant that an emphasis on 'family' could act as an antidote to the fear that medical practice was becoming overly scientific.

Names are symbolic. The conscious and almost universal renaming of 'general practice' as 'family practice' in English-speaking North America was a political as well as an etymological act, with both economic and cultural implications. It can be narrowly located in the late 1960s and is intimately connected to another threatened issue – primary care.

In 1966 Canada enacted a health-care system that was to provide universal access to free or affordable services. Doctors would be paid for all their services, but anonymous taxpayers rather than individual patients would be obligated for medical fees. Confident in the status of their scientific training, pediatricians, obstetricians, and general internists knew that the relative differences in their fees would no longer inhibit patients desirous of their attentions. Surely, demands on their services would and should increase. What more pleasant way to supplement coffers than by looking after people who are not very sick? Already, well-off people in the United States relied on specialists for primary care – pediatricians for children, gynecologists for women, and internists for adults and the aged. The specialist as a primary caregiver became a new and intriguing possibility, occupying increasing space in medical literature.

In Canada, GPs helped to nip this process in the bud in two interesting ways. First, GP-versus-specialist became a matter of fiscal responsibility within the new fee schedules. Taxpayers should not be on the hook for unnecessarily expensive services. To see a specialist, patients would normally need the referral of another physician; without a referral, the specialist would have to accept a lower fee. In Ontario, for example, these restrictions are stated in 'Terms and Definitions' of fee schedules and follow sections on the 'Principles of Ethical Billing.' Suddenly, primary care seemed somewhat less attractive to the specialists in Canada, although it is still hotly debated in the United States.

Second, GPs redefined their enterprise as 'family medicine.' The word 'family' implied all-inclusive practice in a positive way that evoked comfortable images of hearth and home. 'Family' also eliminated – or 'repudiated,' to use Ian McWhinney's term – the negative connotations of that vague word 'general,' which had always seemed to invite the charge of incompetence. How could any doctor be an expert in everything? Unlike 'general,' the word 'family' was not apologetic and needed no justification. It implied that one doctor could serve each person well without forgetting the significant context of the others. Children, women, the elderly – everyone could trust a family doctor to provide primary care.

The renaming of the CCGP as the CCFP formally took place in 1967 just as the residencies were launched. In 1968 Malcolm Hill and colleagues conducted a survey in Hamilton, Ontario, to assess the validity of the term 'family doctor': 86 per cent of respondents representing 600 families in the care of four different doctors reported that one physician looked after the whole family. 'Is family doctor a valid term?' The answer, they concluded, was 'yes.' For our purposes, the date of the survey and the fact that the question needed to be asked at all exemplify a fascinating shift. A similar change soon took place in the United States in 1971 'to reflect more accurately the changing nature of primary health care' (AAFP website) (see table 14.2).

McWhinney predicted that British GPs would resist the trend; in 2010, the British colleges and those of the antipodes still use the term 'general practice.' But in 1984, when Oxford University launched its new journal, the chosen title was *Family Practice.*

Research in Family Medicine: Oxymoron, Phoenix, or Sop?

The Collings Condemnation

My observations have led me to write what is indeed a condemnation of general practice in its present form, but they have also led me to recognize the importance of general practice and the dangers of continuing to pretend it is something which it is not.

– Joseph S. Collings, 'General Practice in England Today – A Reconnaissance,' *Lancet* 255, no. 6604 (1950): 555

Having secured its place in both undergraduate and postgraduate education of many countries, family medicine began to consolidate its position by claiming to provide exceptional research opportunities. The thought of GPs conducting research was ridiculed by many medical professionals. GPs themselves were divided on the issue.

Some feared that research would be self-defeating by detracting from the central purpose of holistic, comprehensive, and continuing clinical care. Research seemed to be an unnecessary concession to the new and hard-won academic status – a concession that would inevitably turn family doctors into specialists by making them experts on tiny topics that lent themselves to scientific investigation. Having successfully resisted the specialists on certification, they saw no reason to offer this sop to the old specialist-dominated structure of academe.

Others, like American leader John P. Geyman, saw tremendous research potential in the very nature of family practice, with its emphasis on continuity and comprehensive care. They argued that consortiums of GPs could use epidemiological methods on their practice records to answer those burning questions that left specialists bored. In Britain, classic works were reprinted on general practice research, describing it as the 'most alluring of occupations.'

One of the earliest general practice research projects was a British epidemiological investigation, published in 1956, which demonstrated that penicillin was of no value in measles. More recently, international committees of WONCA collaborated to create classification systems for assessing functional capacity that can be applied to research into common biological problems. In some places, however, population-based research – especially when it involved patterns of morbidity and mortality – seemed to encroach on the realm of public health experts, who doubted the conceptual and statistical sophistication of their family medicine colleagues.

GPs also turned their research on themselves and their work, or they invited sociologists to do so on their behalf. What assumptions influenced the individuals and services that made up family practice? How could activities be made more efficient? Was solo work better than working in a group? Could a well-equipped office eliminate the need for house calls? Prompted by the famous Collings Report (1950), several British studies made recommendations for changes. In 1963 Kenneth Clute analysed Canadian general practice by comparing two provinces. He identified problems in physician distribution and work-related stress, including lack of time for professional renewal, patients, family, and friends. He predicted that the impending changes in health-care provision would be detrimental. A decade later, Wolfe and Badgley took up the same theme. Studies of the quality and quantity of life and work still constitute a major research issue within the discipline.

Next, family medicine research shifted from epidemiological investigations to behaviourist and psychotherapeutic issues. Disillusionment with statistics may have been one reason for the change. According to Thomas Osborne, GPs perceived limitations in population-based research and were uncomfortable with remote collective surveys. 'Sensitive to singularity,' he said, GPs were trained to focus on individuals and were attuned to a person-centred model. As a result, 'a subjectivizing surveillance of self was substituted for an objectivizing surveillance of morbid populations.' Research came to be motivated by what Osborne called a 'salvationist ideology,' centred on doctor–patient relations, communication, accountability, and introspection.

Fifty years later, research is still a contentious issue in family medicine. GPs have not rushed into scientific investigation, although the university systems of promotion and tenure urge them to do so with tangible rewards. The early 1990s witnessed the advent of 'evidence-based medicine' for validity of practice issues as described by epidemiologists and internists, especially at McMaster University in Hamilton, Ontario (see chapter 5). Family practitioners eyed the new trend with both scepticism and interest. Instead, they turned attention to issues of health care delivery, not only at home but in war-torn parts of the world, such as Bosnia-Herzegovina – places that never had a general practitioner tradition. At the 1992 WONCA meeting in Vancouver, the four thousand delegates were exhorted to preserve global health by promoting peace and protecting the environment. They also experiment with technologies such as computerization and telemedicine, and work on new methods for enhancing physician distribution and assigning credit for continuing education. In some Canadian jurisdictions a primary care reform movement, prompted by government, is bringing family physicians into a new system of salaries based on capitation.

Research also focuses on encouraging graduates to chose family medicine careers. A challenge throughout the developed world in the early twenty-first century is a relative decline in numbers of family doctors. The residency choice for approximately 40 per cent of graduates in Canada in 1990, it attracted only 30 per cent in 2007. The decline has been linked to the sharp increase in medical tuition fees in populous provinces since 1995. In the United States numbers are even smaller; and they declined steadily from a relative two-decade 'high' of nearly 16 per cent in 1995; in 2008, 8.2 per cent of candidates matched to family programs. The choice is influenced by medical school and the origins of the graduates. Primary care delivered by specialists is more costly, but there are not enough family doctors to fill the roles waiting for them. In some places including Japan (1952), Western Australia (1990), Canada (1992), and Sweden (2002), separate associations and journals have formed to support rural practice; in the United States it is promoted through the AAFP, individual states, and many student organizations. Under the auspices of WONCA, the first international conference on rural medicine was held in Shanghai in 1996. With several name changes the function persists as 'Rural Health World,' bringing the concerns of family doctors into the broad public health concerns of the next chapter. WONCA itself grew from an initial eighteen members in 1972 to 97 members representing 79 countries and 200,000 GPs by 2009. Related research issues concern the role and education of foreign-trained physicians who are invited to make up the shortages, and the effect of lifestyle choices of physicians in working fewer hours.

Most recently, family doctors display additional research interests in language and the humanities, writing articles on metaphor, literature, arts, and narration. In 1999, the AAFP launched a National Research Network to empower physicians 'through research to help their communities and the world.' Recognizing that research in the humanities is of value to health care, it also sponsors a Center for the History of Family Medicine in Leawood, Kansas.

Impact of Family Medicine on the Specialties

Family medicine has influenced all medical practice in a wide variety of ways, the most obvious being the importance of Continuing Medical Education (CME) and the need for ongoing evaluation. From its very inception, the CCGP required members to seek a minimum of one hundred hours of postgraduate study every two years. In

> **Vive la différence!**
>
> Academic family medicine has made considerable progress in the last 20 years, yet we still do not fit comfortably into the academic milieu. To gain acceptance, it is said, family medicine must become less pragmatic, more theoretical, and more productive in quantitative research.
>
> I believe that family medicine is marginal because it differs in some fundamental ways from the academic mainstream and that our main value to medicine lies in the differences. Eventually I think the academic mainstream will become more like us than vice versa.
>
> – Ian R. McWhinney, 'The Importance of Being Different,' *Canadian Family Physician* 43 (1997): 193

other words, the historically informed recognition that medicine will continue to change is embedded in the structure of the organization. Patients are assured that a CCFP-certified doctor has met the recognized standard of practice, not once but repeatedly. With its commitment to lifelong learning and public accountability, family medicine has helped to generate a market for the rising industry of CME and has stimulated research in original forms of pedagogic communication. As public mistrust of physicians grew, the enterprise rubbed off on specialist groups concerned about accountability. Thirty years after the founding of the CCGP, the Royal College of Physicians and Surgeons of Canada implemented 'maintenance of competence' programs for Canadian specialists, and similar programs are being considered by specialist groups elsewhere in the world. By 2000, family doctors were deans in several medical faculties.

In trying to promote itself to the well-established schools as an academic discipline, organized family medicine also embarked on the philosophic task of self-definition. Not only did it establish the boundaries for its own identity and pedagogy, but it set criteria that could eventually be applied to the recognition of other newcomers. Having done so, it invited scholars from several nations to develop parameters of evaluation for training programs, for CME, and for evaluation of the evaluations themselves.

The 'miracles' of technology and subspecialization provide yet another justification for the integrative capacity of family medicine. The family practitioner permits the subspecialist to function in a restricted space. Conversely, the chronic problems of an aging population, polypharmacy, iatrogenic illness, and the impersonal face of a medical establishment centred on hospitals have combined to create a continuing role for the family physician. The doctor who actually knows and remembers the patient and her family is essential. Researcher or not, the family doctor *selects, coordinates,* and above all *explains* the specific expertise that will help to diagnose or treat a patient. And with the long-established features of continuity and context, only family medicine can provide the holistic care that an increasingly sceptical public now demands.

Suggestions for Further Reading

At the bibliography website http://histmed.ca.

CHAPTER FIFTEEN

When the Patient Is Plural:
Public and International Health*

The improvement of medicine may eventually prolong human life, but the improvement of social conditions can achieve this result more rapidly and more successfully.

– Rudolf Virchow, *Öffentlichen Medizin* (1879), cited in H. Waitzkin, *Social Medicine* 1 (2006), 7

In this chapter, we explore medical help for collectivities. The oldest and most obvious responses have occurred in times of epidemics, when emergencies dictated policies about freedoms and care (see chapter 7). The laws governing public health (and immigration) are responses to previous outbreaks or threats of disease. They are based on the best guess of what is appropriate according to those holding power in time and place. As a result, they are conditioned by past experience and must needs lag behind the reality of the next problem. Public health operates against the 'medical model' (see chapter 4) in two distinct ways: it aims for prevention rather than treatment, and it concerns groups not individuals. Often it focuses on people who are not sick. With the social and cultural turn in medical history, public and international health has become one of the hottest topics in the field. Some studies are comparative; so far, however, most histories focus on particular countries, colonies, and their interactions.

Without ignoring place, we will slice this story from the perspective

*Learning objectives for this chapter are on p. 457.

of projects that contributed to longer lifespans: plagues, work, water, food, politics, peace, and environment, ending with the international health movement. At least one key contributor is chosen to exemplify the medicalization of each topic. This approach was suggested by my colleagues in community health and epidemiology, who believe that medical students sometimes have difficulty perceiving a future in service to populations for a lack of obvious role models.

Histories of public and international health tend to situate themselves between two extremes: either public health was a noble crusade of philanthropic generosity or it was an evil incursion into vulnerable lives motivated by selfishness or intolerance. The position on this spectrum is conditioned not only by research on the past, but also by the political sentiments of authors in the present.

Disease itself is vulnerable to social perception (see chapter 4). Differences have been construed as pathology, when in reality they represented normal variations in subjected people. Some scholars have used the concept of the 'other' and 'othering' to show how powerful elites turned such difference into disease. Medical action meant eradication of cultures and communities. In most instances, draconian outcomes were unintended consequences.

Plagues

The well-being of towns and migrant groups, such as sailors and armies, could be shattered in days by a new contagion. In their wake, epidemics leave measures intended to preserve health. For example, quarantine was enacted during fourteenth-century plague to protect ports and to force travellers to prove their health; rules also applied to grouping of the sick and dealing with corpses. Municipal sanitary committees or temporary boards of health were struck in disease outbreaks, sometimes persisting when the danger passed, sometimes reconvening if it recurred. Often the rules worked by sacrificing the safety of those considered most vulnerable. For more on responses to epidemics, see chapter 7.

Poverty and Work

Although charitable hospices have a long history with religious communities, publicly funded welfare traces its European origins to the early modern period. In particular, laws providing for the poor and the sick were established in many cities during the sixteenth century. In addition, confraternities to help the underprivileged arose as a form of private philanthropy – sometimes but not always aligned with religion. Poor laws were used in many ways, from simply offering food to confining people in workhouses as a source of cheap labour. Some 'blamed the poor for their own misery and opposed public intervention'; others saw disease as a product of 'miserable conditions of life and sought solutions in public action' (Eyler 1980, 2). Until the nineteenth century and the sanitary movement, however, doctors had little to do with poor relief (see the discussion of Edwin Chadwick below).

In contrast, the idea that people were made sick by their work was only vaguely appreciated before the Italian doctor Bernardino Ramazzini observed the habits of ordinary people. A man fixing a sewer would disappear underground briefly, then resurface gasping before plunging again. When asked why, the labourer explained that the noxious fumes could produce breathing problems and fainting – even death. Fascinated that illiterate workers possessed medical wisdom, Ramazzini began to enumerate all the diseases of workers and how they avoided them. He was laughed at for slumming with the lower classes. In the opening of his *Diseases of Workers* (1700), he apologized should he offend sensibilities by dwelling on such topics (see table 15.1). A masterpiece of considerate observation of people normally ignored, the book clearly defined the employments of his time and place and their risks. Thirteen years later and a year before his death, Ramazzini published an expanded edition.

Occupational health, as a modern specialty, has a quiet, bureaucratic reputation; however, it has the potential to preserve the health of millions of workers from the ravages of fumes, noise, accidents, and long hours. Often the biggest obstacle was not identifying the dangers but convincing the owners of companies and governments to invest in limiting them. Doctors who take on these missions find themselves working for lower wages often in confrontation with powerful opponents in business and politics.

Partly for mutual support, an international association to promote

Table 15.1
'Trades' in Ramazzini, *On Diseases of Workers* (1700 and 1713)

Miners	Grain	*Additions in 1713*
Gilders	Stone cutter	Printers
Mercury therapists	Laundress	Scribes, notaries
Chemists	Flax, hemp, silk	Weavers
Potters	Bathmen	Coppersmiths
Tinsmiths	Salt-makers	Wood work
Glass & mirror	Standing	Razors, lancets
Blacksmiths	Sitting	Brick makers
Gypsum & lime	Jews (sedentary)	Well diggers
Fullers	Grooms	Sailors and rowers
Oil, tanners, cheese	Porters	Hunters
Tobacco	Athletes	Soap makers
Undertakers	Fine work	
Midwives	Voice, singers	
Wet nurses	Farmers	
Vinters, brewers	Fishermen	
Bakers, millers	Camps	
Starch	Learned men (sedentary)	

the study of occupational and environmental health was founded in 1982, called the Collegium Ramazzini. It aims 'to be a bridge between the world of scientific discovery and the social and political centers which must act on the discoveries of science to protect public health.' Governed by 184 fellows representing dozens of countries on six continents, the association arranges conferences, publications, and collective research projects, and it generates scientific statements on hazards and gives awards to significant achievement. Annual meetings are held in Carpi, Ramazzini's home town.

A current initiative of Collegium Ramazzini relates to its 1993 statement on the carcinogenic and pulmonary dangers of chrysotile asbestos. Efforts to seek a world ban on this substance have been repeatedly hampered by the nations that supply it, including Canada. Producers argue that without asbestos, more people would be injured by fires than are harmed with its proper use; other reasons, less often articulated, come from the political and economic risks to workers, industrialists, and politicians in closing the mines.

Extrapolating on concerns for workers, public health reformers in the nineteenth century turned their attention to poverty and the plight of poor children (see chapter 13). The broader medicalization of poverty did not occur until the late 1970s, when demographers proved mathematically that it could be a determinant of mortality at any age (see G.B. Rodgers, *International Journal of Epidemiology* 31 [1979] 2002, 533–8).

Water

Clean and plentiful water is probably the single most important determinant of health, and this knowledge is ancient. Methods for purification of waste were developed by the Egyptians, who used filtration and coagulation. Water quality was a matter of security: Athenians, confronted with a plague in the fifth century B.C., suspected that their Spartan enemy had poisoned the wells (see chapter 7). People also understood how to keep drinking water clean: for example, ancient armies set camps upstream of the horses. Because of this durable wisdom, it is surprising to discover that the water theory of epidemics did not catch on until the mid-nineteenth century. Instead, tainted air, or 'miasma,' was the presumed cause.

The 1850s discovery by John Snow that cholera could be transmitted by water took place three decades before germ theory was established (see chapter 7). Yet the dramatic implications of Snow's elegant detective work around the Broad Street pump were not immediately accepted. Two other Englishmen are relevant to this water story, neither of whom believed Snow at first: one a doctor, the other a lawyer.

William Farr came from a poor family but studied medicine in France and Switzerland thanks to a generous benefactor. In France he learned the numerical medicine of P.C.A. Louis (see chapter 4). Following his wife's death only five years into their marriage, Farr found employment in the General Registrar's office, where he applied medical statistics to identify factors affecting health. His new system for recording deaths extended Ramazzini's lead by permitting comparison of mortality between occupations. For cholera, he accepted the old theory of miasma, finding evidence seemingly in its favour: fewer people contracted cholera the higher they lived above the Thames. Not until later did he accept the water theory.

The London lawyer Edwin Chadwick engaged in reform of the

Poor Laws. Rather than blaming people for their poverty, he argued that their health and ability to work was undermined by squalid living conditions; laws perpetuated the problem. Chadwick thought that it was the business of good government to clean up the world. He too insisted on better statistics, claiming that centralizing the task of recording births and deaths would enhance reliability over the parish records kept by well-intentioned but variably diligent priests. In particular, Chadwick focused on sewers where water and waste stagnated. Without flushing, they had to be cleaned manually by brave labourers like Ramazzini's man. Chadwick's report of 1842 was ignored for five years until another cholera outbreak mobilized action. He then helped design a system of self-flushing sewers, which greatly improved water and air quality and functioned well for decades. Nevertheless, he offended doctors, engineers, politicians, and bureaucrats, some say because of his zeal and personality, and he was forced to resign from the Board of Health in 1854. His 'sanitary idea' did not dissuade him from the miasma theory; indeed, it corresponded well with his observations: better sewers correlated with better cholera statistics. He was knighted a year before his death in 1890.

The sanitarian movement launched by Chadwick moved well beyond England and was supported by ordinary people, especially women, who were attracted by the ancient ideals of hygiene and purity. They exposed 'nuisances' and pressured politicians to value cleanliness. In the 1880s, when germ theory was established (see chapter 4), sanitarians could point to new science to add ballast to their agenda. Their ready-made, energetic organizations helped the new public-health experts accomplish their goals.

Water control was now scientific. Municipalities ignored this responsibility at their peril; henceforth, every illness caused by dirty water could be prevented. Just as nineteenth-century patricians tended to blame the poor for their ailments, now the sick could blame politicians. Temporary boards of health had arisen around epidemics in the 1830s, but the *permanent* governmental structures, boards and laboratories, appeared in the last three decades of the nineteenth century (see table 15.2). At first they focused on seamen and immigrants, who seemed to bring disease with them; however, the principles were soon applied to all citizens. Cold, wet England also

Table 15.2
Some milestones in public health institutions

Britain	
1809, 1831	Board of Health (Central and local) – intermittent
1848	Public Health Act
1854–8	General Board of Health – intermittent
1899	London School of Tropical Medicine
1907	Royal Society of Tropical Medicine and Hygiene
1919	Ministry of Health
Canada	
1830s	Local boards as needed in epidemics
1867	Provincial departments of health – mostly not operative
1882	First permanent Board of Health in Ontario
1919	Dominion Department of Health
1927	School of Hygiene, Toronto
United States	
1830s	Local Boards as needed in epidemics
1871	First Supervising Surgeon of Marine Hospital (later Sugeon General)
1879	National Board of Health – permanent
1887	First federal hygienic laboratory, one room on Staten Island (becomes NIH in 1930)
1890	Chair of Hygiene at the Georgetown Medical School (G. Kober)
1902	Public Health and Marine Hospital Service

developed a special interest in tropical disease because of its many colonies.

By the 1890s, water filtration plants were being built in Europe, the United States, and Canada. Frequently opposed because of concerns over costs, contamination, location, and contracts, their implementation proceeded city by city and was mediated through social activism and private interests. These facilities used improved techniques of coagulation and sand filtration; they also looked for disinfectants, such as chlorine, to actively kill newly discovered bacteria. In 1910 a high incidence of typhoid prompted Canada and the United States to launch a collaborative study of pollution in the Great Lakes for the first, but not the last, time. The mortality rate in America fell more rapidly in the late nineteenth and early twentieth century than at any other time; demographers Cutler and Miller argue that safer water is the most likely explanation.

Keeping water clean requires costly infrastructure, laboratory inspection, and personnel. Even in developed countries, cholera and other infections, especially E. coli, recur if the system is negected or disrupted in earthquakes, floods, and war. An accident in Britain in 1988 resulted in chemical contamination of the water supply for 20,000 homes in Cornwall; more than a hundred residents still complain of sequelae. In 1999, E. coli in a well caused two deaths and hundreds of illnesses among people who attended a New York county fair. Water spoilage by wild pigs may have been the source of E. coli–contaminated spinach across North America in 2006, leaving 200 sick and 3 dead. Neglect of controls produced serious water contamination in Walkerton, Ontario, in 2000, with seven deaths and 2,300 illnesses. The tragedy would have been worse had Medical Officer of Health Murray McQuigge not acted on suspicions and issued a boil-water order. Again water contamination at Kashechewan, in northern Ontario, made national headlines in 2005: after coping with a boil-water advisory for two years, the tiny community had to be evacuated. At the time of writing, in a rich country with one of the world's largest water supplies, approximately one hundred First Nations communities live under boil-water advisories.

The simple goal of clean water is even harder to achieve and preserve on a global scale.

Food

Cicely Williams was born to a British family living in Jamaica. Her father allowed her to study medicine, she said, because she was unlikely to find a husband. After training at Oxford, she went to Africa and Malaysia to research child and maternal health. In west Africa she connected a wasting disease of young children to nutrition and published her classic description of kwashiorkor as protein deficiency in 1935. The name, from a dialect of the African Gold Coast (now Ghana), literally means 'sickness of the deposed baby'; these peoples had long thought of the disease holistically, as a social problem created by a sibling birth (see figure 15.1).

Working near Singapore in February 1942, Williams was captured, along with tens of thousands of Allied troops and nationals, includ-

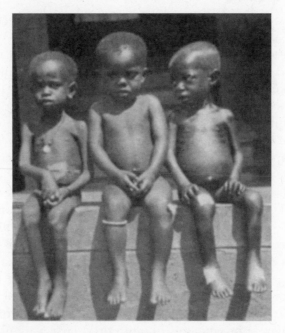

15.1   Kwashiorkor, illness of the displaced child, affects two of the three children. From Williams, *Mother and Child Health*, 1972

ing other doctors. Confined in an internment camp with severe privations, she nearly died; at liberation in August 1945 she was nursed back to health by fellow prisoners and soldiers. Following the war, Williams was invited to lead the Maternal and Child Health division of the new World Health Organization (WHO). Overpopulation was a major concern, but she knew that women in developing countries would not accept birth control until child mortality had been staved. It was important to feed children enough good-quality food.

Food, like water, is essential to life. The ancients knew it and devoted deep attention to dietary manipulation in the face of disease. Somehow the medical achievements of the nineteenth and early twentieth centuries gave doctors permission to leave food quality to homemakers and fledgling nutritionists; its quantity and poor distribution were mechanical problems beneath the radar of scientists. But Williams, like Joseph Goldberger (see chapter 13), demonstrated that conditions like beriberi and pellagra, previously considered con-

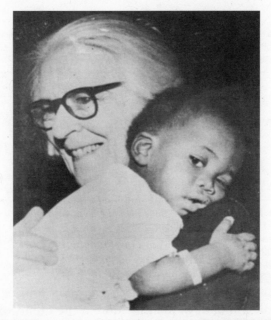

15.2   Cicely D. Williams with child, 1975. From S. Craddock, *Retired Except on Demand: the Life of Dr Cicely D. Williams*, 1983, by permission of Dr Williams's niece, Josephine Cruickshank, and Green Templeton College, Oxford University

tagious, were actually specific deficiencies that had a geographic and cultural basis.

With the discovery of vitamins in the mid-twentieth century (see chapter 13), the elements of healthy diets could now be analysed. In the developed world, science has been preoccupied with food quality and security – keeping it free from chemicals and germs and, most recently, asserting the safety of genetically modified organisms (GMOs). But in developing countries, the lack of sufficient good food is a serious concern, one that has not been medicalized judging by publications. For example, from 1950 to 2008, Medline cites 83,046 articles on obesity; however, many fewer address 'Hunger' or 'Starvation' (just over 11,000), and of those that do, less than 500 recognize 'Food Supply' as a main topic. Scant attention is given to Africa and Asia, the places where food supply really counts (see table 15.3). The

Table 15.3
Number of articles cited in Medline, 1950–2008, using the MeSH headings: Hunger, Starvation (or both), combined with Food Supply, and with Africa, Asia, Canada, Great Britain, or United States

	Hunger	Starvation	Hunger or starvation[a]
	3,389	7,882	11,182
with Food Supply[b]	258	215	463
on Africa	13	21	33
on Asia	4	6	17
on Canada	9	0	9
on UK	2	4	6
on U.S.	65	17	79

[a]The totals in the last column are not simple additions, because some articles use both MeSH headings Hunger and Starvation.
[b]Food supply was an MeSH heading for 5,067 articles of which only 463 pertained to Hunger or Starvation.
Based on a Medline search using MeSH headings, conducted 5 December 2008.

WHO estimates that a billion people are undernourished and 3.5 million people die annually of malnutrition in the twenty-one countries where the problem is chronic. The root causes are political, as well as environmental and biological. It is the greatest health issue in the world, but perhaps because of its political overtones most doctors do not yet see it as their problem.

Politics

What Is Politics?

Medicine is a social science and politics is nothing but medicine on a grand scale.

– Rudolf Virchow (1848), cited in H. Waitzkin, *Social Medicine* 1 (2006): 6

Health-care delivery and public health initiatives are always political because they entail the redistribution of resources from the privileged to the disadvantaged. Political doctors are not rare. At any time in most countries, at least a few politicians or activists hold medical degrees and have practised clinically. However, few doctors join the political left, as did the nineteenth-century pathologist Rudolf Virchow cited above. He lost his job for supporting the 1848 revolution and was later blacklisted by Bismarck for winning an opposition seat in the Prussian legislature.

Unlike Virchow, doctors mostly avoid politics and have trouble seeing its relationship to health-care delivery. Even committed health-care academics will argue that politics is not medical, or that it is unseemly, perhaps unprofessional, and even unethical, for doctors to pronounce on political matters. I made this discovery while researching the history of medical tuition fees: for at least fifty years, doctors have known that their students come from the richest sectors of society; however, broadening access would entail political involvement and that is something doctors are not often prepared to do.

Absence of the medical professions from the debates over health-care delivery are even more striking. Below we sketch a few rare examples of those who dared to enter the fray.

In the political history of medicare systems, doctors were not prominent (see chapter 6). In 1944, when Tommy C. Douglas became premier of Saskatchewan on a promise of free medical care, his staunchest adviser was surgeon Hugh Maclean. A Toronto graduate, Maclean conducted a prairie practice during the Depression and was shocked by the devastation that illness brought to families already on the verge of ruin. Several times, he ran for public office on a socialist ticket – and was never elected. Despised by his colleagues for his leftist sympathies, he retired to California. Douglas sought his help in campaigning, and Maclean's vision for free hospital and medical care with salaried doctors became the blueprint of the government's medical plan.

Within days of his victory, Douglas kept his promise to consult citizens by conducting a survey on needs. He invited the famous Swiss-born physician-historian Henry E. Sigerist of Johns Hopkins University to head it. An erudite man who spoke many languages, Sigerist had studied Russian health systems, visited Canada previously, and graced the cover of *Time* magazine in 1939. With a small

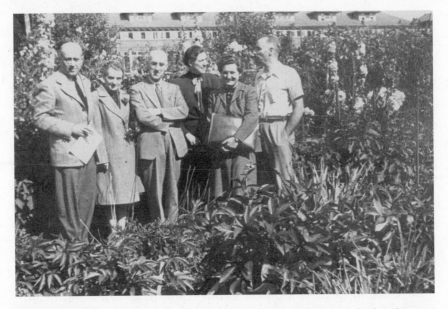

15.3   Henry E. Sigerist with his survey team in Weyburn, Saskatchewan, 1944. Alan Mason Chesney Archive, Johns Hopkins University

team that included a nurse, Sigerist toured the province to conduct the survey (see figure 15.3); his recommendations bore an uncanny resemblance to Maclean's vision. Now, however, it was difficult for alarmed doctors to disagree with a distinguished professor from another country.

Sigerist went home to Baltimore full of admiration for Saskatchewan. For him, medicine advanced only with parallel developments in social as well as technical wisdom; wealthy countries ignored the social side. Soon he fell under suspicion for his left-leaning views and was summoned before the House Un-American Activities Committee. Baffled, wounded, and defeated, he retired to Switzerland, where he died of a stroke in 1957.

Gro Harlem Brundtland trained as a doctor in her native Norway and studied public health in the United States. After working for school children's health, she successfully ran for the socialist Labour Party, becoming minister of the environment. In 1981 at age 41, she became the first woman prime minister of Norway (and the youngest), serving eleven years in that capacity. The term 'sustainable development' was popularized in 1987 with the report of a United Nations commission which she chaired. In 1998 she became Director General of the WHO. During her five-year term, the organization focused on promoting health in developed countries, as well as fighting disease everywhere. She used economic arguments to convince sceptics that investment in health is good for all nations, givers and receivers both.

These distinguished individuals are exceptions. Since their founding, the large professional associations, such as the BMA, CMA, and the AMA, have fought aspects of health-care programs that limit physician income and freedom. They justify their opposition with a political philosophy which holds that state intervention does not improve medical care. However, since the Second World War, groups of students and junior doctors have formed organizations to lobby for improved access to health care, sometimes in opposition to the larger associations. Many founded and served free clinics. The impact of these often short-lived initiatives is difficult to assess.

Doctors who favour improving health-care provision – even if it means lower incomes – organize outside the boundaries of their professional associations. Founded in 1987, Physicians for a National Health Plan is committed to enhancing access to medical care for Americans; it boasts a membership of 15,000 doctors, less than 2 per cent of the total. In late 2008, its members met with president-elect Barack Obama to express their concerns. The history of health activism in America is preserved and promoted at the Health Left History Centre of Philadelphia, founded by physician-activist Walter J. Lear. Even in Canada, physicians have grown worried about increased privatization of services and the absence of protest from the leading professional associations. Canadian Doctors for Medicare formed in 2006 and by 2008 had 1,500 members – again only 2 per cent of the country's total. These trends – small though they are – suggest an increase in the number of doctors who recognize political action as a health-care responsibility.

Wishful Thinking? Prophecy?

One thing that surprised me in a positive way while making this film is how many doctors in the United States now support socialized medicine. That did not use [*sic*] to be the case. They were the biggest fighters and opponents of it. They now realized that they've been had. They supported the HMOs in the beginning. They thought managed care [will] keep the cost down. Insurance companies said 'You'll make more money, we'll make more money, we'll all make more money by providing less care' ... Well, really what the insurance companies were going to do was make sure the doctors didn't get paid either ... Now they've got 5 or 6 [employees] ... doing all the paperwork, on the phone, hear them yelling and screaming at the HMO, fighting to get a twenty-dollar bill paid. Doctors have been ruined by this system. They have been demoralized by this system. Now they are the biggest supporter of real change.

– Michael Moore, 2007 interview for his film *Sicko*, http://www.comingsoon.net/news/movienews.php?id=21257 (accessed 20 June 2009)

The Example of the Third Reich

In this discussion of the worthy contributions of doctors engaged in politics, it is important not to overlook the relationship of the medical profession to National Socialism in Germany. Elected to power in 1933, the Nazi party attracted physicians more than any other profession. It used science to assert the notion of Aryan superiority, relying on the work of geneticist Fritz Lenz, who headed the first department of eugenics. The Reich elaborated a metaphor of public health – 'racial hygiene' – as justification for a 'final solution' of enforced sterilization and genocide of Jews, gypsies, homosexuals, the mentally ill, and the disabled. Doctors joined the party in droves – some argue because it was the only way to ensure a safe living; others suspect that they were lured by the pseudo-scientific rhetoric. More distressingly, doctors committed crimes: murder, torture, confinement, and ghastly 'experiments' without consent.

A special 'doctors' trial' was held at Nuremberg in 1947 to investigate the crimes of twenty-three physicians: sixteen were found guilty; seven were executed. The judges laid out a code of ethical behaviour which led to the Geneva Declaration of 1948 concerning the humanitarian goals of medicine. Many historians have written about medical involvement in the Third Reich, using archives as they came open. Although only twenty-three doctors were tried, thousands more joined the Nazi party, roughly 50 per cent of all German doctors. Many were upstanding members of their communities, before, during, and after the conflict. For example, Lenz continued working after the war, claiming that the Holocaust would set back eugenics research.

Beyond demonizing these individuals, it is important to recognize that they thought that those actions were good for the *collective health* of their nation. And Germany is not an isolated case. 'Racial hygiene' was a precursor for the 1990s 'ethnic cleansing' agenda of another physician-politician, Radovan Karadžić, who, like Hitler before him, invoked medical arguments as a pretext for the genocide of Bosnian Muslims.

Race and Culture as Pathology

Our outrage over the German Third Reich or medically condoned genocide anywhere makes it all too easy to forget that eugenicist notions had currency in North America too (see chapter 13). Furthermore, politically condoned public health efforts to 'help' racially and culturally different communities within our own nations were shown to be attempts to 'cure' the difference by extinguishing it. Critical histories are now being written of the well-intentioned but ultimately damaging missions to help Amerindians, African Americans, Oceanic aboriginals, and colonized peoples everywhere.

Peace

It is often said that Virchow's political opposition to militariza-
tion, had it been successful, might have prevented the Franco-
Prussian War of 1870. Histories of surgery and rehabilitation sometimes emphasize the 'silver lining' – lessons from war that are later
applied during peace. But outright opposition to war was not medicalized as a preventative health measure until the fearsome technology of atomic weapons.

Following the U.S. nuclear attacks on Japan in 1945, the Atomic
Bomb Casualty Commission was sent to study the effects. Its initial
conclusions were horrifying enough, although the long-term effects
were not yet known. Slowly it emerged that people who had not died
in the seconds, minutes, and weeks after the explosion could develop
side effects many years later. Nor was the extent and danger of radioactive fallout fully appreciated in the first postwar decade, when Cold
War powers began testing hundreds of atomic weapons. In 1961,
Physicians for Social Responsibility (PSR) was founded to end atmospheric testing by marshalling scientific evidence on its dangers for
American children. In 1963, Russia, Great Britain, and the United
States moved tests underground, but France and China continued
above-ground testing until 1974 and 1980 respectively.

Among other issues, PSR members studied medical readiness for
war. Eventually, they realized that no medicine could mitigate an
atomic catastrophe; the only public health response was to prevent
nuclear war altogether. To do that, PSR had to become an international movement involving doctors on both sides of the Cold War.
International Physicians for the Prevention of Nuclear War (IPPNW)
was founded at a 1980 meeting in Geneva by two cardiologists – the
American Bernard Lown and the Russian Evgueni Chazov. They
launched a vigorous campaign of public information – nuclear war
would be the final epidemic – and they conducted research to document the short- and long-term effects of nuclear bomb tests in the
atmosphere and underground. The group was awarded the Nobel
Prize for Peace in 1985 (see figure 15.4).

After this award was announced, underground tests continued

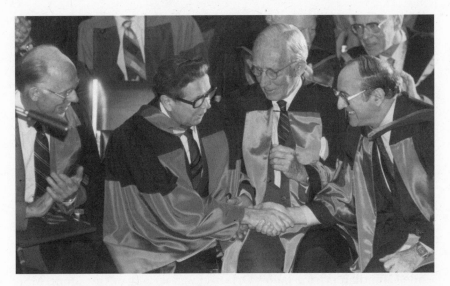

15.4   Shortly after their Nobel Prize had been announced, the founders of IPPNW were given honorary degrees, at Queens University, Kingston, Ontario. From left to right, pediatrician (and IPPNW member) Alex Bryans; E. Chazov; Dean of Medicine E.H. Botterell; and B. Lown, 2 November 1985. By permission of Dr Bryans and Dean David Walker, Faculty of Health Sciences Queen's University

until the five major powers slowly stopped them between 1990 and 1996. India and Pakistan last tested nuclear weapons in 1998, North Korea in 2009. In total, the eight nuclear powers are estimated to have tested at least two thousand weapons. IPPNW continues to lobby for the elimination of nuclear weapons, an end to the 'Star Wars' missile defence system, and a reduction in the harm from conventional weapons. This last goal is a resigned admission that after five thousand years of 'civilization,' people still think that it is a good idea to kill each other; the best hope is damage control.

Without abandoning efforts for peace, some physicians have volunteered to help improve the lives of people in war-ravaged places. The Red Cross filled this mission with nurses and doctors; its efforts were recognized with three Nobel Peace Prizes (see chapter 10). But in the late twentieth century, some criticized the Red Cross for becoming too bureaucratic and too close to national interests. The neediest (and riskiest) places were not given help. Médecins sans frontières (MSF, or Doctors without Borders) was founded in 1971 by French doctors working with journalists, including physician-politician Bernard Kouchner. He is now the French minister of foreign affairs for the current right-wing government, having previously served in socialist governments and as a communist party member. Taking extreme risks to bring high-quality care to the most dangerous and impoverished regions, MSF reserves the right (and knows how) to speak out about abuses wherever they occur. It also claims neutrality. It is in effect a *transnational* group, corresponding to many other examples in the vast civil society movement, which is centred on uncoerced, collective action around shared interests. In 1999, while Canadian doctor James Orbinski was serving as president, MSF won the Nobel Prize for Peace. Currently 27,000 volunteers are working in more than sixty countries.

Many other groups have formed around the need to relieve suffering in war-torn countries. Each must be seen as a solution to a perceived problem created by the inadequacies of its predecessors. All rely on and compete for charitable donations; consequently, their endeavours include publicity. An exhaustive list would be impossible. To offer one example in concluding this section on peace, let us examine War Child. Founded in 1993 by two British filmmakers who were shocked by the plight of children in the former Yugoslavia, War Child has contributed aid during conflicts in more than thirty countries. It has also established an 'international' wing consisting of two 'equal but totally autonomous' national branches: Netherlands (1994) and Canada (1999). The Canadian branch was founded by physicians Eric Hoskins and Samantha Nutt, whose bravery and hard work have brought many awards and much heavier responsibilities.

This labyrinth of helping organizations reminds us that doctor-driven charities are little different from other 'civil society' movements with their own internal contradictions and dependence on generating funds. Although no synthetic history yet exists, an extensive literature from sociology and political science offers insight.

Environment

When the first edition of this book appeared a decade ago, global warming was still controversial. Since then former U.S. vice-president Al Gore and the United Nations panel on climate change won the 2007 Nobel Peace Prize in recognition of their efforts to convince the world of the problem.

But many other aspects of pollution were already well understood. Even Hippocrates knew that good environment was essential to health; his treatise *Airs, Waters, and Places* was a kind of medical geography before the term even existed. Obviously then, people have long known that damage to air, water, food, and climate is destined to have an impact on health; however, finding examples of doctors who made it their problem is difficult. One of the first is Ramazzini, whose contributions were discussed above. But pollution affects everyone, not only workers. This realization dawned slowly through the sanitary movement for clean water (see above) and the Industrial Revolution of the nineteenth century. Plants are both helpers and indicators of population health.

The knowledge that plants produce oxygen from carbon dioxide was worked out in a series of steps involving several observers, including Joseph Priestley and the German doctor Julius Robert Mayer. By 1845, scientists had devised the basic equation in which sunlight converts carbon dioxide to oxygen and water. The more detailed elaboration of the chemical process of photosynthesis came in the early twentieth century. Mayer conceived of the plant world as a 'giant power station' and the planet's most important source of life energy (Rabinowitch).

The American physician Joseph T. Rothrock, who had served in the Civil War and later studied medicine in Philadelphia, turned his attention to this new information about plants and oxygen and recognized the importance of trees for human health – not only for chemical benefits but also for quality of life. By 1873, he was actively campaigning against deforestation – a voice crying in the wilderness (literally). Eighty years later, Pennsylvania set aside a large tract of forest in memory of this little-known doctor-pioneer of environmental health. The medical literature ignores him completely (see figure 15.5).

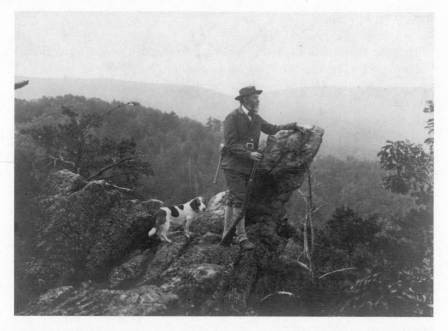

15.5   Joseph T. Rothrock with friend at Eagle's Rock, MG-4B Dock Family Papers, Pennsylvania State Archives

The word 'smog' (smoke and fog) was coined early in the twentieth century to describe the toxic atmosphere of London, England. All industrialized cities had noticed an increase in dangerous airs with greater use of fossil-fuel-burning machines. For some, it merely confirmed the old miasmatic theories. Newly implemented medical statistics charted the effects: when air was especially thick, people died and lung disease increased.

In October 1948, a temperature inversion created toxic smog in Donora, Pennsylvania, resulting in America's worst public health disaster: 5,000 of the town's 7,000 residents fell ill; 400 were hospitalized, and 20 died. Four years later, the 'great smog' of London coincided with an 80 per cent increase in mortality over the previous year. Precise numbers of deaths related to the 1952 smog are still debated. The government blamed a concomitant outbreak of influenza, but recent analyses suggest that even a large influenza outbreak would leave up to 12,000 deaths unaccounted for. These catastrophes promptly resulted in public health investigations and implementation of Clean Air Acts (1955 in the U.S., and 1956 in the UK). More than ever, public health was in direct confrontation with large industry and power stations, the source of employment and collective wealth.

The earliest Medline articles about trees and air quality date from the 1970s; they describe the dangers of pollens and the toxicity of pollutants on vegetation. Only in the mid-1970s did a handful of scientists from eastern Europe and Russia begin to write about trees, not as perpetrators or victims but as allies in the fight against environmental poisoning – something Rothrock had known a century earlier. Around the same time, certain synthetic chemicals were shown to damage the ozone layer of the atmosphere, which blocked harmful ultraviolet radiation; the result would be more skin disease and global warming. This slow, steady process might actually be natural, some argued.

Perhaps the event that finally triggered action, although it was not related directly to the ozone layer, was an industrial disaster in late 1984. Toxic gas leaked from the Union Carbide plant in Bhopal, India, causing between 3,000 and 8,000 deaths and leaving many blind or with lung damage. In the age of satellite television, the human misery was witnessed in real time around the world and could be neither hidden nor ignored. Anger over industry's carelessness deflected attention away from long-standing political indifference and permissiveness, but in the end, people realized that states had to engage.

The Vienna Convention of 1985 was a multi-nation recognition of the dangers to climate, environment, and human health; it resulted in control measures on a list of ozone-depleting substances, spelled out in Montreal two years later. Suddenly, a terrifying spiral of exponentially rising destruction loomed ahead. In the late 1980s, the 'giant power house' of the forest was rediscovered, all eyes turned on the largest and most precious forest in the world: Amazonia, located in one of the poorest countries, where aspirations for independence and improvement collided directly with the future of the entire planet. The rain forest was being destroyed.

Just as in the fight against nuclear weapons, physicians who engaged with these issues realized that medicine cannot combat the effects of climate change. The task is to prevent it in big and little ways. As a result, all the issues discussed above and especially politics enter into the elaborate relationship between business interests, national wealth, personal freedoms, and health.

Although it may not seem like an environmental issue, the attempts to curb smoking are emblematic of this effort and its complexities. Arguments still swirl about who knew what and when, and about the egregious culpability of the tobacco industry in minimizing dangers and luring innocents to their doom. A link to cancer was firmly established in 1950 with the elegant study of British epidemiologist Richard Doll. The understanding of smoking as addiction rather than habit was finally accepted in the 1960s, making the role of industrial advertising all the more important. The wages of second-hand smoke as a major environmental issue became glaringly obvious in the early 1980s, creating a more urgent scenario involving more 'innocent victims.' Smoking-related illnesses killed 100 million people in the twentieth century; a billion deaths are predicted for the twenty-first.

Since the 1970s, public health officials have struggled with legislators to make smoking less accessible and less attractive; the successes occur in tiny, incremental steps. They are most difficult where tobacco is a profitable crop. I remember the ads about the 'brand doctors prefer.' And I vividly recall protests over a 1975 smoking ban in the pulmonary ward of a teaching hospital (where oxygen is used); banishing smoking from the entire hospital came much later. At the time of writing, expulsion of smokers from public buildings, restaurants, and bars is still met with grumbling. The skirmishes are fought municipality by municipality – shades of the medieval past – and the biggest battles lie ahead in the developing world, where, for rich and poor alike, smoking symbolizes achievement, status, and freedom.

Environmental activism was taken on by PSR and IPPNW – a natural choice with their origins in combating nuclear pollution. Various other professional associations, such as the American Academy of Environmental Medicine (founded in 1965), seek to investigate and improve conditions; they work pragmatically through corporate partners. Physician organizations aimed at political lobbying for environmental health are young and small. The British Society for Ecological Medicine began as a 1993 merger of pre-existing specialist groups for nutrition and allergy; the current name dates from 2005. The Canadian Association of Physicians for the Environment was also founded in 1993, held its first meeting two years later, and by 1997 had started a new journal as a vehicle for research, *Healthcare Quarterly*. The *Journal of Political Ecology* is an online, open-access, peer-reviewed publication with international scope, founded in 1994 to feature case studies in history and society; it uses the tools of social science to effect change.

International Health

As should be obvious by now, public health issues do not respect borders; yet humans can deal with them only through available legislative channels. Governments have collaborated on some problems that escape their territory; for example, work on shared rivers is a precedent going back to the nineteenth century. However, collaboration on other health matters has been less successful. As a result, town councils debate smoking bans; states argue over the relative responsibilities for air pollution and environmental cleanup; and international agencies struggle to find ways to make wayward countries behave by spending money they do not have. These measures lack teeth; being vulnerable to economic pressures, they also lack credibility.

The international health movement first began in response to epidemics. Plagues have been crossing borders since before writing began, but people were loath to share information with foreigners. Security was the main reason: the outbreak could be a deliberate enemy attack; if not, announcing its presence was an admission of vulnerability. In modern times, it was also an admission of shameful, social failure. Collaboration on these matters requires peace, stability, and trust.

Following a second wave of cholera in 1848–9 and the dreadful typhus outbreaks among Atlantic immigrants, countries decided to work together. They were prompted by the sanitary movement, the advent of medical statistics, and a general trend towards large international conferences. These meetings began before John Snow had published his observations on water and cholera (see chapter 7). In

1851, the First International Sanitary Conference was held in Paris. Twelve European states, as well as Turkey and Russia, each sent two delegates, one a doctor. The main topics of discussion were twofold: 'Is cholera contagious?' and 'What is the value of quarantine?' The meeting went on for six months without finding consensus on either question. The delegates went home disappointed.

Two years later, in 1853 and still before Snow, the first international conference on medical statistics was held in Brussels. It recommended international classification of causes of death so that states could at least agree on the topic of discussion, the precursor of the International Classification of Disease (ICD). Frightened by yet another wave of cholera and somewhat encouraged by progress on classifying diseases, countries decided to try again. The Second International Sanitary Conference was held in 1859; again the site was Paris (not a bad place for a lengthy meeting); however, this time, doctors were excluded. Delegates discussed the same two topics. Now with the added wisdom of Snow and without the doctors, they generated an agreement, but it was not ratified by host nations.

Sanitary conferences took place at irregular intervals, prompted by outbreaks of disease (cholera for the first four) and hampered by war. The Fifth Conference, motivated by yellow fever, took place in Washington, DC, in 1881. That meeting discussed a recommendation that countries should notify the world about the presence of infections. It failed: perhaps for age-old security reasons, France and the United States were opposed. During the sixth to tenth conferences, some consensus was reached over national behaviours in times of epidemics, especially concerning trade restrictions and quarantine. In particular, it was agreed that quarantine between nations must not be viewed as an act of aggression.

But no permanent body existed to ensure continuity and monitor the implementation of the agreements. Delegates would go home feeling pleased with themselves, but the situation would not change. Greater effort and financial investment were needed for these basic ideals to be attained. Finally, the Eleventh Conference of 1903, held in Washington, recommended a permanent International Office of Public Hygiene (IOPH); member countries would contribute to costs. It opened in 1907 with nine countries, but the total rose quickly to twenty-two by 1911. The goals were to eliminate fleas and rats, newly recognized as vectors of disease, to standardize vaccines, and to establish controls around healthy carriers. Strangely, in 1902, another international organization was proposed, its founders probably acting out of exasperation with the Sanitary Conferences and the desire to redirect the focus from Europe to the Americas. The permanent office of the Pan American Health Organization (PAHA) finally opened in 1921 with an annual budget of $5,000; it still exists as a regional branch of the WHO.

But another war soon interrupted the bloom of cooperation, and all planning stopped. The influenza epidemic of 1918–19 coincided with peace and revived public health cooperation. The name 'Spanish flu' is a misnomer owing to national hesitation over disease notification (see chapter 7). In the interwar period, three different but loosely connected international health organizations struggled to fill the elusive goals defined in the previous century: the PAHA, the IOPH (which collapsed), and the League of Nations. But yet another war stopped all efforts.

Planned from 1946, the World Health Organization (WHO) opened in Geneva two years later as the directing and coordinating authority for health within the United Nations system. It absorbed the PAHA and the IOPH and initially involved fifty-five countries. Hoping to learn from failures of the past, motivated by the recent human tragedies of war, and inspired by the scientific optimism of the age, the WHO took on an unprecedented agenda: in addition to combating infectious diseases, it would fight all disease and aim for health. It now lists 193 member countries.

The first director general of the WHO was Canadian physician G. Brock Chisholm (see figure 15.6). Having moved from general practice into psychiatry, he entered the Second World War as a private and rose through the ranks to head the medical services of the Canadian Army. Controversy surrounded Chisholm's views on childrearing, especially his agnostic stance on religion and his widely publicized opposition to the perpetuation of myths, including Santa Claus. Repeated calls for his resignation from the Canadian bureaucracy were silenced only by his near unanimous election to the WHO leadership.

Chisholm believed that war between nations would persist without conscious and enlightened efforts to develop tolerance and mutual understanding. An active promoter of PSR, he also advocated birth control, acknowledging Cicely Williams's emphasis on the prior need for death control. In concentrating on global health, Chisholm warned against nuclear weapons, overpopulation, and pollution. These preferences marked the future course of the WHO. In retirement on Vancouver Island, Chisholm remained involved in public health, actively promoting sex education, contraception, nuclear disarmament, and clean water initiatives. In 1957, he was one of only two physicians among the twenty-two scientists who participated in the first Pugwash Conference on Science and World Affairs. The Nova Scotia conferences emphasized the need for scientists to take responsibility for their inventions; nearly four decades later, Pugwash shared the 1995 Nobel Prize for Peace. Chisholm died of a stroke in 1971, virtually unknown in his native land.

The WHO does not police action on commitments. Notification of disease now exists as a transparency tool for monitoring states' willingness to help and protect each other; a recent example is the regular reporting on influenza. The efforts of the WHO and other public health organizations are slowly making a difference in the developing world, at least in the realm of disease; smallpox was eradicated and polio is greatly diminished. It also reports a declining incidence in water-borne diseases, most major childhood diseases, and infections controlled with vaccination. But as people begin to live longer, the diseases of a wealthy and sedentary lifestyle are surfacing in countries where once they were rare. This observation has further entrenched the WHO commitment to health promotion as well as disease control.

In 2005, the WHO launched a special commission on the 'social determinants of health' to address wide variations in statistics on mortality and morbidity. Updating the observations of Virchow, Ramazzini, and Farr, the 2006 preliminary report showed, once again, that beyond the wonders of medical science, certain basic priorities are most closely correlated with health: gender, race, literacy, wealth, employment, environment. These principles extend the older concept of 'socioeconomic factors' and have been touted for at least two decades; however, 'social determinants of health' has yet to become

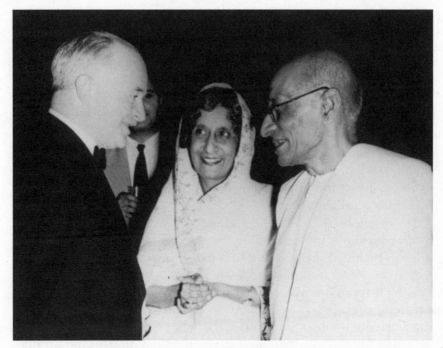

15.6   Brock Chisholm soon to become Director General of WHO with Indian Health Minister Rajkumari Amrit Kaur and Mohandas Karamchand Gandhi, circa 1947. By kind permission of John Farley and Dr Chisholm's daughter, Anne Mentha

a MeSH heading. Medicine remains focused on disease – a worthy cause indeed – but until it recognizes social and political action as a form of medical intervention, global health will remain elusive, and it will not come from doctors.

Making a Difference

Chisholm has had seven distinguished successors in the role of Director General, including Gro Harlem Brundtland. They and the others described in this chapter often worked backwards from the patterns subtended by a typical medical education. They served populations not individuals; they used, but were not exclusively focused on, big science; they earned less money; and they made enemies of the rich and powerful. They even spent a lot of time combating the self-destructive urges of healthy humanity.

But beyond heroic doctors, contributions to global health at home and abroad are effected through many avenues: national, religious, academic, and independent. Here too the resources of government-funded, international initiatives sometimes pale in contrast to the power of private philanthropic foundations, each newcomer organization seeing itself as a solution to the shortcomings of its predecessors. Sometimes the stated motive of these philanthropic foundations was merely a pretext for other more selfish goals. Some have resources in excess of the gross domestic product of entire nations; their influence is undeniable.

For example, the Carnegie Foundation was set up in 1911 to promote education, understanding, peace, and development. Its early mission included the building of public libraries across North America, a prescient recognition of literacy as a social determinant of health. It funded a massive research program on the 'never again' theme to prevent war and made major contributions to developing the academic study of international relations. By 2004 its assets were valued at $1.9 billion. The Rockefeller Foundation, also the product of a wealthy American family, was endowed in 1913 to attack health inequities and eliminate diseases of poverty; in 2001, its assets were in excess of $3 billion. The Bill and Melinda Gates Foundation began in 2000 with a mission to improve health and eliminate poverty. Its special projects have involved vaccination for polio and encephalitis and control of malaria. In 2006, its assets were doubled by Warren Buffet; two years later, its endowment was $35.1 billion. The amount it spends on health care each year is roughly equivalent to the budget of the WHO. Yet poverty rates fall slowly: in developing countries one person in every five lives on less than a dollar a day; in parts of sub-Saharan Africa rates are increasing.

Literally thousands of other charitable organizations participate in the task of improving health at home and abroad. Sometimes it is difficult to understand why so many agencies are necessary, and how much must be wasted in duplicating the functions of administration and fundraising. But it is hard to criticize the good-hearted drive for food and warm clothing held in the town hall basement.

Perhaps the historian must be resigned to the inexplicability of the present. In whatever ways these groups manage to do their work with, around, and in spite of each other, she can only hope that they attain the worthiest and most ancient of medical goals: to help and to do no harm.

Suggestions for Further Reading

At the bibliography website http://histmed.ca.

CHAPTER SIXTEEN

*Sleuthing and Science: How to Research a Question in Medical History**

I love these little things, this pointillist approach to verisimilitude, the correction of detail that cumulatively gives such satisfaction ... Like policemen in a search team, we go on hands and knees and crawl our way towards the truth.

– Ian McEwan, *Atonement* (Toronto: Vintage Canada, 2001), 359

History as a simple recitation of names and dates is dusty, boring stuff. But questions about why we do what we do, or think what we think, are compelling. So is the search for answers to questions about why people *used to* think or do certain things, especially if those thoughts or deeds are now considered wrong. Historians can enjoy all the excitement and intrigue of detective work with a much lower risk of getting shot.

Bad medical history gives the entire enterprise an undeservedly poor reputation; it may explain why teaching history to health-care students seems to require self-justification. Anatomy, physiology, and pharmacology do not apologize for their presence in the curriculum. Good history is directly relevant to health-care education. It revolves around a fundamental truth: things change – at different rates in different times and places, and for different reasons. Exploring the dimensions of past changes in any aspect of health care, in any culture at any time, is meaningful for the present. Historical investigation

*Learning objectives for this chapter are on p. 458.

relates to the much-touted goals of lifelong learning and evidence-based choice, which are essential for competent practice. Furthermore, good historical research resembles the scientific enterprise in many ways; it is about questions and answers.

This chapter contains my advice for conducting historical research. It is a subjective product of personal trial and error. I make no claims for originality. A history project can be approached in countless other ways. My method was and still is being shaped by my professors in medicine and history, and by colleagues, writers, editors, and especially students. Since I am unable to perceive its weaknesses and biases, I advise you to use these ideas with care.

Framing a Clear Question

> The question is like the hypothesis in a scientific experiment.

The would-be investigator of history must understand exactly what she is looking for and why. Presenting rounds, preparing a report or an after-dinner speech, contemplating a change in practice, developing a policy, or simply being curious are some of the many reasons that lead students and practitioners to ask historical questions. The question will be refined by the available sources of information, by the results, and by the individual conducting the investigation. The final form of the question may bear little resemblance to the original. In other words, you may find an answer to an entirely different question – one you had not imagined at the outset.

At all times, the investigator should have in mind an honest and concise statement of the current question. Sophisticated questions take into account theoretical explanations generated by other scholars for similar problems; however, simple questions are not intrinsically boring, nor does anything preclude creating a new theory.

Thoughout the process, the historian must acknowledge his or her role as a participant in the project – in matters of taste pertaining to the selection of subject, in the choice of research avenues that appeal, and in the neglect of pathways that seem less promising.

Identifying Sources

Sources are like the materials in a scientific experiment.

The evidence for statements about the past are the sources. In general, sources are of two types – primary and secondary – but they may overlap. Sometimes it is simpler to begin with the secondary sources, histories already written, where you may quickly find an answer to your question. The webpage on resources and research tools introduces general secondary sources on various subjects. But answers derived from secondary sources should be handled with caution. The best evidence comes from primary sources.

Primary Sources

Primary sources are documents or objects produced during the period under investigation or by the subject of the study. Sometimes – for example, in the case of a newly discovered manuscript – they become the question, because their origin and purpose are unknown. If the project focuses on a person, the primary sources encompass that individual's publications and manuscript papers, including diplomas, practice records, laboratory notebooks, diaries, letters written and received, and scrapbooks. Primary sources also include other collections of manuscripts, contemporary books, journals, and newspapers. If the subject is a disease, a treatment, or a technology, the primary sources might include original descriptions, subsequent modifications, commentary, and possibly extant artefacts used in treatment and care. If the subject is an institution, a period, or a place, the primary materials are found in anything emerging from that institution, period, or place. To learn about the health of populations, it is essential to consult government documents, census statistics, and agency surveys.

In defining primary sources, context is important. A historian must strive to situate the topic in time and place. No medical subject – be it a person, a practice, an institution, a technology, or an idea – can be fully explored without also studying its political, social, economic, and cultural environment. Sometimes, the environmental conditions are revealed by comparing them with those elsewhere. For example, revolution or famine in one country will influence its medicine, while the medicine of another country that is enjoying peace and prosperity will be different.

History – itself made up of writing – has traditionally placed a special value on the written word as the ultimate form of evidence. But this practice can obscure or skew the past by excluding the testimony of those who were not able to publish, read, or write – women, children, patients, and illiterate or disadvantaged peoples. Moreover, just because something was written does not make it accurate. Historical documents are powerful witnesses, but they have certain problems: only some survive; they reflect the authors' priorities; and their contents may be flawed. In recent decades, historical emphasis shifted away from great men, great discoveries, and great nations. Consequently, primary sources have become more eclectic and include 'oral histories' (the result of interviews), paleopathology, pictures, films, novels, art, music, comic books, and objects.

In the search for printed primary sources, the historian must rely on libraries – the bigger the better – and on bibliographies and indexes; happily, most are now online and many early works are digitized. For example, when dealing with a subject from antiquity, claims and quotations found in a secondary source must be verified with scholarly editions (e.g., the Loeb Classical Library or the Corpus Medicorum Grecorum). Do not cite Hippocrates or Galen from *JAMA*. With electronic resources, it is possible to stay at home and browse the catalogues of great institutions, such as the Wellcome Library, the National Library of Medicine (NLM), or McGill's Osler Library. Online catalogues of most national libraries –for example of France's Bibliothèque Nationale, the British Library, the Vatican Library, and the United States Library of Congress can be searched individually and collectively.

Books can be found through the online catalogues, and Medline helps to trace articles back to 1950. But finding historical journal articles prior to 1950 can be a challenge. A useful tool is the *Index Catalogue of the Library of the Surgeon General's Office*: in several multi-volume series from 1880, it listed the holdings of what is now the NLM, providing references to a host of journal articles dating back centuries to the earliest periodicals. Since the first edition of this book, it has been digitized and is available on the internet (http://www.index cat.nlm.nih.gov). At the time of writing you may be obliged to go to a library or use interlibrary loans to obtain the actual articles cited there; however, no study of topics in nineteenth- or early twentieth-century medical history can be considered complete without use of this resource.

For recent topics, both Medline and periodical literature indexes, including newspaper archives, provide a start (such as *The New York Times Index*, *The Times Index*, and *Canadian Periodical Index*). But they have limitations (see below). Morton's *Bibliography* is an attempt to list the most significant contributions to Western medicine, and several other recent books feature great medical works, fewer in number but with more commentary. (See Resources, 2, at the bibliography website http://histmed.ca.)

Tracing unpublished primary sources is usually more complicated. Historians are rarely confident that they have examined every scrap of paper that could be seen. Archives exist in a surprising variety of forms and places. National and institutional archives are good places to begin. Published and online catalogues of holdings are helpful, but the Web – though extremely useful – is insufficient for conducting this work. Only a tiny fraction of holdings and search tools are digitized (at least so far), and the selection is inevitably skewed towards someone's version of a tale to be told. Specific collections are often indexed in unpublished guides called 'Finding Aids.' Archivists will usually respond to questions by mail or email. But the scholar must know (or imagine) that an archive exists in order to find it. Again, local archivists can be of assistance.

In a perfect world, all important papers would be kept in archives. Government and institutional documents are ordered by law to be preserved. Every country, every province or state, many cities, all universities, and most hospitals, organizations, and associations maintain records. In reality, however, complete preservation is rare. Even when you are confident that the papers must reside in a particular archive, locating them there through a baffling classification system can be daunting. Having found the 'official' government records, you must remember that they are precisely that – official. They tell the story of a bureaucrat. Unknown quantities of papers may have been lost or deliberately destroyed. Indeed, the most salacious, controversial, and intriguing aspects in the life of an individual or institution can be forever excised in this way. Some papers may belong to friends, relatives, or descendants who refuse to open them to historians. Still others are withdrawn from scholarship, having become the property of private dealers and investors. Occasionally, an obituary or an entry in a biographical or national dictionary will indicate where the papers of an individual are kept. Looking for papers is time-consuming and frustrating, but it is also deeply rewarding. For this kind of discovery – a small piece of evidence to support an idea – the historian shouts, 'Eureka!' (Okay, we don't get out much.)

Secondary Sources

Secondary sources are produced by fellow historians, living or dead. Like a scientific review of the literature, the historian must find all attempts to explore the same or similar questions. The authors may be other practitioners, historians, sociologists, or philosophers; they may also be contemporaries of the subject, such as colleagues, eulogists, and descendants.

Sometimes, the secondary source will provide an immediate and satisfying answer to your question; however, before accepting such information at face value, it is wise to contemplate the nine tasks described in the box below.

When I am asked for help with a research question, like everyone else, I now start with the amazing Web-based resources like Google or Wikipedia. But it is important to emphasize that nothing found in this manner can be accepted without consideration of the list of tasks in the box. Things have changed rapidly. In direct contrast to just a decade ago, historians are now confronted with far too much information rather than too little. But most of this information is not peer-reviewed. Students sometimes seem unable to distinguish between scholarship and junk: if it crops up at the top of a Google search, they think it must be true. But truth is not decided by

On Secondary Sources: Beware!

1 Assume someone else has already asked (and answered) your question.
2 Find out who, when, and where, and do not neglect books.
3 If you find no predecessors, be creative and search in tangential fields.
4 Exploit others' footnotes for leads to additional primary and secondary sources.
5 Be aware that you are not obliged to agree with your predecessors.
6 Find reviews of the sources on which you rely heavily. Is your opinion shared by experts? Is your confidence well placed?
7 Do not trust history without references, aka 'scholarly apparatus.'
8 Believe nothing you read if it does not refer to primary sources.
9 Believe nothing you read if you cannot understand why it was written.

majority. As a result, it is important to cross-check all information gathered in this way with scholarly work lurking in the less visible peer-reviewed literature. How do we find that?

Medline (or Pubmed) is an excellent guide to peer-reviewed secondary sources (as well as primary sources for topics since 1950). The Medical Subject Heading (MeSH) system includes many subject headings for 'History,' organized by century and period. But separate entries on the history of *any* MeSH topic can be located simply by adding a '/hi' subheading (e.g., 'nursing/hi'). To narrow a search, a strategic combination with keywords must be made. However, do not rely on Medline alone. It indexes thousands of periodicals, but only a handful of those that cover history. It does not always assign historical subject headings or keywords to articles with historical information. It contains very little published prior to 1950. And above all, it ignores books and edited volumes (unless they happen to have enjoyed essay reviews in journals). It is extremely embarrassing for a would-be historian to do a thorough Medline search and fail to notice a key book on the very topic under study. It happens.

The literature review should extend beyond the obvious healthcare tools. Relevant information may have appeared in periodicals devoted to philosophy, anthropology, history, sociology, literature, economics, geography, political studies, women's studies, law, and public administration. Databases similar to Medline are available for the scholarly literature in the humanities and social sciences, and for newspapers and other periodicals. More reliably than Medline, these tools will include books. Ask a reference librarian for help.

The distinction between primary and secondary sources can blur in several situations. For example, an obituary can be both a primary and a secondary source. Similarly, a history written at the time of the subject under study can be a primary as well as a secondary source. A survey of several volumes of a journal counting the frequency of articles on a certain topic through time will turn a primary source into a secondary source, or vice versa, as the numerical results raise new questions. Analysis of what other historians have said about a topic transforms secondary sources into primary sources, as part of the fascinating enterprise of historiography. Historiography examines trends, problems, methods, gaps, and interpretive styles. It can help to orient confused enthusiasts (again, see the online Suggestions for Further Reading at the bibliography website http://histmed.ca).

Method and Interpretation

For figures in the past, including other historians, the most important question is this: How did writers come to know what (they thought) they knew? In other words, how did they justify their beliefs?

– Mirko Grmek, physician and historian

Analysis of the sources reveals the evidence, or 'argument,' to support the answer to your question. Historical methods are the direct cognate of methods in scientific experiments. Reading may be their basis, but this work also entails selection, interpretation, and manipulation – actions strongly influenced both by the taste and imagination of the investigator and by current standards and fashions of historical practice (see 'History Has Its Own History' p. 440).

In gathering evidence, it is ideal to examine all relevant primary and secondary sources. Sometimes, however, an overwhelming abundance of information – for example, in the case of hospital records – can be dealt with only by devising a sampling system. Microcomputers have revolutionized historical research and enhanced the potential of voluminous collections, but this technology demands selection. Decisions to rely on some data and reject others must be made with care, as you confront any biases that you the historian may introduce.

Secondary sources must be analysed too. Just as in a scientific literature review, this analysis connects your research – questions and answers – to other histories. Being human, historians like to see their work cited – but citation is much more than a sop to vanity or a homage to reputation. It distinguishes good history from bad. Here's how it works:

Good historical product is not only information about the past; it situates itself within the domain described by historian predecessors. It may support existing ideas with new data, or, even better, it may introduce original ideas to explain the past. Exciting new theories about why and how things came to be, or to change, can be applied and tested in future projects. In other words – and still drawing parallels to science – a thorough history project may conclude with more questions to guide future research.

The political and philosophical leanings of an investigator colour the interpretation of data, just as they enter into framing the research question. Marxists, capitalists, socialists, feminists, chauvinists, racists, creationists, scientists, Baptists, atheists, deconstructionists, midwives, nurses, physicians, surgeons, and patients will find radically different explanations to account for the same past (see chapter 11).

> We are forever slaying old paradigms. Instead of standing on the shoulders of our predecessors, we take an ax to their knees. As each new approach goes after its precursors with an ax, the social sciences have come to resemble, as Eric Wolf so poignantly phrased it, "a project in intellectual deforestation." The problem, of course, is that while knowledge is socially produced, to launch professional careers, it must be individually appropriated.
>
> – J.B. Greenberg and T.K. Park, 'Political Ecology,'
> *Journal of Political Ecology* 1 (1994): 1

The laudable, positivistic aim of controlling all subjective variables, which dominates laboratory work, is simply not attainable in history, nor may it be in science. Unlike scientists, however, historians admit it – although, for a short time earlier in the twentieth century, they too strove for elusive objectivity. Instead, historians deal with interpretive bias by recognizing it and by bolstering their arguments with convincing evidence comprising a swathe of sources chosen by complete and/or systematic sampling in a openly reproducible fashion. An eclectic array of sources, selected simply because it supports an investigator's hypothesis, does not inspire confidence. A project that ignores mainstream historical thought may be entertaining, stimulating, plausible, and well written, but it is simply not history; it is journalism, editorializing or proselytizing. These principles are reflected in the writing process.

Writing It Up

> Acknowledge your biases, but do not judge the past by the standards of the present.

Even if publication is not your goal, recording your findings in summary notes or a bibliography is a good idea. Names and dates are easily forgotten or confused; sources are tricky to recall; and ideas – even brilliant ones – prove evanescent. Retracing one's steps in historical research should be unnecessary, but all too often historians come to check their references and find holes or mistakes. A passage which ·seemed trivial on first reading can suddenly loom crucially large after further research sparks a related idea. Finding it again can be daunting. Even if your work was only for an introduction to case rounds, keep your notes and slides; you have become an expert, but you are no good without your evidence.

For health-care professionals, writing history is inhibiting. Like scientific reporting, however, the best composition is not a solid, seamless block of narrative – it needs a structure. The 'steps' included in the box outline the process I generally use, its sequence, and the reasons for it. Many other procedures exist, but starting at the beginning and writing to the end is perhaps the least popular approach.

> An original idea. That can't be too hard. The library must be full of them.
>
> – Stephen Fry, *The Liar* (1991)

Publication of historical research, just like that of scientific research, demands originality. A rehash of other work is not usually very interesting. Again as in science, there is vast scope for originality in topics, questions, sources, methods, analysis, and conclusions.

New topics are constantly being discovered. For example, the rise of feminism brought women practitioners and patients to the fore; shifts in political views revealed gaps in knowledge about alternative medicines, postcolonial relationships, and the experience of patients. Even well-studied topics merit re-examination in the light of new sources, histories, methods, theories, and questions. Because questions about the past emerge from the present, it is often said that all history needs to be rewritten in each generation.

Historical writing is distinguished from scientific writing by the relative permissibility of the first person and the active voice. By conven-

Steps for Writing History

1 Start in the middle with the results of your research, i.e., the evidence and argument, a description of primary sources, method, and interpretation.
2 Next, draft the conclusion. Once you have set down the argument in step 1, the conclusion (hopefully) becomes obvious. It contains the answer to the question used to guide the work. Sometimes the question is (re)discovered at this point.
3 Next, write the introduction. In it, review the secondary literature and present the final version of your question. In other words, (re)compose your question *after* you have decided on its answer. Sometimes, the most intriguing version of the question will not have been discovered until after the research is done and the answer (conclusion) found.
4 You may then return to the conclusion, modifying it with commentary on how your question and your findings differ from those of your secondary-source predecessors. Historians are often excited by the unanticipated discovery that their research on a tiny topic challenges existing ideas about the past on a much broader scale. Another historiographic 'Eureka!' is possible here too.
5 Document by leaving traceable references to the sources for everything you write.

tion, scientific reports use the passive voice and the third person to reflect the positivistic ideals of experimentation: 'The blood was let, then it was boiled.' In clinical reports, patients become 'cases' who do not take pills but are passively 'treated.' Rarely, and usually only in the conclusion, does the first person 'I' or 'we' appear.

Here, history is different from science. Modesty and style may dictate sparing use of the first person and the active voice, but their relative acceptability reminds authors of their own creative role at each

step of the project: 'I took the blood, then I boiled it.' This acknowledged subjectivity is the open recognition that history is not limited
to information about the past: history is also made up of the writing
that expresses it, thereby marking it as a humanities discipline akin
to art, music, and literature.

History Has Its Own History

Periodicals devoted to the history of medicine and science go
back to the early twentieth century. At first they were edited by
erudite physicians, scientists, and librarians. Journals devoted
to history of medicine as opposed to science began to appear
in the 1930s and 1940s; various national and international societies gradually founded their own as vehicles for research on
their specific parts of the world. A burst of social history activity in the late 1960s transformed medicine into a cultural topic
for 'professional' (PhD) historians – people who are paid for
doing history. The 1970s and 1980s resulted in the creation
of new journals to accommodate their work because older periodicals rejected it for missing the science or displaying hostility to doctors. By 1993 the *Journal of Medical Biography* was
founded almost as a reaction to the social turn, because life
writing was being excluded from established journals as passé;
now in a process of rediscovery, scholars warn not to throw the
biographical baby out with the social tide.

Every new journal is the solution to a (perceived) problem.
The founding editorial of the journal tells a story about why.

Pitfalls of Crossing Boundaries

The meetings of the national and international societies for the history of medicine are sometimes dominated by two artificial solitudes:
doctors (generally older and often male) congregating in one room,
historians (generally younger and more often female) in another.

Sometimes plenary sessions will force one group to listen to the other, and much mutual grumbling will follow. Editorials proclaim who should be doing history and how. This particular dichotomy – a woeful intellectual apartheid – is not the only controversy in a fractious field, but it is perhaps the most counterproductive. It derives, I believe, from intolerance and a failure to communicate. If I could bestow one gift on my discipline, I would chose to heal this rift. Neither group functions well without the other.

Doctors complain that historians are boring, abstract, divorced from clinical reality, absorbed with minutiae, and too frequently hostile to the medical profession. They know that medicine is not perfect, but they respect it, and like generations of their predecessors, they strive to do no harm. They resent history being used for political purposes; for them, history is a collection of 'facts' or 'truths.' They do not salivate over effete references to obscure historians. At the mention of Foucault – or, worse, his cognate adjective, Foucauldian – their eyes glaze over.

Historians are not boring to each other; theory turns them on. They celebrate the creativity of humanities writing, thinking, and speaking. They love convincing arguments and imaginative yet well-reasoned interpretations anchored in detailed examinations of sources, inevitably constrained by time and space. For them, 'facts' do not exist and 'truth' is relative. They are suspicious of a medical preoccupation with what has survived, misinterpreting it either as unwillingness to face up to past mistakes or as a desire to glorify present practice. Trained in, and by, 'the word,' historians are baffled by doctors' love of images, which they find distracting, especially when the 'pictures' are made up entirely of bullet points on a screen. For them, images trivialize communication, turning history into entertainment, a slide show, a travelogue; worse, they convey their own messages that may distract from or destroy the argument. And if historians do not mention Foucault, some clever listener, reader, or editor will punish them by archly pointing out the omission. The trick is to refer to important theorists first – nod in the direction of common ground – and carry on. Some historians dislike the medical profession – a few may even be motivated by hatred for it – but editors try to assess quality by evidence and argument, not by opinion.

Historians complain that doctors who attempt history are bumbling amateurs or devout antiquarians, dabbling in a professional discipline that they neither respect nor understand. They invoke an obvious analogy – that retired historians do not take up brain surgery. How dare these rich interlopers think that age and experience alone can turn them into historians?

On either side of this useless debate, the criticisms are both valid and unjust. Beyond jealousy and intolerance, there is a happy mean. From practitioners, historians could learn how to challenge their hostile assumptions and communicate their findings – indeed, far more historians now deign to use slides at conferences than in the past. Here, however, I will concentrate on the problems of health-care providers who want to write history. How do you convince an anonymous, sceptical, academic historian that your work is worth publishing?

> History is ... fiction with footnotes.
>
> – Roderick A. Macdonald

Common Problems and How to Avoid Them

With pressures stemming from the 'publish-or-perish' mentality, editors of quality medical journals turn increasingly to professional historians for advice on submissions. Rejection letters can be baffling as well as disappointing. The criticisms cite 'problems' that appear to be inconsequential or mysterious to clinicians. Yet these faults are rarely insurmountable. To overcome them, the first step is to understand them. The second step, accepting them, is often more difficult, but it helps to set aside the readers' reports for a few weeks before responding. Whether or not you agree with the comments, it is foolish to ignore them. If you hope to carry on with this editor (or another), you are obliged to reframe your work in a manner that addresses the criticisms with respect. The most common faults of doctor-written history are summarized as follows:

1 Failure to ask a question. An assemblage of names, dates, and

events set out in chronological 'thick description' is not history. The editor will wonder, 'Why should I or the readers care?' Enthusiastic historians who have done their research well should have no difficulty supplying a question, but they must remember to write it. Sometimes, the problem is remedied with a simple statement of why you yourself are interested in the topic, or why others ought to share that interest, or why now. More attractive questions will feature the originality of your work.

2 Failure to use primary sources or to reveal the method used to exploit them – a serious flaw in much of the history once published in medical journals. One variation of this ubiquitous problem is the exclusive use of translations, something many of us are obliged to do when it comes to using ancient, medieval, or Asian sources. It may be unavoidable, but it should be acknowledged with humility. Translations inevitably contain interpretations.

3 Failure to contextualize a subject in time or place. Research that ignores social factors is often called 'internalist.' The topic is examined from within – inside the boundaries of medical knowledge – a narrow process that is inappropriately equated with history of ideas (intellectual history). As a result 'external' issues or social factors, which may be of equal importance, are overlooked, leading the author into anachronistic assumptions. The reverse criticism, 'externalist,' could be applied to some social history writing, although critical doctors do not resort to that word because they don't know it. Instead, they deride it as 'medical history without the medicine.' Just as doctors and historians need each other, historical accounts either of an idea or of a social phenomenon are incomplete without the context provided by the other.

4 Failure to cite relevant secondary literature. This failing has two vast dimensions. The first relates to the nature of history; situating the work within the body of ideas defined by fellow historical writers is an important part of the process. The second is common sense; the reader who is invited to assess your work will most likely be a person who has already published on the same topic or a related one. How would you react if you were asked to evaluate an essay by some young upstart (or old codger) who proposed to publish in your area of expertise without having read your brilliant book?

5 Overreliance on secondary literature. Why should any article be printed if it merely rehashes what has already been published elsewhere? Explicitly state the originality of your work. Be honest. If it is not original, why do you think it deserves to be published? It may be difficult, though not impossible, to justify its publication. For example, perhaps you are the first to bring two bodies of secondary literature together; or maybe you can enhance your research by going back to primary sources to test the claims of the secondary sources that you used. Sometimes such an exercise may surprise you by showing errors made by the other historians on whom you relied. It may also provide you with a new question. Do not allow yourself to perpetuate the mistakes of others. Expert readers will notice and trace the genealogy of your research to a certain second-rate history rather than to a credible primary source.

6 Journal mismatch (see 'History Has Its Own History' above).

7 Presentism and whiggism (see below).

Presentism and Whiggism

> We are not obliged to forget what we know, if we use it with care.

Presentism and whiggism are serious flaws from a historical perspective – they could even be called sins or crimes. Presentism is the tendency to judge the past by the standards of the present. It is unfair and anachronistic to blame predecessors for not saying, seeing, or knowing what could not yet be said, seen, or known. It is better history (and more interesting) to understand why they saw things as they did. 'Whiggism,' a term directly related to the progressive political philosophy of the British Liberal Party, is similar; it portrays the past as a series of events progressing to a better present. The assumption is that things change by improving and that progress has brought us to where we are now.

Historians are wary of 'progress.' The very word sets off mental alarms and shrieking whistles. Are things *really* getting better? Many technologies and treatments were once touted as miracle cures only to be rejected because of unforeseen side effects. Even the most ingenious discovery may have negative ecological considerations when the passage of centuries is taken into account. Not only is it premature to judge our own practices, but it is simplistic to reduce the past to a mere preparation for the future (a.k.a. our own glorious present). For postmodern scholars, progress, like facts, may no longer exist. Progress, in the sense of desirable improvement, is certainly problematic when those doing the labelling are also its proponents. We can be curious about the present without believing in its immutable superiority.

What to do? Never use the word 'progress.' If you feel an urge to do so, ask yourself why you think it is necessary and what you might really be avoiding. Take a deep breath, and if that doesn't work, take a Valium. Think carefully before you resort to words like 'advance' or 'setback' – they bespeak agendas that may have existed only in retrospect.

For health-care professionals, presentism and whiggism are the most difficult problems to avoid, since our questions emerge from a present anchored in clinical practice. Since we work in that present, it is appropriate that we believe it is better than the past and that we lapse into 'medicalese' as a vehicle for our ideas. We cannot suppress our awareness of current medicine. Pretending that we do not know what we do know is dishonest posturing. To that extent, Marxists, feminists, deconstructionists, and a host of other theoreticians also use questions, interpretations, and language that emerge from their present. Indeed, their works are presentist too. But somehow they manage to avoid the charge. I think the key is language. Medical verbiage should be kept to a minimum, because words convey ideas – and words that did not yet exist at a certain time will inevitably convey ideas that did not yet exist too, making your statements seem anachronistic. For non-practitioners, it is exclusionary jargon, a red flag; and even for fellow practitioners, it can mask a superficial understanding of the past.

An Example: Hypothetical Histories of Bloodletting

All authors below have carefully researched how and when bleeding was done, when it worked, failed, or appeared to work in situations that we might now think of as disastrous. But individual writers produce different histories, some better than others.

The presentist history suggests that some applications were more 'rational' than others, because bleeding 'works' or is still used now in a few cognate conditions (e.g., polycythemia, hemochromatosis, or heart failure) – none of which were diagnosed in the period under study.

The whiggish account of bloodletting is governed by the assumption that less bleeding is better. It extols a noble (but non-existent) crusade marching into the present, intent on eradicating phlebotomy.

A pseudo-historian may trot out numerous entertaining examples of famous people who died after being bled – without looking for the many who survived, or the reasons doctors and patients thought that it worked.

Here's where it gets tricky. A medically trained historian might explain the popularity of bleeding by appealing to neurovascular responses to depletion – a red-faced, hot individual turns pale, cool, and clammy – thus providing immediate positive feedback for the practice. Such use of modern concepts is neither presentist nor whiggish, but it makes some non-medical reviewers nervous.

Sometimes accusations of presentism are unjust. They are inspired by the ideas we use or the way we write. If you must resort to current medical ideas or terminology, provide a footnote to explain your choice and deal directly with the potential criticism of presentism or whiggism. Make it clear that you understand the flaw and explain why you think it does not apply in your case. Show that you know what you are doing.

The Last Word

Have fun. Remember that these ideas are far from infallible. I have a drawer full of unpublished papers. If you know an editor who might like to see them, please let me know.

Suggestions for Further Reading

At the bibliography website http://histmed.ca.

Learning Objectives of This Book

1: Introduction: Heroes and Villains in the History of Medicine

The overall educational objectives of this book are:

- to raise awareness of history (and the humanities as a whole) as a research discipline that enriches understanding of present-day medicine
- to instil a sense of scepticism with regard to the 'dogma' of the rest of the medical curriculum

The objectives of each chapter are given below.

2: The Fabricated Body: History of Anatomy

To recognize the historical evolution of

- anatomy as an important component of medicine
- the views of different societies on dissection

To identify

- the relationship between art and anatomy
- the importance and impact of the work of Andreas Vesalius

To know that

- applications of anatomical knowledge entered physiology prior to medicine

- medical students and professors resorted to grave-robbing and murder
- the study of anatomy has social as well as biological functions
- even today, not all diseases can be linked to a physical change

3: Interrogating Life: History of Physiology

To recognize the historical evolution of

- ideas concerning the nature of life
- the uses of animals in physiological research
- quality-of-life research

To identify

- the meaning of vitalism, mechanism, empiricism, teleology, positivism, professionalization
- the reasons for and significance of the discovery of circulation of blood
- the role and limitations of chance in scientific discovery

To analyse

- how positivism influences modern methods of experimental physiology
- how experimentation demarcated physiology as a distinct science

4: Science of Suffering: History of Pathology

To recognize the historical evolution of

- concepts of disease
- anatomical causes of disease
- germ theory and bacteriology
- the role of the doctor in diagnosis
- genetics

To analyse

- the potential in distinguishing between 'disease' as idea and 'illness' as suffering

To identify

- pathology as a link between medicine and science

- uses of paleopathology in investigation of the past
- reasons for the rise of narrative medicine

To know

- two pairs theories of disease about patients and causes of disease
- the meaning and criticisms of the 'medical model' of disease
- the meaning of 'social construction' of disease (also chapter 7)

5: First Do No Harm: History of Treatment, Pharmacology, and Pharmaceuticals

To recognize the historical evolution of

- remedies, from plants, to metals, to purifications, to designer drugs
- drug classifications, from side effects to chemical action
- clinical trials and Evidence-Based Medicine
- recent scepticism resulting from the failure of remedies, such as thalidomide

To analyse

- the role of social factors in perceived need for remedies
- the impact and problems of 'magic bullets' (vitamins, hormones, and antibiotics)
- the role of the pharmaceutical industry in defining disease and treatment choices
- ethical issues of patent protection and drug development

To know

- that most therapies have been discovered by empirical methods
- that many therapeutic 'discoveries' have non-scientific precursors
- the life cycle of drugs

6: On Becoming and Being a Doctor: Education, Licensing, Payment, and Bioethics

To recognize the historical evolution of

- physician-patient relations, as a contract of expectations and privileges

- patient expectations, from hope for relief to demand for cure
- health-care systems, as mechanisms for medical payment and poor relief
- professional bioethics and palliative care, in improving physician-patient relations

To analyse

- doctors' strikes as triggered by matters of third-party payment

To know that

- medical education has always been socially and culturally conditioned
- an increase in information does not mean an increase in knowledge
- medical privileges are threatened by past mistakes and by present-day scepticism

7: Plagues and Peoples: Epidemic Diseases in History

To recognize the historical evolution of

- public health measures, as the product and legacy of prior epidemics
- germ theory and antibiotics, and their roles in control of epidemics

To analyse how

- 'new' diseases appear
- incidence of infectious disease relates to changes in wealth, hygiene, and nutrition
- 'social construction' affects public health responses (also chapter 4)

To identify

- the impact of epidemics on populations, including the economic, social, intellectual, and political aspects of life
- the implications of the term 'innocent victim'

To know that

- breakdown of social order typifies human reactions to epidemic disease
- nineteenth-century cholera was linked to water
- knowledge of a microbial cause is not essential for preventing infectious disease

- with vaccination, smallpox became the first human disease to be eradicated

8: Why Is Blood Special? Changing Concepts of a Vital Humour

To recognize the historical evolution of

- blood in theories of life and disease, from the ancient humours to cellular and humoral immunity, to molecular medicine
- the link between blood, respiration, and oxygen
- blood as treatment (transfusion) from early modern times to the present

To analyse

- the cultural and political significance of hemophilia
- bloodletting as one of the most ancient and durable of all remedies

To identify

- the special status of blood in anthropological, social, mystical, and intellectual terms
- the importance of microscopy for discoveries in blood cells
- the role of mixing studies in defining clotting-factor deficiencies

To know

- the main dangers of transfusion and their solutions

9: Technology and Disease: Stethoscopes, Hospitals, and Other Gadgets

To recognize the historical evolution of

- technologies, as ways of measuring previously immeasurable phenomena, e.g., thermometers, kymographs
- auscultation and microscopy
- X-rays and other imaging technologies
- molecular biotechnology
- hospitals as sites and forms of technology

To analyse

- how changes in social factors and disease concepts prompt new technologies

- how technologies, in turn, alter disease concepts and society

To identify

- the role of individuals in the context of 'inevitable' discoveries

To know that

- technology aims to introduce diagnostic acumen and objectivity
- technology tends to distance the patient from the doctor

10: Work of the Hand: History of Surgery

To recognize the historical evolution of

- surgical practices, from prehistory to modern times
- wound care, including Paré's accidental discovery
- anesthesia
- antisepsis
- operative interventions

To analyse

- pain and infection as obstacles to the development of surgical techniques
- the role of antisepsis and anesthesia in surgical innovation
- how surgical practices are modified by economic and epidemiological factors

To identify

- some surgical techniques developed to deal with the trauma of war

To know that

- some elective operations are of great antiquity, e.g., trephination and circumcision
- some ancient and folk recipes for wound dressing were (and are) beneficial
- anesthesia was promoted by dentists before it was adopted by surgeons

11: Women's Medicine and Medicine's Women: History of Obstetrics, Gynecology, and Women

To recognize the historical evolution of

- birthing, from the exclusive domain of non-medical women to its early modern medicalization
- scientific ideas concerning reproduction
- Cesarean delivery
- obstetrical forceps
- nursing in relation to socially conditioned notions of gender and class
- midwifery as it is revived in developed countries
- women in nursing, medicine, and other health-care professions

To analyse

- the past as a variety of interpretations all 'true' in their context
- how control of bleeding and infection improved perinatal mortality
- the controversy surrounding the first uses of anesthesia in birthing
- the controversies surrounding modern reproductive technology and birth control

To identify

- Paré's description of podalic version
- the impact of increased use of forceps, ergotamine, and anesthesia
- the meaning of medicalization

To know that

- history is about the present as well as the past
- birthing women can die of bleeding and infection
- doctors could transmit infections to birthing mothers
- gynecological surgery was used to treat mental distress

12: Wrestling with Demons: History of Psychiatry

To recognize the historical evolution of

- humane measures to care for the insane

- asylums
- the classification of mental diseases
- physical treatments in the twentieth century
- 'decarceration' movements and community care
- antipsychiatry movements

To analyse

- the long tradition of linking mental disorders to physical causes
- the social construction of mental disease
- the stigma of mental illness
- how homosexuality was medicalized and demedicalized

To identify

- ancient words for diseases of the psyche, such as melancholia, hysteria, and mania
- the pervasive impact of Freud's theories of the unconscious

To know that

- mental illness relies on a conceptual separation of mind and body

13: No Baby, No Nation: History of Pediatrics

To recognize the historical evolution of

- child care, as related to social attitudes toward childhood and children
- childhood diseases
- surgical, hormonal, and dietary treatments for child health
- eugenics

To analyse

- the recognition of child mortality, as a force in the creation of pediatrics
- prevention of disease in children, as one of the first welfare initiatives
- eugenics as it was widely practised in the twentieth century

To identify

- problems and diseases that contribute to child mortality around the world

To know that
- experts' advice on child care is often later considered wrong
- medical recognition of child abuse appeared in the twentieth century

14: A Many-Faceted Gem: The Decline and Rebirth of Family Medicine

To recognize the historical evolution of
- 'general practice' and family medicine

To analyse
- the challenge of research in academic family medicine

To identify
- the influence of family medicine on health-care delivery and training, certification, and continuing education in other fields

15: When the Patient Is Plural: Public and International Health

To recognize the historical evolution of
- medical statistics
- international health collaboration
- the World Health Organization

To analyse
- the bias of the medical model against collective health
- examples of doctors in service of collectives in public health and work on water, food, politics, peace, and environment
- how a multiplicity of philanthropic organizations also strive for public health
- the ambivalence of medicine to sociopolitical action

To identify
- the role of clean water in population health
- the social determinants of health

16: Sleuthing and Science: How to Research a Question in Medical History

To identify

- conceptual and methodological issues in medico-historical research and writing
- common pitfalls in medico-historical research and writing and how to avoid them

Index